# The Big Book of Kombucha

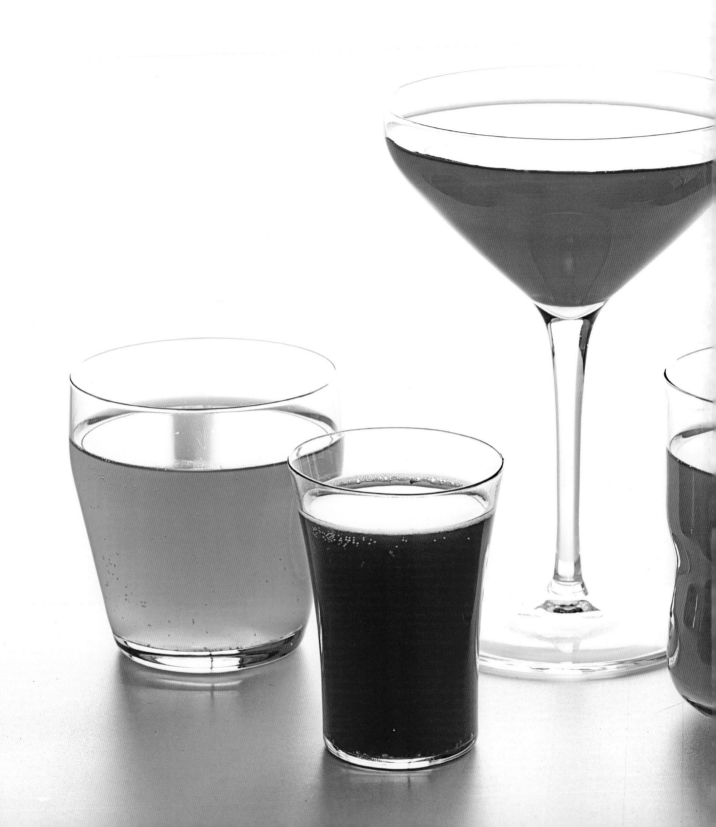

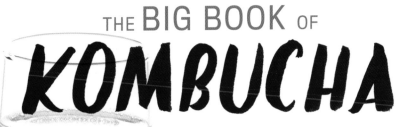

THE BIG BOOK OF

# KOMBUCHA

Brewing, Flavoring,
and Enjoying the Health Benefits of
**Fermented Tea**

*Hannah Crum & Alex LaGory*
FOREWORD BY SANDOR ELLIX KATZ

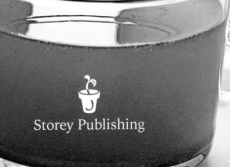

Storey Publishing

*The mission of Storey Publishing is to serve our customers by
publishing practical information that encourages
personal independence in harmony with the environment.*

Edited by Margaret Sutherland and Lisa Hiley
Art direction, book design, and lettering by
   Alethea Morrison
Text production by Jennifer Jepson Smith
Indexed by Christine R. Lindemer, Boston Road
   Communications

Cover photography by © Matt Armendariz
Cover illustrations by © Yao Cheng Design, LLC (spine)
   and © Katie Eberts (back)

Interior illustrations by © Georgina Luck (spots), © Yao
Cheng Design, LLC (chapter openers), and © Katie Eberts
(watercolor washes)

Interior photography by © Matt Armendariz (with excep-
tions noted below)

2004 Stijn Ghesquiere/ Wikimedia Commons, 338; ©
2010 Bloomberg/Getty Images, 63; A. Kniesel/Wikipedia,
337; courtesy of the authors, 35 (row 2 center), 171 (row 1
right, row 2 left & center, row 3 left & center); courtesy of
GT's Kombucha, 340; © CSA Images/Mod Art Collection/
Getty Images, 295; Dan Budnik/Wikimedia Commons,
339; © De Agostini / G. Dagli Orti, 275; © DEA/A. DAGLI
ORTI/Getty Images, 8, 174, 275; © Fuse/Getty Images,
71; © Heritage Image Partnership Ltd./Alamy, 96; ©
ImageBROKER/Alamy, 160; © Imagemore Co., Ltd./
Alamy, 121; © Ingrid Kessler, 162; © John Henshall/
Alamy, 9; © Jonathan Kingston/Getty Images, 55; Julius
Schnorr von Carolsfeld/Wikimedia Commons, 334 (left);
Mars Vilaubi, 44, 45, 53, 59, 67, 173; © Matthew Williams-
Ellis/Getty Images, 73; © Michael S. Yamashita/Getty
Images, 51; © Philip Kubarev, 336; Sean Minteh, courtesy
of Sandor Katz, 341; © Sergio Momo/Dorling Kindersley/
Getty Images, 334 (right); © Staci Valentine, 187, 199,
209, 213, 219, 226, 229, 232, 235, 237, 239, 243, 244; © Tom
Nulens/iStockphoto.com, xii, 32, 82, 140, 355

© 2016 by Hannah Crum and Alex M. LaGory

Be sure to read all instructions thoroughly before using
any of the techniques or recipes in this book and follow
all safety guidelines.

This publication is intended to provide information on
the covered subject. It is not intended to take the place of
personalized medical counseling, diagnosis, or treatment
from a trained health professional.

   Storey books are available for special premium and
promotional uses and for customized editions. For further
information, please call 1-800-793-9396.

**Storey Publishing**
210 MASS MoCA Way
North Adams, MA 01247
*www.storey.com*

Printed in China by Toppan Leefung Printing Ltd.
20 19 18 17 16 15 14 13 12 11 10 9 8

Library of Congress Cataloging-in-Publication Data

Names: Crum, Hannah, author. | LaGory, Alex, author.
Title: The big book of kombucha : brewing, flavoring, and enjoy-
ing the health benefits of fermented tea / Hannah Crum and Alex
LaGory.
Description: North Adams, MA : Storey Publishing, [2016] |
   Includes bibliographical references and index.
   Identifiers: LCCN 2015039360
ISBN 9781612124339 (pbk. : alk. paper)
ISBN 9781612124346 (hardcover : alk. paper)
ISBN 9781612124353 (ebook)
Subjects:  LCSH: Kombucha tea.
Classification: LCC TP650 .C78 2016 | DDC 663/.94—dc23 LC
record available at http://lccn.loc.gov/2015039360

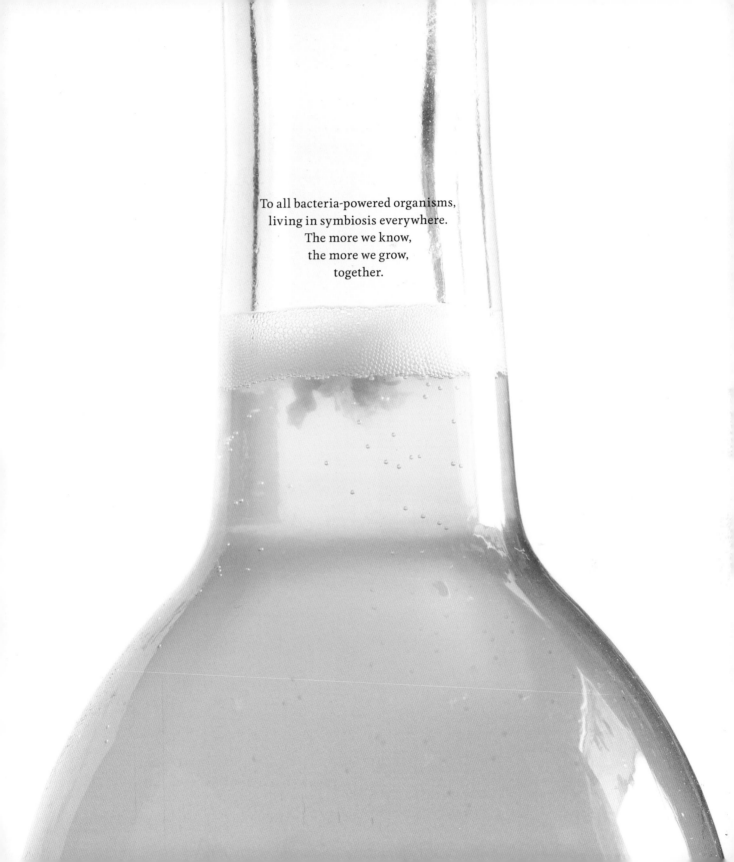

To all bacteria-powered organisms,
living in symbiosis everywhere.
The more we know,
the more we grow,
together.

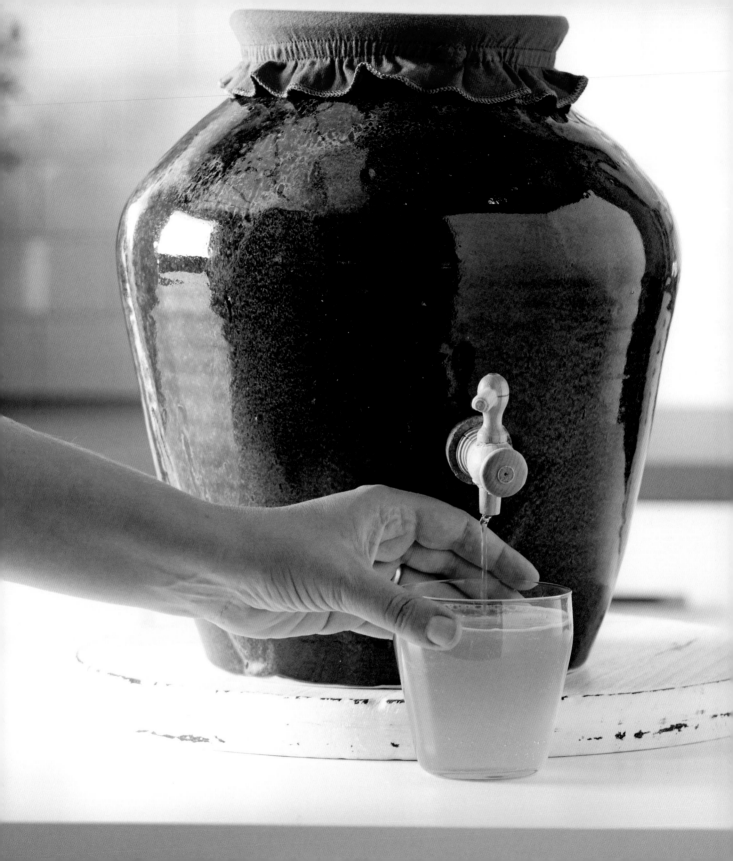

# -CONTENTS-

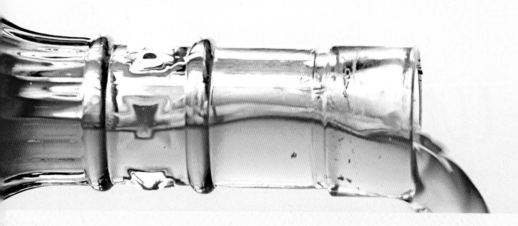

# A NOTE FROM GT DAVE

Kombucha came into my life over 20 years ago and changed me forever. My parents, who received a kombucha culture from a close family friend, began making and drinking kombucha in our home. I noticed how they quickly fell in love with how good it made them feel and look. But it wasn't until my mom's battle with breast cancer that I truly realized the magnitude of kombucha's health properties. Her doctors marveled and I observed firsthand how it kept her strong and resilient all the way through her recovery. It was then that I became convinced that kombucha was a gift that had blessed my family and that it needed to be shared with the world.

Hannah and I have both experienced that it is an understatement to say that kombucha is a "life changer." It restores balance in the digestion, rejuvenates the immune system, and revitalizes the mind. It unlocks an enlightened way of thinking and living by putting you back in touch with your body.

Kombucha is also an instrument for finding more ways to be healthier and therefore happier. Through its symbiotic cycle of life with the mother and baby SCOBY, it's a constant reminder that we need to seek the life force in all our food and to surround ourselves with love and positive energy. Whether you make your own kombucha or have it made for you, within this book you'll discover the impact that it can have on your life; it may change you forever.

**– GT DAVE**
Founder and President of GT's Kombucha

# FOREWORD

Kombucha, fermented sweet tea, has become the drink of the new millennium. Not that it's new, because it isn't. Like all fermented foods and beverages, it is ancient and its specific origins are murky. But until the dawn of the new millennium, it was not commercially available, and it was spread exclusively through grassroots channels.

The starter for kombucha is a rubbery disk known as the mother, a symbiotic culture of bacteria and yeast (SCOBY), which grows a new layer and thickens with each batch. As enthusiasts grew more and more mothers, they sought to share them, often with evangelical zeal.

I first encountered kombucha around 1994, when a friend with AIDS, who was dealing with a major health crisis, got drawn into kombucha for its reputed immune benefits. Soon he had a stack of mothers and started giving them to his friends to take home.

The grassroots spread of kombucha continues, but it has also spawned an industry, with U.S. annual sales now estimated at $600 million and steadily growing. This book is written by two people who have devoted themselves to kombucha's continued success. Hannah and Alex teach workshops, sell kombucha mothers and kits, and organize small producers, and now they have written this book.

*The Big Book of Kombucha* will certainly alleviate any fears you might have about making your own kombucha. It is full of ideas for innovative ways to flavor kombucha and has a very thorough troubleshooting section. The authors promote kombucha as a healing tonic, but do so in a balanced way, backed by citations to research (in contrast to some unsubstantiated hype). As much as I love kombucha (and sauerkraut and kefir and many other ferments), it is not reasonable to expect any single food or beverage to cure specific diseases.

I bring up these other ferments because kombucha exists in a much broader context of foods and beverages transformed by the action of microorganisms. According to one estimate, one-third of all food that human beings consume has been fermented before we eat it. Bread, cheese, and cured meats are fermented. Sauerkraut, kimchi, olives, and certain styles of pickles are fermented. So are soy sauce, fish sauce, and the vinegar found in most other condiments. Coffee, chocolate, and vanilla are fermented, as are wines and beers. Flavors of fermentation are prominent not only in Western cuisines but also around the world. In many diverse locales ferments are essential everyday foods. I have been unable to find a single example of a culinary tradition that does not incorporate fermentation.

Fermentation preserves food, makes it more flavorful and digestible, makes nutrients more bioavailable, breaks down certain toxic compounds, and produces others that are beneficial. I hope that as this book is your gateway to kombucha; kombucha will be your gateway to fermentation.

Welcome to the fermentation revival!
**– SANDOR ELLIX KATZ**
Author of *The Art of Fermentation* and
*Wild Fermentation*

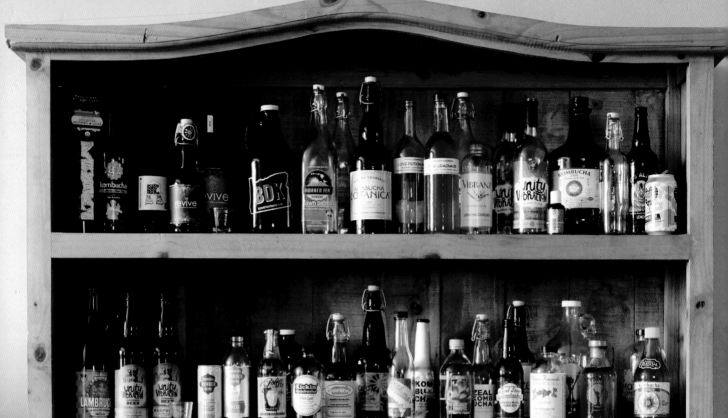
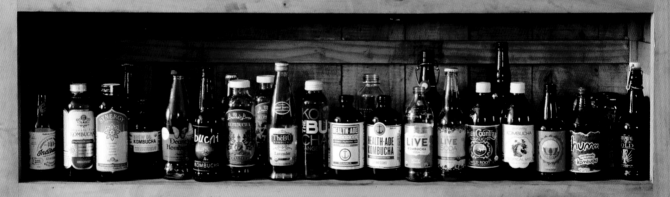
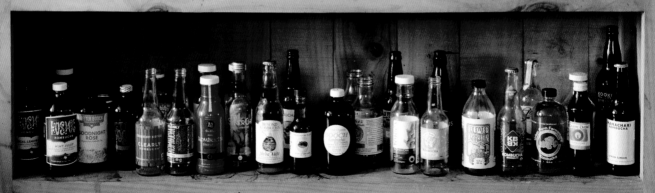

# Our Kombucha Journey

## — from Hannah —

"Kombucha Kismet" — whenever people ask how I first discovered kombucha, that is how I describe the experience. In Turkish, *kismet* means "fate" or "your lot in life" and is derived from the Arabic root word *qasama* (to divide). As someone who enjoys digging into the root of problems, words, and mysteries (I'm a total word nerd!), looking back it makes sense that my first experience with kombucha in 2003 marked a clear divide in my life path. At the time, it was simply a curious stop on a fun tour of a college friend's groovy San Francisco apartment, full of neat things I hadn't considered: a filter on the shower head (of course, get the chlorine off your skin!), pink Himalayan salt (salt is good for you?), and kombucha. While Alex and I didn't even taste their homebrew (not ready yet), my appetite to learn more had been piqued.

Not until a week later, when I purchased a couple of bottles at the West LA Whole Foods, did I even get my first taste. The bright-white lights of the display case illuminated the neat rows of amber and jewel-toned liquid, complete with similar floating globs to the jars I had spied in San Francisco. I couldn't wait to finally sip this mysterious brew, so I popped a bottle right there in the aisle before checking out, and when the tangy GT's Gingerade hit my tongue, wow! It was electric! Every nerve ending in my body instantly lit up, and in hindsight, I do recall angels in heaven singing hallelujah as divine light shone around me and the kombucha — LOVE at first sip!

(True confession: when I was a kid, Mom would often admonish me for sneaking slugs of sour, briny pickle juice right from the jar, even before the pickles were gone! She was worried it was bad for me, but the salty tang was irresistible.)

The Chinese say, "A journey of a thousand miles begins with a single step." For me, that first sip of kombucha was my "single step" on a journey of evolution and transformation, more than a decade long, that continues to this day.

My store-bought kombucha thirst quickly escalated beyond my budget, and getting my own "magic" jars and brewing at home became a necessity. For a girl whose idea of cooking was pressing the start button on the microwave, taking up a kitchen hobby might have seemed counterintuitive, but I trusted my gut and went hunting for a kombucha culture, which I sourced locally through the interweb. A friend was kind enough to pick it up for me, but I realized too late that I had forgotten to tell her exactly what a kombucha "baby" was. I felt bad but it was entertaining to see her face when she arrived at my doorstep, white as a sheet, holding the plastic baggie at arm's length and demanding, "What the heck is this? An alien blob? A placenta?"

I began brewing right away, eager to make my own delicious nectar. Reinvigorated by the kombucha process and inspired by an Artist's Way workshop, it was not long before I started teaching others how to make this tasty transformative brew. Kombucha Kamp, an in-person workshop at our tiny LA guesthouse. A few years later, disheartened by the lack of quality information on the Internet, I started blogging to spread the word and sending out cultures upon request. Soon after, Alex's background in documentary film was put to use in producing video content for the blog.

That quickly progressed to relaunching as a comprehensive website with all new updated content at KombuchaKamp.com, as well as a full webstore to serve the whole world. Our mission has always been to empower people by providing quality information, quality supplies, and quality support so everyone can find what they need for their own successful kombucha journey, from buying it at the store to brewing it at home to starting their own kombucha company.

Along the way, the process of brewing and the habit of drinking kombucha have gradually revealed many truths about our very nature as human beings. One of the most important and imperative to reclaiming our immunity is that we are "bacteriosapiens": we have a vital relationship with bacteria. In fact, when you get down to the most basic level, every living thing on this planet — from plants to fish to birds to humans — is powered by bacteria. Without bacteria, none of us could exist. Embracing this knowledge offers insight into how profoundly we are affected by not only the bacteria, but also the antibiotics in our food and environment. We are literally living in a bacterial world!

These pages collect the details of kombucha's history, evolution, and secrets. Our best practices for simple and efficient kombucha brewing, recipes, and flavor combinations have been developed over a decade, and we share a myriad of practical applications from beauty products to animal feed supplements and soil amendments to vegan leather substitute. We hope these pages inspire you to begin or expand your own kombucha journey!

## *from Alex*

It was not love at first sip for me and kombucha. I was there when Hannah saw the blob for the first time in San Francisco, and I was there when her friend brought a "kombucha baby" back for Hannah's first batch. But for many years, aside from a polite taste now and again, I wanted no part of her burgeoning hobby. As time passed, I saw her enjoying making and drinking the kombucha, and more and more people came by for classes and cultures. Eventually Hannah developed a knack for flavoring, and soon after, Pink Lemonade was born. The blend of strawberry, lemon, and thyme, bottled at just the right stage and then perfectly fermented for a second time, resulted in such a delicious glass of icy kombucha that I was finally convinced to give up my morning Gatorade. For me, that was the first step to freeing myself from the chains of the standard American diet (SAD).

Over the next 18 months, my regular kombucha consumption coincided with a variety of health-related breakthroughs that had eluded me for many years. First and foremost, I suffered from acid reflux and was taking an antacid essentially every night. After a few weeks of drinking kombucha daily, even without changing my diet much otherwise, I found that the need for those pills disappeared, and I could go to bed each night without any ill effects.

Without any specific plan, I fell into a morning regimen that included an 8-ounce glass of kombucha over ice followed by an 8-ounce glass of raw milk. Soon, either because I was drinking the kombucha or just because I was ready for change, my other choices evolved as well. Sometimes these changes were immediate, such as eliminating certain fast food or prepared foods that I knew — based on how I felt after eating them — had significant negative impacts on my body.

Other changes were gradual, such as consuming less bread and pasta, incorporating more vegetables and fermented foods into my diet, and in general just thinking more about the source and even the farmer, focusing on "real food" choices.

Could the kombucha bacteria have been changing my thinking and making me more open-minded to consuming their fermented, probiotic, and real-food friends? Perhaps that type of quorum sensing is the future of nutrition therapy? I imagine a future where "microbiome bacteriotherapy" — the mapping of one's personal gut bacteria as a starting point for all medical and nutritional decisions — is standard practice.

No matter the reason, the results followed: I lost about 40 pounds in that year and a half. More important, I felt great and I was eating satisfying food. The process of cleaning up my diet has taken years, and that's fine with me. It took years to become toxic, and my body had to be ready to let go of those bad habits in a gradual, healthy way. But in my mind, there's no doubt that kombucha helped make those transitions easier.

Maybe I'd have found another way into these choices, but kombucha was a great gateway for me. I continue to try to improve my everyday choices, but I never feel too bad about splurging on one of my old "treats." I know I can always use kombucha to help soothe the aftereffects of my chosen poison. Life's too short to worry about every single thing we eat or drink, but in the end I know that I've made enough good choices to trust my gut.

## Our Kombucha Lifestyle

When we met in 2002, our diet was dramatically different than it is now. Chips and dips, microwave popcorn, frozen pizza, and packaged ramen were staples; corn syrup–filled sports drinks and sodas stocked the refrigerator; cheap fast food was a regular indulgence.

We knew that many of these foods were negatively affecting our health, so we mixed in some "healthier" foods now and then; while it relieved our consciences, it didn't do much to make our bodies feel better. We were having juice for lunch once a week, eating raw food once or twice a month, and doing three-day cleanses every now and again, but we still found ourselves feeling bloated and heavy.

Unsatisfied, we searched for answers, experimenting with vegetarian, vegan, South Beach, Master Cleanse, and many other diets and lifestyles. Each path brought different results but also other issues. Losing weight was easy, but when former habits returned, the results of weeks or months of self-imposed suffering vaporized.

ONE GOOD CHOICE LEADS TO OTHERS. So we gave up on the formal experiments and went back to eating whatever we felt like, but both of us were now regularly consuming kombucha, and gradually we found that making good dietary choices became easier. Foods that we had once considered treats began to taste more "chemical-ly" and were significantly less satisfying. We became sensitive to added sweeteners and quickly realized that nearly every processed food was loaded with them.

Kombucha Kismet led us in 2010 to the Weston A. Price Foundation, an organization dedicated to the promotion of traditional diets, including ferments like kombucha. That education completely transformed the way we thought about, selected, and prepared our food.

Expanding the blog into a website was another huge step for us. Researching and writing about fermented foods and nutrition for KombuchaKamp.com, and documenting the kombucha industry as beverage journalists accelerated the process for us. The incredible platform of the Internet and our little corner of it allowed us to grow in ways we never imagined.

To connect with other food bloggers; to meet and consult for (and often supply cultures to) people all over the country and the world who were starting kombucha brands or other food businesses; and most important, to connect with readers facing health challenges and succeeding, people whose lives had been transformed much more than our own: these experiences showed us the power of the movement we had joined, which inspired us to work that much harder to help more people.

We didn't change everything all at once, but over time the preponderance of our choices improved. And whenever we splurged on some terrible food, we just accepted that moment of indulgence and tried to make a better choice next time. There is, of course, no perfect diet. "Eating perfectly" presents an onerous and stressful path, not to mention it's pretty much impossible. We've found that a healthy relationship with food involves balance and variety, including the occasional high-calorie dessert or late-night snack if our bodies demand.

As kombucha became a regular component of our diet, our body's demands changed. We found ourselves craving less of the over-processed junk food we had been accustomed to eating and more of the nourishing, nutrient-dense food that better supported our individual well-being. Over time, we came to live by our simple mantra: trust your gut.

## *Where Will the Gateway Lead You?*

We consider kombucha to be a gateway food. In the literal sense, a gateway is simply a passage from one place to another. In the figurative sense, it leads to a path of new experiences and inspirations. Gateway foods introduce us to new ways of thinking about, preparing, and consuming food.

In our modern society, fraught with confusing and conflicting messages, it can be difficult to weed out what is important versus what is just noise. Fad diets come and go. "Miraculous" nutritional benefits are claimed, debated, and disproved. But kombucha, like all ferments, is neither a diet nor a miracle food; it is a time-honored tradition with proven nutritional components and long-lasting health benefits.

When people drink kombucha — or as often happens, brew their own and eventually make kefir and sauerkraut and whatever else tickles their fancy — they engage in ancient practices that unite them with generations past and those yet to come, stepping through a gateway toward trusting their gut and connecting to their bacteriosapien nature. The process of brewing and the influx of beneficial bacteria can be much like enlightenment, a rebirth with vision broad and senses keen. For some it is a rolling back of the clock, as the joy of the hobby mixes with the pleasure of deep nutrition, an exciting blend of science and art last experienced in youth.

No matter if kombucha is just an occasional grab-and-go from the local store or a brewing obsession that drives you to create your own new brand, we hope your journey is as rewarding as ours.

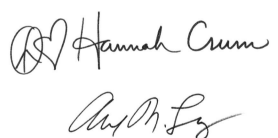

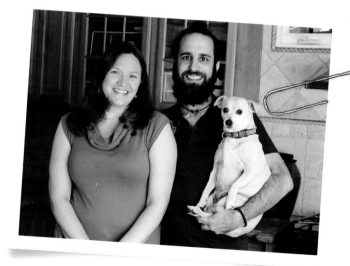

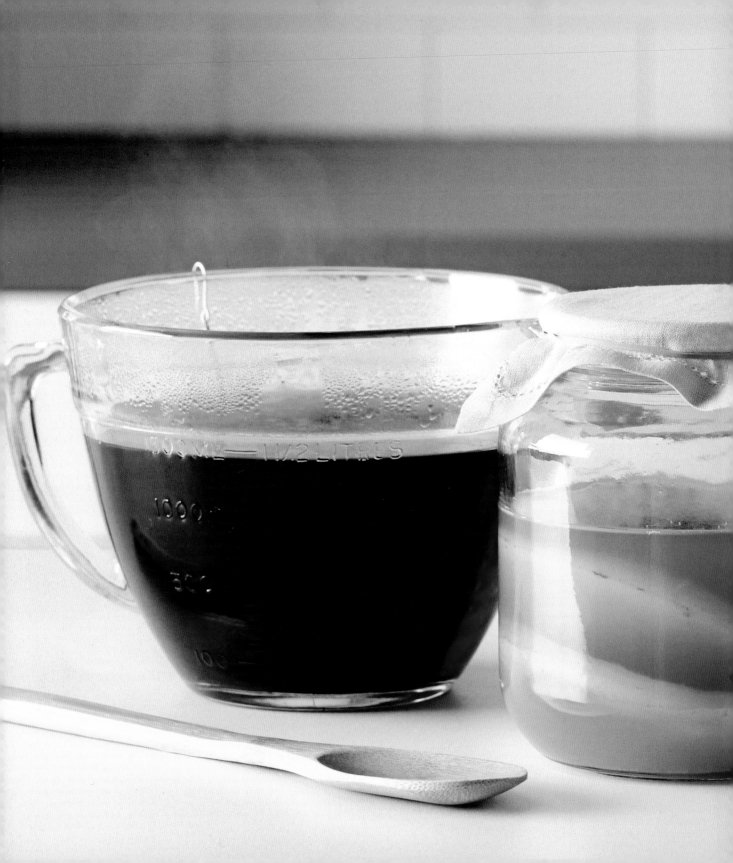

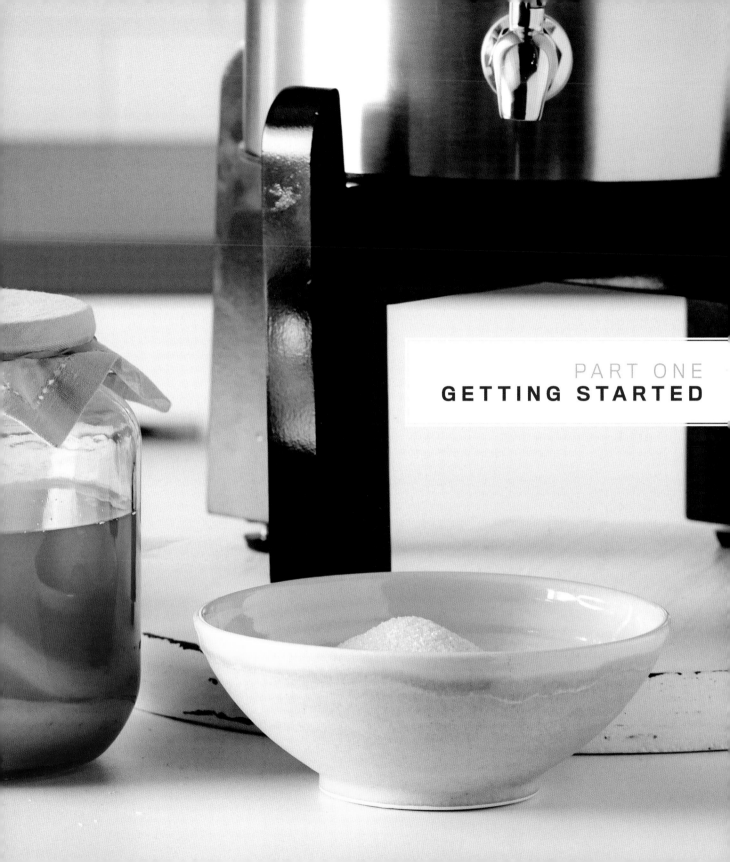

PART ONE
**GETTING STARTED**

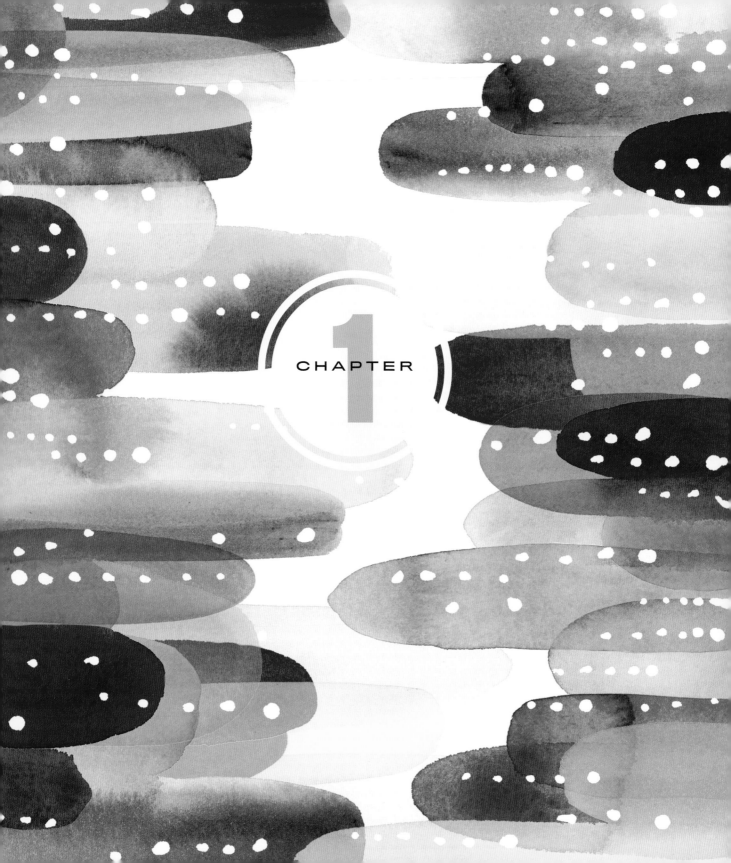

CHAPTER **1**

# Fermentation

## NATURE'S NUTRITIONAL GIFT

The simplest description of kombucha is that it is fermented tea. Sure, we all know what tea is, but what exactly is fermentation? And how could a whole generation of Americans have been raised thinking "fermented" means "rotten and moldy" or "alcoholic" when for millennia fermentation has been inextricably linked to human survival? The good news is that fermentation's stock is on the rise, and kombucha is a big reason why.

"Who wants to drink moldy tea?" You may hear this and similar questions should you begin offering your very own homebrewed kombucha to friends and family. You can either dazzle them with your knowledge of fermentation or just ignore their petty insults. Either will work because, as you may already know, kombucha tastes delicious and they'll soon be begging you for more.

How has the ancient and once essential tradition of fermentation come to be so misunderstood and maligned in the modern world? To fully understand this vital symbiosis between microorganisms and humans, we need to take a closer look at our bacterial brethren.

# We Are Our Bacteria

Humans and bacteria coevolved over millions of years. As the cosmic dust from the formation of the universe cooled, bacteria shuffled strands of DNA, evolving from single-celled organisms into multicellular beings and developing more efficient and sophisticated symbiotic relationships. Humans are supra-organisms, which means that several different types of organisms — human cells, bacteria, yeast, viruses, parasites — live in symbiosis on and within our pliable skin covering.

Research conducted over the past few decades has completely transformed the way in which we see bacteria. Crowd-sourced science experiments designed to map the living contents of our digestive systems are proving that we are essentially bacteria-powered organisms — or, as we like to say, "bacteriosapiens."

*WORD NERD:* **Ferment**

*One of the key visual clues that a ferment is working is to look for bubbles, so it's no surprise that the root comes from the Latin word* fevere, *which means "to boil." It makes sense: the action of the yeast converting sugars into* $CO_2$ *creates a layer of foam that looks exactly like the bubbles created by boiling water.*

The mind-blowing truth is that bacteria cover every surface on the planet. That includes the external surface of the human body, as well as every internal surface. If you were to turn yourself inside out, you'd still be completely covered in bacteria!

## BACTERIA FACTERIA

- Bacteria are found in even the most extreme environments, including volcanoes and Antarctica and in radioactive waste!
- 1 milliliter of fresh water contains 1 million bacterial cells.
- 1 gram of soil contains 40 million bacterial cells.
- It is estimated that bacteria are responsible for generating at least half of the oxygen used in the environment — without bacteria we wouldn't be able to breathe!
- The human body comprises 10 trillion human cells and 90 trillion bacterial cells.

- All of the bacteria in your body collectively weigh about 4 pounds.
- Researchers have discovered 2,375 species of bacteria in belly buttons (1,500 of them previously unknown!).
- The human gut microbiome — the ecological community of microorganisms that occupy our digestive tract — contains more than 1,000 types of bacteria.

# The Benefits of Fermented Foods

Being covered in bacteria may sound creepy, but when we consider that most bacteria are our allies, not our enemies, the meaning of "bacteria powered" becomes easier to appreciate. And it makes sense that consuming foods containing those beneficial bacteria can help support the bacteria in and on our bodies.

Here is where fermentation comes into play: fermented foods are rich sources of probiotics — that is, those beneficial bacteria. And they are ubiquitous! Most people can find fermented foods lurking in their fridges right now. These familiar foods all undergo fermentation:

- Most cheeses (cheddar, blue, Brie, etc.)
- Cured meats (prosciutto, salami, etc.)
- Yogurt
- Pickles
- Miso
- Tempeh
- Kimchi

When done right, fermentation of food helps with nutrient absorption, vitamin synthesis, breaking down proteins, alkalizing pH, restoring homeostasis, boosting immunity, and producing immunoglobulins. When we consume this somewhat predigested food, our bodies do less work for more gain, something that keeps us coming back for more. Fermentation not only provides superior nutrition, it acts as nature's fridge, allowing us to preserve food through long cold winters when the land is fallow. And it allows us to extract nutrition from foods that would otherwise be toxic, such as

when the process removes cyanide from cassava or destroys phytic acid in grains.

The real genius of fermentation is the way in which it naturally evolved with our needs. Take sauerkraut as an example. Like any fruit or vegetable, cabbage has its own contingent of bacteria, especially on its outer leaves, which come from the soil. Humans can nurture these bacteria by providing a low-pH environment in the form of brine, similar to (but not as sour as) the human stomach — and then letting the bacteria do their thing.

The healthy acids created by the bacterial digestive process (that is, fermentation) break the cabbage leaves down into their nutritional components, at the same time creating a unique new flavor and smell. By trusting *their* guts, early humans learned that creating a pro-bacteria environment not only led to improved immunity and mood, but also provided a means of survival, especially during harsher months when food was scarce.

Weston A. Price, pioneering nutrition researcher of the early twentieth century and founder of the American Dental Association, meticulously documented the native dietaries of indigenous people from all parts of the earth. He found, over and over, that adults of childbearing age — both women and men, but especially pregnant women — were fed the most highly prized nutrient-dense foods and

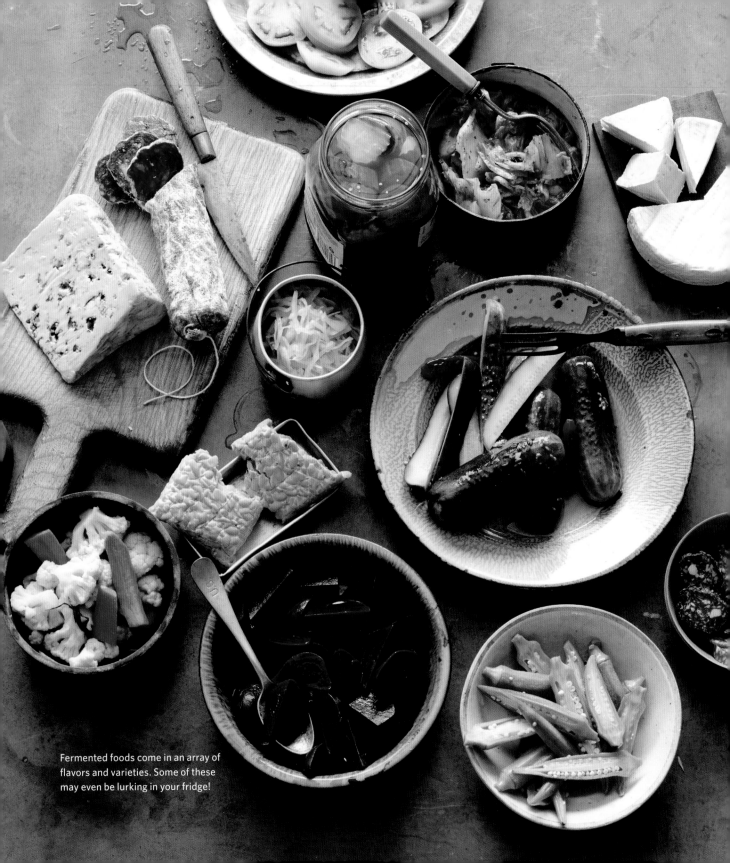

Fermented foods come in an array of flavors and varieties. Some of these may even be lurking in your fridge!

ferments to nourish themselves, from before procreation to pregnancy all the way through nursing, thus ensuring healthier newborns, maximum milk production, and increased nutrient density in that breast milk.

Sandor Katz, author of *The Art of Fermentation* and godfather of the modern fermentation revival, has made, consumed, and studied fermented foods for many decades. His work attests that every human society on earth includes ferments in their diet.

# Two Brains Are Better Than One

In addition to the brain in your head, the one you've been told does all the work, you have a brain in your gut, too, called the enteric nervous system. Consisting of neurons that line the digestive tract from esophagus to colon, your enteric brain carries out complex processes and is capable of learning and remembering, just like the one in your head. It is the seat of what we call "gut instinct."

As a fetus develops, its enteric system and brain are formed from the same tissue. Connected by the vagus nerve, which acts as the core of the gut-brain axis, these two brains send and receive signals that control heart rate, sweating, and speech, among other behaviors. When the mind experiences nervousness, that feeling travels down the vagus nerve, causing blood to pump faster, palms to sweat, "butterflies" to arise in the stomach, even a nervous stammer. Nearly 90 percent of all stimulation of the vagus nerve originates in the gut, making it a key pathway of communication to the brain.

What a revelation this can be! Knowing that the brain in our head and the brain in our belly are intimately connected illuminates why and how the foods we eat have an impact not only on our physical well-being but also on our mental and emotional well-being. Seemingly disparate conditions from food allergies to autism and irritable bowel syndrome to mental illness have been tied to the relationship between the neurological and gastrointestinal systems and the bacterial diversity of the gut.

Understanding this relationship can drastically change our approach to resolving various neurological and gastrointestinal ailments, whether through individualized diet plans or healing treatments. For the latest research, check out the Human Microbiome Project or American Gut project.

# The Fermentation of Tea

Through the alchemy of fermentation, tea, the most popular beverage in the world, becomes a healthy, bubbly brew. Just as in other types of fermentation, a SCOBY (Symbiotic Culture of Bacteria and Yeast) and an inoculant (starter liquid) are added to the substrate (sweet tea) for a period of primary fermentation that typically lasts seven or more days. After that time, the sweet and tart liquid is often flavored with fruit, herbs, and/or spices and is bottle-aged or secondary fermented to create additional carbonation and flavor. This dynamic health duo — tea and fermentation — packs a nutritional punch that improves digestion and boosts immunity in one tasty quaff.

# Fermented Beverages of the Ancient World

One of fermentation's most important uses is turning questionable drinking water into delicious, nutritious, low-alcohol drinks — think ginger "ale" and root "beer" — suitable for children and adults alike via the addition of herbs and barks. Modern sodas try to cheaply imitate the sweet-tart flavor of living ferments by combining table sugar with man-made acids and bubbles, failing miserably but profiting nonetheless.

Perhaps the very first fermented beverages were prehistoric accidents involving berries, trees, honey, standing water, and wild yeast. Ever since, humans have found countless applications, from medicinal to nutritional to social, and archaeologists have long understood that the fermentation of beverages played a vital role in the development of human society.

One of the most important and prolific categories of ferments from a nutritional, food-storage, and medicinal standpoint is vinegar, which humans have long consumed in combination with other herbals. Here are some traditional vinegar beverages from throughout history.

**Chomez.** A mixture of vinegar, oil, and dates, *chomez* likely was the vinegar beverage that Ruth of the Old Testament (Ruth 2:14) was said to have consumed. It is still popular in the Middle East to this day, a refreshing beverage in the heat of the desert.

**Oxymel.** Oxymel is a combination of vinegar and honey boiled down to a thick syrup, the benefits of which were described by Hippocrates as far back as 400 BCE and included treatment of acute illness. The Romans revered it as a panacea. The Arabic version of oxymel, *sekanjabin* (a Persian drink with mint), is traditionally made with sugar and was first mentioned in texts dating back to the tenth century.

**Posca.** Adding vinegar to water is an ancient practice that not only made the water potable but also imbued it with a refreshing flavor. The Romans called this drink *posca*, and soldiers from many cultures sipped it to increase strength and stamina and to stave off disease.

**Shrubs.** Shrubs are sweetened fruit syrups preserved in vinegar. Developed as a method of preserving the harvest and popular in the United States during colonial times, they saved countless sailors from scurvy on long voyages across the ocean. (See page 236 for more on shrubs.)

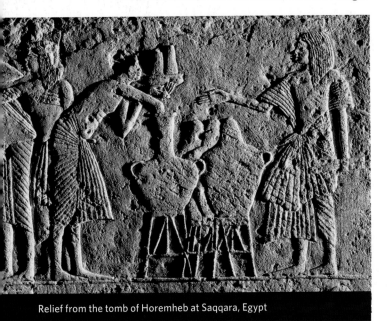

Relief from the tomb of Horemheb at Saqqara, Egypt

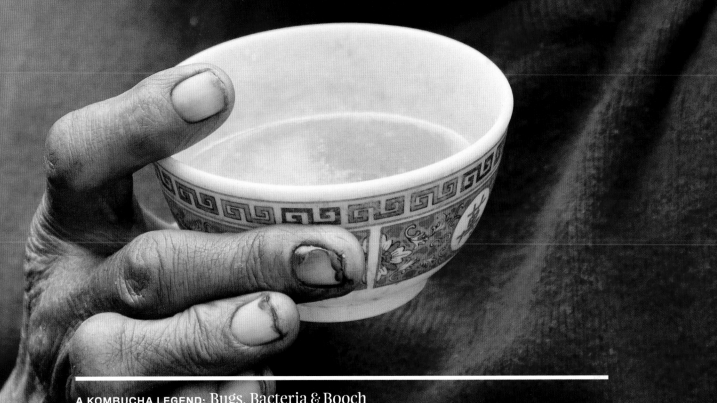

## A KOMBUCHA LEGEND: Bugs, Bacteria & Booch

So where did the original kombucha culture come from? Theories abound (see page 332), but one of the most compelling and simplest of explanations could be that when bacteria-carrying insects landed in a cup of sweet tea forgotten on a windowsill, a culture was able to form. According to one Tibetan legend, a slumbering monk inadvertently allowed a fresh pot of tea to be infiltrated this way. After discovering the wonderful properties of this happy accident, he shared his good fortune with friends, and the rest is history.

A Russian fable involves a monk with healing powers who was summoned to help an ailing emperor. The monk promises to treat the emperor's sickness with an ant, and then drops it in the emperor's tea, advising him to wait for the jellyfish to grow and transform the tea to a healing potion before drinking it. The emperor followed the monk's advice and was healed. Could this have been Dr. Kombu? (See page 332.)

Bachinskaya, the Russian scientist who first studied kombucha at the turn of the twentieth century (see page 336), based her origin theory on the fact that fruit flies (which, granted, don't look much like ants) can turn a batch of wine or beer to vinegar simply by landing in it. When the *Acetobacter* bacteria that live on the flies' legs are transferred to the liquid, they quickly begin multiplying and converting the sugars into acetic acid.

All of these legends carry a kernel of truth at their heart, which is that kombucha comes from nature. A fly, an ant, an observant and curious human, ideal brewing conditions — all of these factors combined to create the original kombucha mother that has been nurtured, treasured, and passed down for generations.

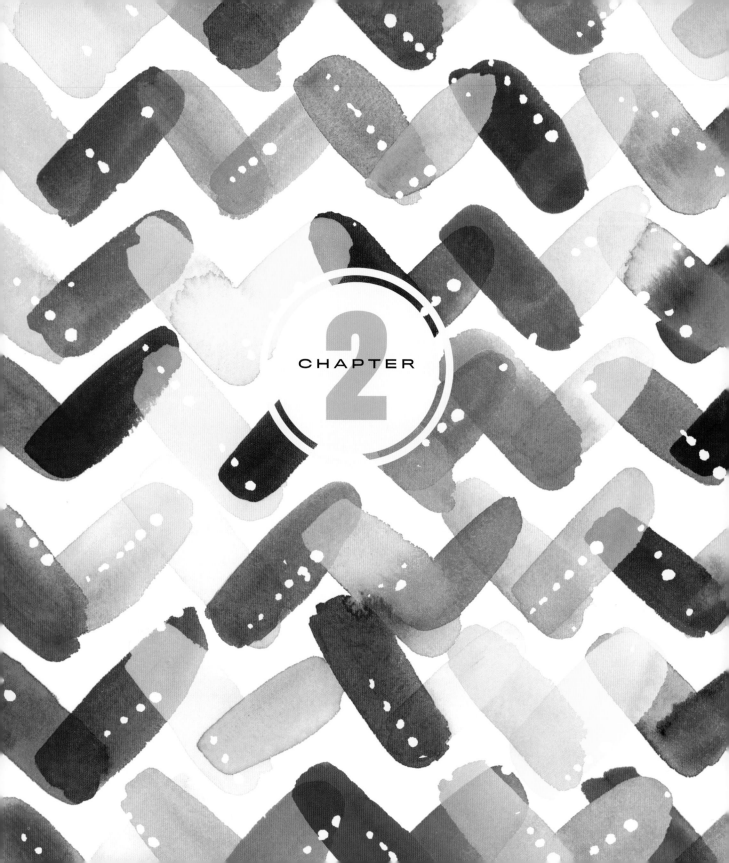

CHAPTER

2

# Why Kombucha Tea?

All fermented foods offer nutrition as well as beneficial bacteria and yeast, so why drink kombucha? The answer is both obvious and a mystery. It is obvious because kombucha is the most versatile ferment in the world. Consumed at all times of day, it can be brewed as sweet or sour as desired, is equally delicious with savory flavorings and sweet ones, and pairs just as well with a salty slice of pizza as with a chunk of chocolate. In many homes around the world, it replaces sodas, carbonated waters, alcohol, and other store-bought drinks with an inexpensive, homemade option.

Kombucha has left its mark in countries on every (inhabited) continent and is suitable for any type of diet. Safe and easy to brew and flavor at home, it can even be used in place of products sold for the kitchen, bathroom, pantry, cleaning closet, garden, and more. For these reasons and more, kombucha's appeal is obvious.

Yet kombucha's appeal is also a mystery — some people never acquire the taste for it, others have a hard time saying why they enjoy it, and many people drink it every day, yet would never brew their own. People discover kombucha for a variety of reasons, but they almost always remember the first time they had it (Kombucha Kismet!).

Many decide to try kombucha because they've heard it can ease or alleviate a variety of ailments, and indeed, when they begin drinking kombucha, they often experience positive results in a short time. However, kombucha doesn't cure specific ailments; rather, it gives the body the opportunity to return to balance so that the immune and other physiological systems function more efficiently.

Kombucha is often referred to as a gateway food, because this one health-promoting choice can lead to a whole host of others, bringing balance to body, diet, and lifestyle. With regular consumption, kombucha can be part of deep, positive changes in all aspects of life.

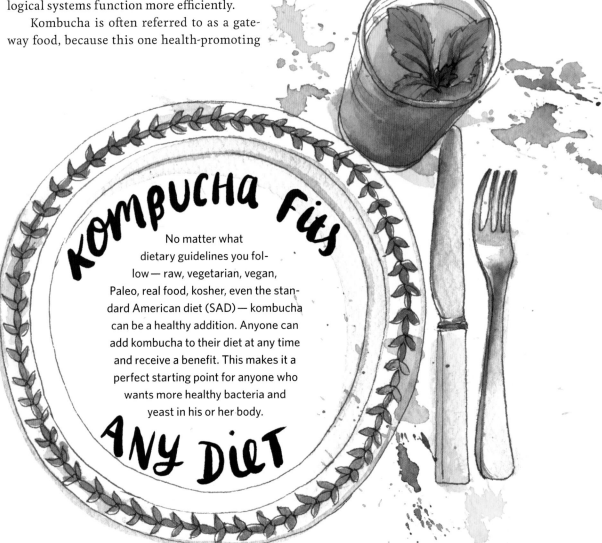

## KOMBUCHA FiTS ANY DiET

No matter what dietary guidelines you follow — raw, vegetarian, vegan, Paleo, real food, kosher, even the standard American diet (SAD) — kombucha can be a healthy addition. Anyone can add kombucha to their diet at any time and receive a benefit. This makes it a perfect starting point for anyone who wants more healthy bacteria and yeast in his or her body.

# Reconnect to the Gut with Kombucha

Too often people regularly consume toxic foods while complaining about how sick and tired they feel without drawing the connection: "Garbage in, garbage out." The rebalancing effect of regular kombucha consumption often sparks a reconnection to the gut by "closing the loop," allowing one to make informed choices based on how the body experiences different inputs.

Drinking kombucha on an empty stomach is a great way to feel its effects on the body. Starting with 4 ounces or less first thing in the morning gives you a chance to more keenly observe how it makes your body feel. As the gut adjusts to a regular influx of living bacteria and yeast, as well as healthful acids that stimulate the body, it will communicate which foods support health and which don't.

Some who are new to fermented foods may feel energized and crave more, while others could spend the day in bed or the bathroom experiencing a Herxheimer reaction (see page 20). There is no wrong way to determine which foods support your individual system.

## What Can Kombucha Do?

The health issues that can purportedly be relieved by kombucha read like a laundry list of modern ailments. Here are some of the benefits that have been observed:

- Promotes healthy bacteria in the gut
- Rebalances homeostasis in the body
- Supports healthy liver function
- Boosts metabolism
- Improves digestion and bowel function
- Rebuilds connective tissue
- Boosts energy
- Reduces blood pressure
- Relieves headache and migraine
- Reduces occurrence and size of kidney stones
- Destroys free radicals, which are known to cause cell damage
- Aids healthy cell regeneration
- Improves eyesight
- Heals eczema
- Prevents arteriosclerosis
- Speeds healing of ulcers
- Helps clear up candidiasis (i.e., yeast infections)
- Lowers glucose levels (prevents energy spikes)

How can one beverage possibly be good for so many seemingly different problems? These are the types of claims that cause some people to refer to kombucha as a "panacea" and others to call it "snake oil" — but both are wrong. It's just a healthy food that doesn't cure or prevent any disease.

However, the more we understand the effects of diet and stress on our human organism, the more it becomes obvious why kombucha is of such great benefit for so many of our modern diseases. When experiencing digestive or systemic imbalances, the body generates signals of stress that indicate impending failure. These signals are the symptoms of disease. Unlike over-the-counter or prescription medications, kombucha does not aim

# TOP 5 WAYS KOMBUCHA RELIEVES STRESS

The stress response is one of the body's most valuable defense mechanisms. When our body perceives a threat, a snap decision must be made — fight or flight. Adrenaline and cortisol are released to increase heart rate, sharpen the senses, and prepare muscles for quick action. This is exactly what we need when surviving in the wild.

The modern human, however, confronts multiple stressors — almost always non-life-threatening — on a daily basis, and this overactivation of the stress response has proven detrimental to our health, creating a host of adverse effects on the body.

While many medications and treatments can alleviate the symptoms of chronic overstimulation of the stress response, they don't tend to address the source of the problem, which is that modern humans are stressed out to the max. There are solutions: making time for exercise, getting enough sleep, enjoying the company of good friends, communing with nature, taking time to unplug from the doom-and-gloom news and electronic media. Adding kombucha to the mix can help too! Here are five ways kombucha relieves stress.

## 1.
### Kombucha is an adaptogen.

An adaptogen is a plant or plant-based derivative (fermented tea in this case) that normalizes and balances the body, benefiting the entire physiology rather than a specific organ or system. Adaptogens are generally very good sources of antioxidants, which eliminate free radicals that cause oxidative stress. They also provide liver protection, reduce cravings for sugar and alcohol, and boost immunity, energy, and stamina.

## 2.
### Kombucha supports healthy digestion.

Kombucha regulates the digestive system by increasing the acidity of the gut. Gut acidity is crucial for easing digestion and absorbing nutrients from food. Stress often manifests in the gut as irritable bowel syndrome or ulcers, both of which are aided by improved digestion and acidity.

## 3.
### Kombucha contains B vitamins and vitamin C.

Kombucha contains vitamins $B_1$ (thiamine), $B_6$, and $B_{12}$, all of which are known to help the body fight depression, stabilize mood, and improve concentration. It also contains vitamin C, which suppresses the release of cortisol (one of the stress hormones). Higher levels of cortisol in the blood contribute to hypertension, depression, and impaired mental clarity.

Moreover, while these vitamins are found in kombucha in trace amounts, they are bioavailable — that is, they are in a form that the body has evolved to assimilate instantly. In contrast, oftentimes the vitamins in supplements are not easily assimilated by the body; they lack the cofactors or enzymes found in whole foods that are needed to catalyze the absorption process.

## 4.

### Drinking kombucha can reduce caffeine and sugar intake.

Choosing kombucha over coffee as your morning eye-opener means less caffeine in your system. And the L-theanine in tea counteracts the harmful effects of caffeine, providing focused, calm energy.

## 5.

### Low amounts of alcohol have a beneficial effect on the body.

Kombucha is not an alcoholic ferment like beer or wine, but it does contain trace amounts of alcohol. These naturally occurring low levels of alcohol increase feelings of well-being and decrease stress. Numerous studies show that moderate consumption of alcohol has many positive benefits. (Learn more about the alcohol content of kombucha on page 18.)

to simply alleviate the symptoms of disease; it empowers the body to get to work on the root cause.

While large-scale, double-blind human trials may still be out of reach, a growing body of in vitro and in vivo research demonstrates the potential mechanisms by which kombucha can correct systemic imbalances. This research, in conjunction with the body of anecdotal information from millions of kombucha consumers, generates the kind of interest that will lead to the type of studies needed for Western medical proof. (See What's in Kombucha, page 357, and Highlights of Kombucha Benefits Research, page 364.)

## Getting Started with Kombucha

When first introducing kombucha to your diet, start slowly. Drink just 2 to 4 ounces, perhaps mixed with water, first thing in the morning on an empty stomach. Then wait to see how your body reacts over the next few hours. Observing how food makes your body feel is a powerful tool for truly learning to trust *your* gut.

If your body reacts well or even craves more, gradually increase your consumption, but remember that too much too fast can lead to detoxification symptoms and a healing crisis (see page 20). If this happens, reduce intake and drink more water, then ease back into the booch as your body recalibrates.

You might feel ravenous for kombucha when you first begin drinking it. This is normal, and it likely indicates that the kombucha is supplying some nutrient that your body needs to correct a deficiency. Kombucha is a tonic, so for greatest effect it is best consumed in small amounts regularly rather than in large amounts every once in a while. Once your gut tells you that it's ready for a regular regimen of kombucha, most people find that consuming eight ounces of kombucha, one to three times a day provides the flavor and nutrition they seek. Then again, you might drink a gallon today and none tomorrow. There's no wrong way to consume kombucha if it makes you feel good.

## Introducing Kombucha to Newbies

We all know people who could use some kombucha in their life. But most people dislike getting a lecture about their health, especially if they didn't ask for advice in the first place! To avoid sounding like a nag, here are a few tricks that might tip the balance.

1. Bring your kombucha to a party or potluck, perhaps labeled "Flavored Tea" or something else innocuous, and leave it on the table for others to discover. Stake out a vantage point, and enjoy the show as people react to the flavor (look for the "Kombucha Face"). Soon they will be enlisting others to give it a try, and once you reveal that you make this delicious beverage at home, you may find yourself answering a lot of questions!

2. For the reluctant taster, offer it with a splash of water or over ice. Just as it enhances the experience of drinking scotch, a little water opens up the more complex notes of the kombucha and mellows the bite of acetic acid.

3. For soda and juice addicts, dilute kombucha by half with their favorite beverage. They'll receive the full benefit of the kombucha, but the fermented flavor will be mostly masked by the added sweeteners

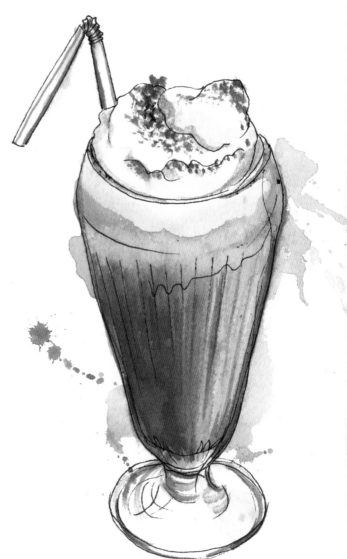

in their chosen beverage. If they're intrigued, they can gradually increase the amount of kombucha as their addictions subside.

4. Offer people who spurn "health talk" a kombucha kocktail from chapter 13. A little bit of kombucha balances the alcohol and supports healthy liver function.

5. Even someone who's tried it and "doesn't like it" might say yes to a kombucha float! A scoop of vanilla ice cream plopped in a tall glass of delicious, tangy booch is a match made in heaven! (See Chocolate Cherry Kombucha Float, page 228.)

### The Lemon Test

"When I first started drinking kombucha, my body chemistry was very different. I couldn't taste how much sugar was in the processed foods that were a regular part of my diet. As I drank more, the pH of my body shifted, and processed foods started to be too sweet for my palate. This led me to incorporate a variety of new foods into my diet, including other fermented foods, grapefruit juice (used to hate it!), and other sour, bitter, and salty flavors formerly offensive to my over-sugarfied palate.

Now, if I want to test if my pH is in balance, I lick a cut lemon. If I've been eating too much sugar, it will taste sour to me and I'll make a face. If I've been drinking enough kombucha, the lemon might even taste sweet. Give it a try and see what kind of face you make!"

# Why Kombucha "Works"

Poor dietary choices and chronic stress are the root causes of many modern diseases. Both diet and stress can trigger physiological imbalances and degradation, particularly in the immune system. As an adaptogenic tonic, kombucha contains elements that offer nutritional and digestive support, strengthen the immune system, and assist in removing impurities from the blood and organs.

Kombucha has several "good guys" in its corner that contribute to the body's ability to restore physiological balance and support the immune system: tea, sugar, healthy bacteria and yeast, and low levels of alcohol. In the brewing process, a kind of alchemy takes place, transforming these common elements into an extraordinary nutritive tonic, producing a sum greater than the parts.

We may not ever understand every single acid and vitamin interaction in the human gut, but we know that what we eat matters and that fermented foods can help most people.

## Nutritional and Digestive Support

Positioned at the center of the body, the gut is truly the human engine, and it requires the right fuel and maintenance. Kombucha can help populate the gut with good bacteria and B-vitamin–rich yeast, lower the pH of the stomach, and jump-start digestion and nutrition absorption with a number of healthy acids and enzymes.

Acetic acid provides flavor and antimicrobial power; gluconic, butyric, and lactic acids rebuild the lining of the gut, balance pH, and destroy *Candida* overgrowth; and the enzymes invertase and phytase cleave longer sugar molecules into shorter ones, reducing the impact on the digestive system (see page 361).

## Immune Support

The body's first line of defense comes directly from the gut, where immunoglobulins and other protective compounds are synthesized from the foods we consume. Kombucha's immune-boosting properties begin with digestive function support in the form of living organisms and healthy acids, enabling the body to more effectively protect itself. From there, kombucha's antioxidant activity, which cleans the body of free radicals, can begin the breakdown of polyphenols and the production of powerhouses such as vitamin C and DSL (D-saccharic acid-1,4-lactone).

The variety and quality of the B vitamins produced by the yeast along with glutamic acid, an amino acid important in balancing the immune system, also play a role. Anecdotally, kombucha drinkers find that once they begin consuming booch, the frequency and duration of common illnesses decrease.

## Detoxification

Toxicants enter our bodies daily from air, water, food, and other external sources, but the body also produces toxins as a natural by-product of several metabolic processes. No matter how they got there, these toxicants must be removed for optimal functioning.

Gluconic acid and glucuronic acids bond with toxins in the liver, transforming them from fat soluble to water soluble so they can be flushed out through the urine.

Amino acids like glutamic acid and proline, as well as benzoic acid, assist in this process while, as previously mentioned, powerful antioxidants assist detoxification by eliminating free radicals, which can damage tissue or lead to tumor formation.

## Adaptogenic Tonic

Adaptogens are natural nontoxic herbs or compounds that adhere to the pharmacological concept of encouraging homeostasis (balance), which in turn improves the body's ability to reduce the negative impact of normal stressors, be they biological or psychological. Generally adaptogens — kombucha, ashwagandha, and ginseng, to name a few — provide antioxidants, protect the liver, and reduce cravings for sugar and alcohol, as well as boost immunity, energy, and stamina.

# The Role of Healthy Low Alcohol

"Healthy alcohol" might seem like an oxymoron, but when we examine the roots of alcohol consumption, it is easy to understand the key role it plays in human health. Alcohol was humanity's earliest medicine.

Our ancestors infused herbs in alcohol to make cough syrups and healing tinctures. The health benefits inherent in the herbs were enhanced by the fermentation process and easily conferred upon the imbiber, as alcohol also thins the blood for speedy absorption.

As human knowledge of flora has grown, so too has our consumption of herb-infused tonics, whether alcoholic or not. In the case of kombucha, the trace amounts of alcohol serve a dual function: it draws out the nutritive and healing constituents from the herbs and other ingredients and it acts as a preservative.

Kombucha is a traditional "soft" drink — a naturally low-alcohol fermented beverage. Fermented soft drinks may top out between 1 and 2% ABV (alcohol by volume), usually less, and are non-inebriating. Once consumed the world over by old and young alike, they have been largely displaced by sodas and energy drinks.

Sally Fallon, author of *Nourishing Traditions*, theorizes that "the craving for both alcohol and soft drinks stems from an ancient collective memory of the kind of lacto-fermented beverages still found in traditional societies. These beverages give a lift to the tired body by supplying mineral ions depleted

## CAN RECOVERING ALCOHOLICS DRINK KOMBUCHA?

Alcoholism is a complex issue with emotional as well as physical components. Individuals who struggle with this disease ultimately must decide for themselves if kombucha is right for them. As discussed, a slight amount of alcohol is a natural by-product of fermentation, but the exact amount in a given batch depends on many factors. The trace amounts present in a properly fermented kombucha are non-inebriating, and in contrast to the effects of "hard" liquor, kombucha supports healthy liver function.

Some people who drink kombucha do report sometimes feeling a slight buzz that is similar to the feeling many experience after receiving a vitamin B injection. Whether the body is being affected by trace amounts of alcohol or simply enjoying a nutritional buzz, it is up to each person to interpret their own experience.

Many individuals who quit drinking alcohol report that kombucha actually helps reduce their cravings or has no effect on their recovery, perhaps because the kombucha delivers nutrition as well as relaxation from the trace amounts of alcohol. A recent study showed that recovering alcoholics with greater gut bacteria diversity were more successful at maintaining sobriety than those with less diversity, another potential application for bacteriotherapy. (See study cited on page 370.)

Others in recovery do not feel comfortable consuming a beverage with any alcohol content. It is worth noting that kombucha is considered halal and is consumed by Muslims, whose faith proscribes drinking alcohol.

For those who remain unsure, remember that kombucha is a tonic that is intended to be consumed in small amounts, limiting the alcohol intake from the beginning. Diluting a serving by half with water or juice has the added benefit of helping to hydrate and flush away anything released by the body. While alcohol levels rarely rise above 2 percent, there are ways to reduce even those low levels (see page 151 for details).

through perspiration and contribute to easy and thorough assimilation of our food by supplying lactobacilli, lactic-acid and enzymes." Her words echo our own theory that humans instinctually crave carbonation because it is synonymous with nutrition. (See Is Kombucha a Soft Drink?, page 348.)

# The Detoxification Process

When the body is out of balance, introducing healthy bacteria and other probiotic flora initiates a process of detoxification that can cause unpleasant side effects. In fact, incorporating kombucha, especially into a diet that doesn't include many fermented foods, may stimulate what's known as a healing crisis, also called a Herxheimer reaction.

As beneficial flora gradually take control of the gut, usually by ending the overgrowth of yeast and bad bacteria, the dying organisms release various endotoxins. At the same time, kombucha's nutritive and immune-supportive properties encourage the body to release long-held toxins that have built up. This toxic release may cause some people to initially feel worse, not better.

This is an example of things being darkest just before dawn, but as the body returns to balance, symptoms taper off. A healing crisis is most likely to occur in those who have a history of ill health or weakened immunity (acne, rashes, arthritis, and so on). Temporary intensification of current or past symptoms of ill health as well as muscle aches, breakouts, rashes, headache, upset stomach, and loose stool are all common side effects that usually pass within hours or days.

Kombucha has introduced probiotics and healthy detoxifying acids to a system that may need it badly, prompting a period of kicking out bad stuff on the way to getting healthy!

## Recognizing a Healing Crisis

Healing crises are not exclusive to kombucha. Many other fermented foods, probiotic supplements, and holistic or naturopathic treatments intended to bring on the detoxification process can induce the same symptoms, especially if they are introduced too rapidly or in overly large amounts. Potential symptoms caused by a healing crisis include the following:

- Joint pain and inflammation
- Muscle soreness
- Difficulty sleeping
- Tiredness/headache/irritability
- Stuffy nose
- Fever or chills
- Acne
- Loose stool or constipation
- Candidiasis flare-up

## How to Handle a Healing Crisis

If a healing crisis has taken hold, do not panic. Reducing consumption to very small amounts or even stopping for a brief time — a couple of days — will help reduce symptoms, and following the tips below will minimize the potential for recurrence:

- Hydrate well with water and herbal teas.
- Get plenty of rest.
- Get as much sun and fresh air as possible.

- Take baths; they aid in detoxification. Use salts, oils, and herbs in baths to support the detox process.
- Keep pores clear. Pores can be an important channel of elimination for toxins, and they can become clogged during a healing crisis. Light exercise, saunas, and hot showers can help unclog them.
- Eliminate all processed foods.
- Stay away from chemical cleaners and artificial scents.

Most people feel better after reducing intake, but if symptoms persist for more than a few days after stopping consumption, seek advice from your health-care provider.

**KOMBUCHA MAMMA SEZ**

## My Own Healing Crisis

"Since incorporating kombucha into my life, I've experienced a number of healing crises. From changes in elimination habits to bouts of acne, I've healed in stages. Kombucha has assisted in removing built-up toxins in a gentle, gradual fashion. It has not only helped me detox internally, but externally as well.

A few years after I started drinking kombucha, while hiking in the woods I foolishly assumed that poison oak couldn't possibly hang down from a tree. That error in judgment resulted in a painful case of poison oak that covered the majority of my body in red, painful sores and blisters. While I immediately applied kombucha cultures to the affected areas, it provided only minimal relief by reducing the swelling but did not alleviate the intense pain and discomfort. It took steroids, lots of hot showers to release the histamines, and bottles of calamine slathered on my skin to finally calm the rash.

Fast-forward three years to when I was working as master brewer for a local restaurant and I began having extensive contact with large amounts of kombucha culture and tea. After a couple of weeks I noticed a rash on my hand and arm that looked an awful lot like poison oak. Knowing that I had not been exposed, I racked my brain for the cause. Was it foods I was eating or a new laundry detergent? Within a few days the rash subsided, only to recur the following week. Finally it dawned on me that the close contact with the kombucha was pulling out the poison oak toxins through my skin.

Over time the symptoms continued to emerge and recede, less intensely with each occurrence, until eventually they disappeared altogether. Those poisons are now gone forever instead of lingering in my body, dragging me down a little at a time.

That's an example of dramatic and obvious detoxification. The skin is a conduit for absorbing and releasing anything applied topically. In the case of kombucha, it can be used for eczema, psoriasis, and any other inflammations of the skin. Adding kombucha vinegar or extra SCOBYs to a bath or a foot soak is a terrific way to eliminate toxins through the skin.

Most often kombucha detoxification is not as clear-cut as my experience, but can be felt in the form of a headache, body aches, sore throat, or other mild reactions. It does demonstrate, however, that like peeling the layers from an onion, the detox process happens in multiple, gradual stages."

# When to Be Cautious with Kombucha

There are no known contraindications for kombucha, and it has no known adverse interactions with medications, either over-the-counter or prescription. However, it is always prudent for people with compromised or susceptible immune systems to exercise caution when initiating any dietary or lifestyle changes; this applies to fermented foods that contain beneficial bacteria and yeast.

Some of those warned to proceed with caution include pregnant or nursing women, infants, and those with illnesses related to weakened immunity. If you have any questions, it never hurts to consult with a primary care provider. That said, many sick people consume living foods successfully and receive healing support from the nutrition. Only the individual can make the final choice.

## Pregnant or Nursing Women

Pregnancy, childbirth, and nursing, especially for first-time mothers, has become overrun with anxiety and stress around "doing everything right." New moms or moms-to-be often wonder if kombucha is helpful or harmful, and our answer is predictable: trust *your* gut.

In general, if you are already a kombucha drinker, there's no reason to give it up when you become pregnant. If kombucha is new to you, then pregnancy may not be the best time to begin drinking it. As we've discussed, anyone who begins to drink kombucha may experience a healing crisis, and a mother's symptoms may or may not affect the baby. Regardless, as with all beginning kombucha drinkers, a pregnant or nursing mother should not consume more than a couple of ounces of kombucha at a time.

It's interesting to note that some pregnant women, even ones who have enjoyed kombucha before pregnancy, report finding the smell and/or taste of kombucha revolting. After giving birth, they find that they once again enjoy it. Isn't that wonderful? The body, which may normally love and crave the kombucha, sends a message, for whatever reason, to those women to avoid it and then lets them know when it's okay to drink it again — an amazing example of "trust *your* gut" in action.

Conversely, many women report that they crave kombucha throughout their pregnancy and beyond. That's no surprise, as there are a variety of ways in which kombucha can be helpful in addressing some common pregnancy issues. Throughout pregnancy, women experience an influx of hormones that support the growing fetus and prepare the body for childbirth. In many women these hormones also stimulate unwelcome physiological side effects, and kombucha can be helpful in soothing them. They include the following:

***Difficulty sleeping/fatigue.*** During pregnancy, the body expends a great deal of energy supporting the growing child, and fatigue is normal. Kombucha boosts energy naturally by delivering microdoses of B vitamins and small amounts of caffeine, both of which energize without the crash and burn cycle of coffee. The excitement and attendant anxiety around childbirth can also lead to insomnia. Kombucha's adaptogenic properties make it easier for the body to deal with stress; those qualities are amplified when it is flavored with lavender, chamomile, or other relaxing herbs.

*Constipation, heartburn, and indigestion.* During pregnancy the esophagus relaxes, increasing the likelihood of heartburn. Digestive muscles also relax, which decreases peristaltic movements and contributes to constipation. Kombucha is a well-known remedy for constipation, indigestion, heartburn, and other digestive issues. Regularly drinking a few ounces of kombucha in a large glass of water not only passes on the health benefits of the kombucha but also hydrates the body.

*Hemorrhoids.* Increased blood flow during pregnancy causes the veins to expand. Couple that with constipation and pressure from the expanding uterus and pop go the hemorrhoids. Kombucha reduces topical inflammation, so a small piece of SCOBY or a compress soaked in kombucha and positioned over the affected area can bring relief. Repeat as needed.

*Leg cramps.* Some pregnant women experience leg cramps, and there is some speculation that the cramping may be due to shifts in how much calcium is used by the body. If you take calcium supplements, drinking kombucha can increase the amount of calcium your body absorbs. If you brew your own kombucha, you can add crushed eggshells to the ferment, which not only adds calcium but also mellows the flavor and increases carbonation. (See page 150).

*Stretch marks and other skin changes.* The skin is an amazing organ that stretches to accommodate the growing baby. Applying kombucha cultures topically can be effective at minimizing stretch marks and other pregnancy-related changes to the skin. (See the recipe for Soothing SCOBY Cream on page 314.)

*Breast-milk flow.* The stress of caring for an infant coupled with inexperience can often frustrate new mothers as they learn to breast-feed. In Europe new mothers are often provided unfiltered (or "raw") beer to help them relax and encourage a good flow of breast milk. The trace amounts of alcohol and nutrition in kombucha provide a similar benefit.

## KOMBUCHA'S EFFECT ON THE FEMALE CYCLE

When systems are out of balance, they may not function properly; the effects could be digestive, menstrual, or emotional. This means that when balance is restored, those systems might start working again.

Kombucha's gentle balancing and detoxifying properties may have particular benefit for women who are struggling with infertility. If the human organism is not receiving the nutrition it needs to thrive or is bogged down with toxins or harmful bacteria and yeast, then it will not be in an optimal position to reproduce. Gentle, gradual detoxification and rebalancing may assist the body's efforts to create a suitable environment for reproduction.

Some women also report that their period starts again after menopause while others have noted changes in their menstrual flow. All bodies are different, so each woman's experience will be unique.

## Infants and Young Children

Determining when to begin offering kombucha to children is a personal choice. Contrary to what many adults think, kids often love the taste of kombucha right away. Perhaps exposure to sodas and other overly processed foods has not taken full effect on their body's chemistry and taste preferences? Whatever the reason, even if they make a sour face at first taste, kids will often ask for more booch!

Some parenting sources question giving any fermented food to children under 12 months old for various reasons, usually related to concerns about underdeveloped immune systems or fears of allergic reactions. Most agree that introducing foods like kombucha to children after that is fine, but others recommend waiting until they are toddlers.

We have heard from parents who served kombucha and other ferments like kefir to their infant children, and in countries around the world, the question of whether or not to feed ferments to children would be met with confused looks. "Of course, it's nutritious!" would be a likely answer. Yet somehow vitamins in a bottle are considered safer and superior? Talk about crazy!

As with anyone new to kombucha, children should consume very small amounts at first (1 to 2 ounces), mixed with or followed by water. If the response is positive, gradually increase consumption. This allows the parent to observe how the kombucha works in the child's system. Biofeedback signals include stool (frequency, size, smell), elimination habits, and digestive response (gas or bloating).

We hear from proud parents all the time that their kids have become booch pros, helping with the weekly decant and brew.

## People with Compromised Immune Systems

Generally, people facing serious health challenges involving the immune system must exercise caution when introducing living fermented foods into their compromised internal environment. At the same time, fermented foods and/or probiotics can improve health and encourage recovery for many people suffering from exactly this type of health challenge. They are a great option for many people with health issues but can be problematic for an unpredictable few. People with specific immunological ailments should monitor their biofeedback signals to observe how the kombucha interacts with their body.

That said, patients prescribed a combination of medications intended to treat multiple conditions are well advised to consult closely with their health-care professional and to consume only small amounts of kombucha until the effect on the body can be assessed completely. Those with liver issues may specifically want to monitor their progress with the assistance of a primary care physician as they begin a kombucha consumption routine.

# THE KOMBUCHA BOGEYMEN

There are some wild claims about kombucha out there, but the craziest one has to be that people have died from drinking it. Let's start with this: As a natural remedy, kombucha has a documented history of use around the world, stretching back well over one hundred years. Scientific studies have been conducted during that entire time, and millions of homebrewers have made batch after batch, yet there is not a single case of fatality from kombucha on record. Zero. Nada. A big goose egg.

That is not to say that nobody has ever felt sick from drinking kombucha or that it's not possible for kombucha to negatively affect an already ill person's system due to an inability to process the beverage. That is no different from any other fermented food, which anyone with a compromised immune system should consume with caution.

And then there are otherwise healthful and accepted foods such as peanuts, which are responsible for up to one hundred deaths per year in the United States alone. In fact, our government-approved food supply is responsible for about three thousand deaths per year; prescription drugs, also regulated by the government, contribute to over one hundred thousand deaths annually.

Even so, several "bogeyman" stories persist on the Internet. The scariest, and the only one involving a death, goes back to 1995, before the modern kombucha research boom and the ready availability of information online. Unfortunately, an older woman who was making and consuming kombucha at home developed sepsis from a perforated intestine and then passed away from a heart attack. Two weeks later, another woman in the same town who was also brewing kombucha began suffering major problems with her lungs and heart that likely led to elevated acid levels (see Myth: Kombucha Makes Your Body Acidic, page 27). She was treated and survived.

Because the doctors had never heard of kombucha but knew that both women were brewing it, they contacted the government. In response, the FDA was dispatched to collect samples and the CDC issued a standard statement saying kombucha was "possibly associated" with the illnesses. In that bulletin, test results provided for the cultures show no pathogens, and no connection or medical explanation was provided.

Additionally, none of the more than one hundred other people in the same town who were all brewing with related kombucha SCOBYs experienced any issues. In short, an unfortunate coincidence was blamed on kombucha. If only the myriad of wonderful studies that have been conducted on kombucha since then were as easy to find in Web searches as this myth!

Another persistent story involves an AIDS patient who, in 2007, checked into the emergency room with dizziness and shortness of breath after reportedly consuming a store-bought kombucha. No testing was conducted on either the beverage or the individual to demonstrate any potential connection, but once again the reporting doctor, unfamiliar with kombucha, assumed it to be the cause of the patient's symptoms.

And that pretty much wraps up the haunted house of "Death by Kombucha," though there is this one other scare story that pops up: It has been reported that a batch of kombucha brewed in Iran sometime in the 1990s developed anthrax. While being brewed in a barn. Right next to cows infected with anthrax. So whatever you do, don't brew your kombucha next to anthrax-infected cows!

# KOMBUCHA MYTH-BUSTING

The fairly recent resurgence of interest in traditional methods of food cultivation and preparation and the attendant fascination with fermenting and brewing make kombucha nearly irresistible. When ignorance and excitement combine, however, factual information often becomes jumbled with the fantastical and the fearful. As knowledge of kombucha has grown and more information has become available, old myths have been outgrown but unfortunately not always discarded.

While mostly harmless, misinformation masquerading as fact too often confuses the homebrewer and disrupts proper brewing techniques. Here are some myths we'd like to bust for good.

## Myth: Kombucha Is a Mushroom

This widely held belief most likely arises from the obvious resemblance of the SCOBY to a large mushroom cap. The kombucha culture, as you know by now, is in fact a symbiotic culture of bacteria and yeast. Although the taxonomy for kombucha has not yet been formalized, mushrooms are fungi and so are yeast, so in that regard kombucha cultures and mushrooms are in the same family. But they are distant cousins, not siblings.

Adding to the confusion is that some of the old names in other languages called it a "mushroom." When those terms were translated into English, "kombucha mushroom" became a catchy name for the culture.

## Myth: Metal Will "Kill" Kombucha

Due to kombucha's powerful detoxifying properties, dire warnings to avoid even a few seconds of metal-to-kombucha contact are overblown. Brief contact with something like a strainer or a pair of scissors will not lead to a toxic SCOBY or tainted brew. However, the only type of metal that is safe for actually brewing kombucha is stainless steel, 304 grade or better, to prevent leaching potentially harmful contaminants into the brew. (See page 76 for more information.)

## Myth: SCOBYs Should Be Refrigerated

This nasty nugget is widespread and often passed along by well-meaning brewers with the explanation, "So they won't rot" or "It just puts them to sleep." In fact, SCOBYs never "go bad" when properly stored. In cold temperatures the bacteria and yeast, which keep the SCOBY healthy and protect the brew, become inactive and are unable to put up a defense against mold. When a SCOBY that has been refrigerated is activated, the first batch or two may (or may not) turn out okay, but eventually mold is likely to appear in the brew. (See page 157 for more about refrigerated cultures.)

## Myth: Dehydrated SCOBYs Are Viable

The issues are the same as with refrigeration; only this time the bacteria and yeast are too weak from dehydration to protect against mold. If the culture is deprived of the protective pH of the starter liquid, which kills harmful organisms on contact, it becomes vulnerable to mold, and the bacteria in kombucha do not perform well after dehydration. Additionally, it can take up to six weeks to rehydrate a dried-out culture before attempting the first batch. No point in wasting the time for a likely-to-fail experience.

## Myth: Kombucha Makes the Body Acidic

The body is a complex and marvelous organism, masterful at maintaining health through homeostasis. Significant shifts of internal pH indicate illness or, rarely, impending death. In order to maintain the correct pH at all times, our bodies employ several detoxification and buffering systems — such as the lungs, kidneys, and digestive system — to process acidic ash, the residue generated by the consumption of certain foods and also present in the body as the by-product of metabolic processes.

There is a debate over whether so-called acid/alkaline diets are beneficial to health, but we do know that when food is digested in the gut, its components leave residues that are either acid forming or alkali forming. The body suffers from ill effects at either extreme, so the key, according to proponents of these diets, is to strive for balance rather than focusing on consuming only one type of food or another.

So what about drinking kombucha? Won't the low pH make the body more acidic (something you've probably been told to avoid)? The answer is no. While it is true that kombucha has a low pH

(2.5–3.5), the residue (ash) is alkaline-forming rather than acidic, and has an effect similar to lemon juice and apple cider vinegar.

## Myth: Brewing Kombucha at Home Is Unsafe

When brewing kombucha at home, you pretty much have only one major issue to worry about: mold. And mold is obvious — it's the blue, black, or white fuzz growing on top of the culture. If you see it, simply toss the brew, just like you would a moldy piece of bread, cheese, or fruit. Otherwise, if you have a quality culture and strong starter liquid, and you follow the proper procedures, success is virtually guaranteed.

## Myth: Kombucha Is a Cure-All

Let's get this straight once and for all: *Kombucha is not a panacea.* In fact, it doesn't *cure* anything! Kombucha gradually detoxifies the body so that the immune system can function properly. Think of it as a filter cleaner, where the filter is your liver.

Kombucha is an adaptogen. Adaptogens are plants or compounds that satisfy three important criteria — they are nontoxic, they are nonspecific (they work on the whole body, rather than a particular part or system), and they help the body maintain homeostasis. This means that if you need to lose weight, kombucha may help you to do so, and if you need to gain weight, kombucha may help with that also.

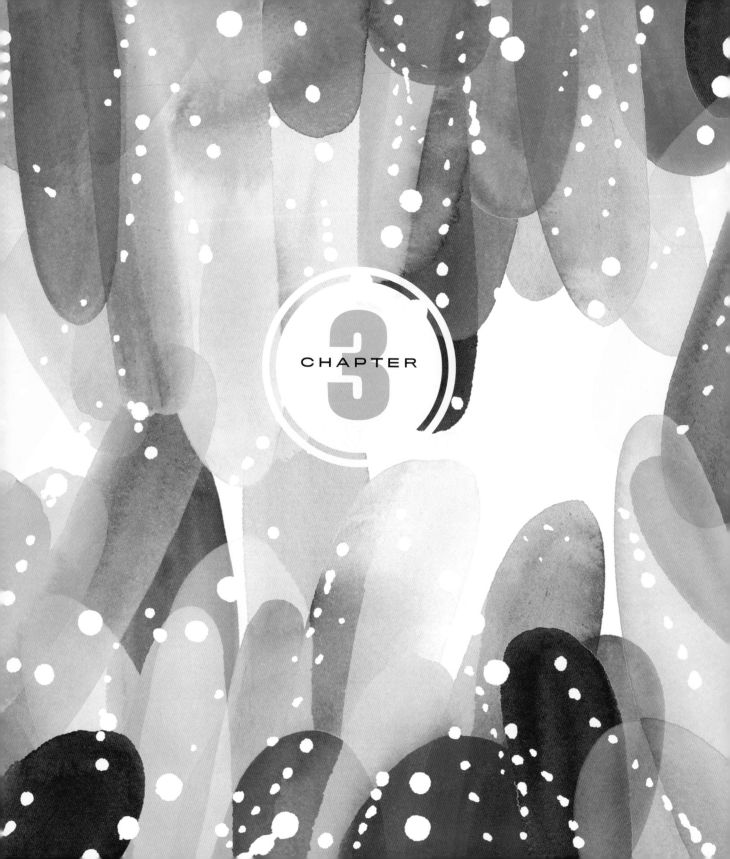

CHAPTER

3

# It All Starts with the SCOBY

The kombucha culture — which is the living material that drives the fermentation — is called a *SCOBY* (symbiotic culture of bacteria and yeast). It is a living contradiction: at once beautiful and ugly, hardy yet delicate, both mother and baby, it springs forth anew with each batch, a physical manifestation of a successful brew that also protects against contamination and prevents evaporation.

Coined by Len Porzio, a member of the Original Kombucha List on Yahoo in the mid-1990s, the term *SCOBY* originated as a means to distinguish finished brew from mother culture (read more about Len on page 353.) As the name literally states, the culture and its starter liquid, both populated with yeast and bacteria, are a dynamic symbiosis, two taxonomic kingdoms competing and cooperating like few things on earth.

The balance and interplay between the bacteria and yeast in this living culture drives the fermentation process and the production of healthy acids. But not all SCOBYs comprise the same mix of bacteria and yeast, nor are all SCOBYs of equal quality; as a result, some naturally produce a more consistent or delicious beverage than others.

This variation in composition mirrors the diversity found in all living organisms. Just as two siblings born of the same parents and reared in the same environment may grow up to be very different people, two identically prepared batches of kombucha may taste or look different. We can never perfectly control the kombucha brew, and that is part of the joy of fermentation: it is a living process.

# What Exactly Is a SCOBY?

The SCOBY is a zoogleal mat — that is, a mass of bacteria and yeast, tied together with cellulose nanofibers. The primary bacteria in a SCOBY is *Komatagaeibacter xylinum* (aka *Acetobacter xylinum*), which produces copious amounts of cellulose, although there could also be any of several other strains. The bacteria and yeast in a SCOBY depend on each other, in that the by-products of the yeast fermentation feed the bacteria and the by-products of the bacteria fermentation feed the yeast.

They build the matlike cellulose structure to make working together easier. Think of the SCOBY as an apartment building with the yeast living on some floors and bacteria on others. The mat protects the fermenting tea — their food source — against infiltration by wild bacteria and yeast.

It also reduces evaporation of the liquid while holding in more of the naturally occurring carbonation as the batch progresses. And the mat makes it extremely easy for kombucha brewers to transfer the bacteria and yeast from one batch to the next, ensuring continued propagation of select strains and species.

The symbiosis between the bacteria and yeast acts like a double karate chop to pathogenic organisms that might try to invade the sweet tea solution. The low pH of the starter liquid and culture disrupts the cell membranes of unwanted bacteria, while several of the healthy organic acids that create the low pH in the first place demonstrate specific antibacterial, antiviral, and other antimicrobial properties. This dual function makes kombucha even more effective as a health tonic because it reduces the already small likelihood that the brew will develop any toxins.

The SCOBY is the mother ship to millions of microorganisms, all working together to support their continued existence. Let's begin with a basic introduction to these component organisms, which will provide the necessary context for understanding the nuances of the symbiotic relationship.

---

**KOMBUCHA MAMMA SEZ**

### Trust All Your Senses

"Brewing and drinking kombucha is a full sensory experience. You can expect the following:

- **TASTE:** It is sweet and tart, with complex notes that change over time.
- **SMELL:** The aroma should have a sharp tang indicating a healthy ferment.
- **SIGHT:** The SCOBY is often creamy white with brown yeast strands and may be pockmarked with blowholes to release carbon dioxide. Bubbles play beneath the surface of the culture.
- **TOUCH:** The SCOBY feels smooth and soft.
- **SOUND:** The happy burbling sounds of gently popping bubbles indicate a healthy brew.

How does your experience of kombucha match up?"

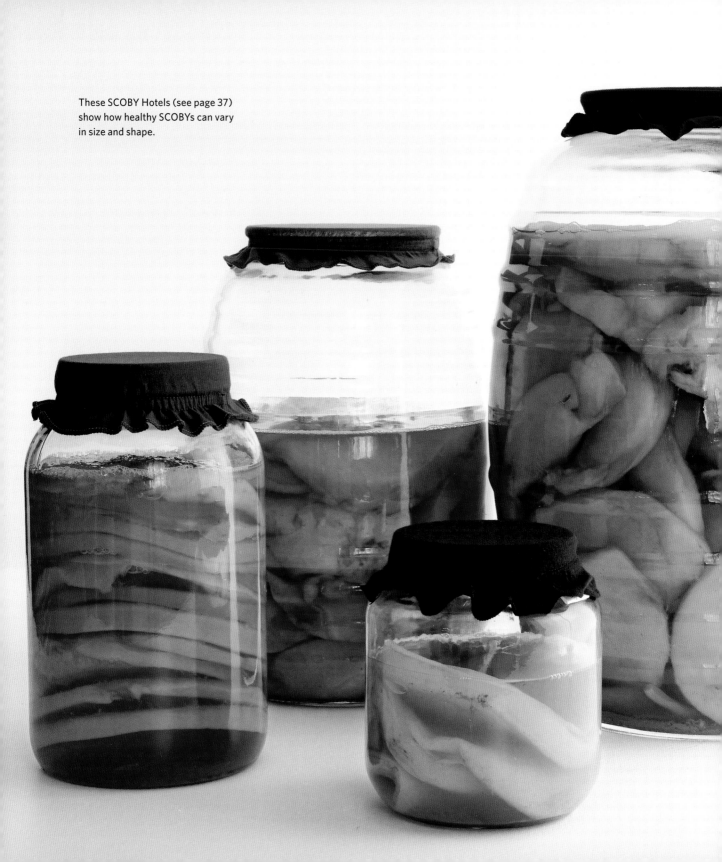

These SCOBY Hotels (see page 37) show how healthy SCOBYs can vary in size and shape.

## What Are Bacteria?

Unfortunately, bacteria have gotten a bad rap in our germaphobic society. There is no question that cleanliness is important in food preparation, but our "War on Bacteria" — too many unnecessary prescriptions for antibiotics, antibiotics added to our food supply, and antibacterial soaps and hand sanitizers in every bathroom — has upset the natural balance of "good" and "bad" bacteria that our bodies have evolved with. Research is finally coming to grips with the negative effects of this mind-set.

Bacteria are single-celled prokaryotic microorganisms. As prokaryotes, their cells lack a distinct nucleus and membrane-bound organelles, which sets them apart from the more complex eukaryotes, which include yeast, mushrooms, and human beings (amazingly, we are more like mushrooms than bacteria!). Though extremely simple organisms, bacteria are prolific, vastly diverse, and essential to life on this planet. Their very simplicity makes them vital to the healthy functioning of every living organism. As vehicles of evolution, transporting DNA to and from, turning on and off genes, bacteria are intimately involved in cellular reproduction.

Kombucha cultures always contain a preponderance of acetic-acid bacteria, which, in addition to producing the cellulose that the SCOBY is made from, convert ethanol (produced by yeast) into acetic acid. Though *Komagataeibacter xylinus* is dominant in kombucha cultures, each culture will also have unique species and strains of bacteria,

*WORD NERD* **Bacteria**

*In 1838, German naturalist Christian Gottfried Ehrenberg, a pioneer in the field of microscopic research and identification of microorganisms, saw a rod-shaped figure in his microscope. He named the organism* bacterium *from the Greek* baktērion, *meaning "staff" or "cane."*

depending on the parent culture and on local wild populations of bacteria. (See a complete list of potential bacteria, on opposite page.) In addition to building the SCOBY, the bacteria are responsible for converting the ethanol produced by the yeast into healthy acids.

## What Are Yeast?

Yeast are single-celled fungal organisms that have been faithful companions of humans since the dawn of time. Without our good buddy yeast, we would not be able to bake much or ferment at all. Yeast consume sugar and release carbon dioxide, along with either ethanol (in fermentation) or water (in respiration). The carbon dioxide causes bread to rise and gives fermented drinks their natural fizz. As we just discussed, the ethanol produced by yeast in a SCOBY in turn becomes food for bacteria, which convert the ethanol to acetic acid.

Yeast are visible to the naked eye when they collect as brown strands or strings that float through the kombucha, making it murkier as the yeast reproduce, attach to the underside of the SCOBY, and collect at the bottom of

# BACTERIA AND YEAST FOUND IN KOMBUCHA CULTURES

The nearly infinite types of bacteria are constantly being reexamined and renamed as new distinctions are recognized. This happened to the *Gluconacetobacters* in 2013, when Dr. Kazuo Komagata, of the University of Tokyo's Institute of Applied Microbiology, used DNA sequencing to study acetic-acid bacteria. Categorical differences were easier to classify, and the data clearly demonstrated phylogenetic, phenotypic, and ecological differences. Consequently, a number of bacteria were renamed *Komagataeibacter*. However, since the name change is recent, many older studies still have the old names. We have included the updated names with the older names in parenthesis.

Saccharomyces; Saccharomyces apiculatus varieties; Saccharomyces cerevisiae; Saccharomycodes ludwigii

Zygosaccharomyces; Zygosaccharomyces bailii; Zygosaccharomyces bisporus; Zygosaccharomyces kombuchaensis; Zygosaccharomyces rouxii

Candida albicans; Candida kefyr; Candida stellata

Brettanomyces anomalus (aka *Dekkera anomala*); Brettanomyces bruxellensis (aka *Dekkera bruxellensis* or *Brettanomyces custersii*); Brettanomyces clausenii; Brettanomyces lambicus

**YEAST**

Schizosaccharomyces pombe

Torulaspora delbrueckii (aka *Saccharomyces delbrueckii* or *Saccharomyces fermentati*); Torulopsis spp.

Kregervanrija fluxuum (aka *Pichia fluxuum*)

Bacterium katogenum

**BACTERIA**

Komagataeibacter saccharivorans (aka *Gluconacetobacter saccharivorans*)

Komagataeibacter xylinus (aka *Acetobacter pasteurianus, Acetobacter xylinum, Bacterium xylinum* or *Bacterium xylinoides*)

Gluconacetobacter; Gluconacetobacter spp.; Gluconobacter oxydans (aka *Bacterium gluconicum*)

Hanseniaspora uvarum (aka *Kloeckera apiculata*)

Pichia fermentans

Acetobacter aceti (aka *Acetobacter ketogenum*)

Komagataeibacter sucrofermentans (aka *Gluconacetobacter xylinus sucrofermentans*)

Acetobacter tropicalis

Komagataeibacter hansenii (aka *Gluconacetobacter kombuchae* sp.)

Rhodotorula; Rhodotorula mucilaginosa

Pseudomonas; Pseudomonas putida

Acetobacter nitrogenifigens, sp. nov.

Komagataeibacter intermedius (aka *Gluconacetobacter intermedius* or *Acetobacter intermedius*)

the jar. The exact mix and type present will vary based on different cultures as well as local yeast populations, but the most commonly found dominant strains include *Saccharomyces*, *Brettanomyces*, and *Zygosaccharomyces* spp.

## How Does the Symbiosis Work?

Symbiosis is a beautiful dance between organisms — bacteria and yeast, mother and child, human and environment. While we all experience symbiosis in daily life, taking time to reflect on the deep interconnectedness of all things is not always foremost in our minds. Brewing kombucha is a way to physically engage with symbiosis while allowing the

*WORD NERD:* **Yeast**

*To the ancient mind, the bubbles created by the fermentation process looked similar to the bubbles created by boiling water. The word yeast is derived from the Proto-Indo-European word* jes, *meaning "to boil, foam, froth." It passed to English via the Proto-Germanic word* jest *(j's are pronounced like y's in German).*

mind and spirit to feel deeply connected to our true nature as symbiotic beings.

The yeast and bacteria in a kombucha culture maintain an intricate web of interdependence. When the culture and starter liquid

## BACTERIA & YEAST
### *Party Planners vs. Party Animals*

Every good party has the right balance of party planners to party animals, and our kombucha brewing party is no different. As we all know, there is no shortage of people who like to be party animals, while party planners are scarcer. In kombucha, the yeast are the party animals, being the first to eat when food arrives and tending to reproduce rapidly if everyone is having a good time. To balance the brew, we generally need to take measures to keep the yeast in check.

These techniques include taking starter liquid from the top of the brew, which is rich with bacteria, rather than the bottom of the brew, where the yeast love to congregate. To correct persistent yeast issues from batch to batch, that starter

liquid can be filtered to remove more yeast (the much smaller bacteria pass through the filter).

And while the yeast can thrive in a much wider temperature range, the 75 to 85°F (24–30°C) range for kombucha is designed specifically to favor the health and reproduction of the bacteria, our party planners. Heating from the side rather than from the bottom also favors the bacteria by delivering warmth to where they reside in the brew and allowing the yeast to come to rest at the bottom of the vessel. There, those passed-out party animals can do no harm while the party planners clean up and finish the delicious brew for our enjoyment!

# GALLERY OF YEAST

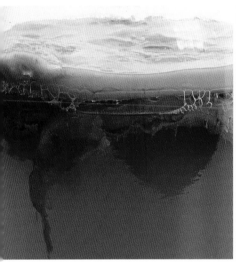

Yeast strands hang from the mother culture throughout the fermentation process.

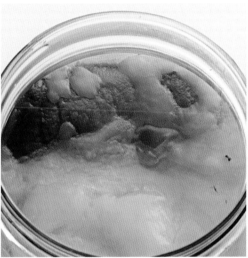

As new culture forms, some yeast bodies may become trapped in or under the cellulose, visible as brown, black, and/or blue areas or flecks.

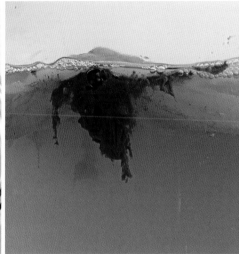

A large but normal collection of yeast hovers close to the oxygen-rich surface early in the fermentation process.

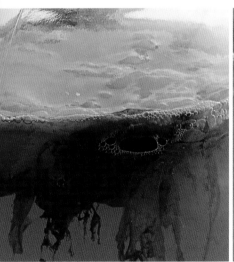

Carbon dioxide bubbles collect between the glass and culture during anaerobic fermentation under a fully formed SCOBY.

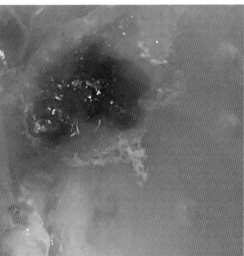

A glob of yeast trapped under new SCOBY growth may look like mold but is perfectly normal and harmless.

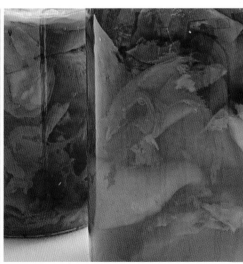

In the SCOBY Hotel, yeast may be attached to the culture, floating free, or accumulated on the bottom of the vessel.

are first added to a fresh batch of sweet tea, the yeast get right to work breaking down the weak chemical bonds of the sucrose molecule, cleaving it into its components of fructose and glucose.

At this stage, where oxygen is readily available, the yeast engage in respiration, creating carbon dioxide and water, and the yeast globs hover near the surface of the liquid. As the yeast break down the sugar, the bacteria utilize the glucose as energy to spin nanofibers of cellulose, constructing the new layer over the top of the brew.

Once the new SCOBY completely covers the surface of the brewing vessel, oxygen levels decrease, causing the yeast to switch from respiration to fermentation. Now they begin to produce carbon dioxide and ethanol, which the bacteria use to synthesize the acids that give kombucha its sour flavor and contribute to its health benefits. At this point some of the spent yeast cells fall to the bottom of the vessel, creating a layer of brown sludge. Here they rest until more fuel (sugar) is provided.

## Fermentation vs. Respiration

Fermentation and respiration are the two processes by which yeast metabolize (break down) carbohydrates. Fermentation takes place under anaerobic (without oxygen) conditions and is the process by which yeast break down sugars into carbon dioxide and ethanol.

Respiration takes place under aerobic (with oxygen) conditions and converts sugars into carbon dioxide and water. Kombucha is a unique ferment in that it employs both processes at different times in the brewing cycle.

## Balance Is Key

As we've seen, the symbiosis between the bacteria and yeast has a specific rhythm, like a dance, that leads to positive benefits for all parties. Our role in the process is to provide the highest-quality ingredients and to oversee the balance between the different organisms. Maintaining an appropriate balance makes the difference between a well-rounded sweet-tart brew and one that tastes like a mouthful of sour dirt.

It also means the difference between positive proliferation or lopsided growth for the bacteria and yeast. If there is too much yeast in the brew, the bacteria may struggle; the other way around and the brew will have little to no fizz.

Being aware of the individual players and how they contribute to the bigger picture provides key insight for keeping the brew in balance. (See Rebalancing the Brew, page 166, for specific tips.)

# Obtaining Your First SCOBY

The adage "You get what you pay for" applies to food as much as anything, and that includes a kombucha culture. There is a long tradition of passing SCOBYs along, which can be a good option if you connect with a friend or local homebrewer who meets the criteria of a reliable supplier (see page 37), and who is actively brewing, so the cultures and starter liquid are very fresh and strong.

But for peace of mind — not to mention full and detailed instructions, fast delivery, and a guaranteed brew the very first time — sourcing a SCOBY from a highly rated, reliable supplier is often the best option. But be aware that any SCOBY, whether gifted or purchased, can be of poor quality. Some suppliers advise refrigerator storage and some ship dehydrated or partially hydrated (no starter liquid) cultures, or tiny or test tube–sized cultures, saving the shipper additional expense but robbing the brew of power and flavor.

For a great brewing experience the very first time, choose a SCOBY supplier that meets the following criteria:

- Is an experienced kombucha brewer with accurate information
- Provides detailed instructions and follow-up support throughout the process
- Regularly ships or provides large SCOBYs, at least 5 inches wide
- Includes well-aged but fresh starter liquid, 6 weeks old is best, at least 1 full cup
- Does *not* recommend refrigerating cultures, covering the brew with cheesecloth, or using what's left at the bottom of the jar as starter liquid

**KOMBUCHA MAMMA SEZ**

## Get a Good SCOBY

❝All SCOBYs are not the same! Here are some tips for finding a good source.

- **EXCELLENT CHOICE:** Order a fresh, full-sized culture from a reputable supplier.
- **GOOD CHOICE:** Obtain a healthy one from a knowledgeable friend or local homebrewer.
- **AVOID:** Any SCOBY that is dehydrated, refrigerated, test tube sized, or grown from a commercial bottle."

This advice comes from over a decade spent assisting tens of thousands of homebrewers who have written or called for help while struggling with cultures that just won't make tasty booch or even reproduce. After sipping and dumping weeks or months of unsuccessful batches from a poorly sourced SCOBY, they switched to a high-quality culture and within 7 to 10 days they had exactly the brew they had always wanted.

If a culture does not perform as expected, it's probably not your fault. It may be weak or compromised due to storage, freshness, or origin. Don't waste time and money, get a guaranteed culture and instead start "worrying" about what flavors to make!

Then, when friends ask for a SCOBY, make sure to meet all the criteria above so they have a great start too, or just send them to your supplier if that's easier.

A single SCOBY is generally viable for at least 10 brewing cycles in a row before it tires, atrophies, or fails to reproduce — though some homebrewers claim to use the same SCOBY for years. We normally brew with younger SCOBYs and use older SCOBYs for experiments or eating (really! — see chapter 16). If they become mushy or grow jellylike on the edges, compost them.

## Growing and Storing SCOBYs: The SCOBY Hotel

With every batch of brew, the original SCOBY "mother" produces a "daughter" or "baby" growth, usually as another layer that forms a sort of pancake (it can be thick or thin, depending on the conditions). After a while, the daughters can be separated to start their own batches of brew or used for other purposes (see chapter 17).

Extra SCOBYs can be given away to friends or used for experimental brews — it's a good idea to have them on hand and a simple storage solution is a SCOBY Hotel. Learn all about creating and maintaining a SCOBY Hotel in chapter 6.

## Cultures to Avoid

You definitely don't want to use any of the following types of SCOBY.

*Dehydrated.* Some types of cultures, such as kefir grains, may remain viable when dehydrated (though fresh ones always brew faster and make a tastier product with more diversity of organisms), but a kombucha SCOBY is a poor candidate for this process. More often than not, the brew from a dehydrated SCOBY becomes moldy, but even if it does not, the SCOBY seldom reproduces, a sign that bacterial activity is negligible. You may believe you are making kombucha, but it is likely only a yeast drink. A dehydrated SCOBY really isn't good for much else besides being used as a chew toy for the dog! (See page 326 for more on that.)

*Refrigerated or frozen.* The kombucha SCOBY is a hardy culture that can withstand wide fluctuations in temperature as well as other less-than-ideal conditions, but only for a few hours to a few days. If stored for long periods, colder temperatures put the acetic-acid bacteria to sleep more permanently. When a new batch is started, the bacteria are sluggish and cannot protect the brew, often leading to mold within the first couple of cycles.

*Test tube or miniature.* Brewing success requires a large enough culture and strong enough starter liquid to properly acidify the sweet tea. Providers offering nuggets of SCOBYs packaged in test tubes or small jars are cutting costs at the expense of quality.

## CHILLY SCOBY? NO BIGGIE!

SCOBYs are hardy organisms that can tolerate brief periods of extreme temperatures and survive to brew again. At Kombucha Kamp, we ship cultures all over the world year-round, which means a fair share of SCOBYs end up very cold or even freezing solid for short periods en route.

So is the SCOBY dead? No! Will it still work? Yes! While refrigerating a SCOBY for many weeks will put it to sleep, a few hours or days in cold transit is not long enough to damage the culture.

However, before tossing that briefly frozen or cold culture into sweet tea, it is important to revive the SCOBY for at least a couple of days so it can do its job. Fortunately, reviving is easy! First, bring the culture back to room temperature by letting it rest in the package in a warm spot until the temperature has normalized. Give it another 12 to 24 hours for the bacteria and yeast to fully regain their fermentation mojo, then brew as you normally would!

## Growing a SCOBY from Commercial Kombucha

While some sources recommend growing a culture from a bottle of commercial kombucha, there are a number of reasons why sourcing a genuine SCOBY with full-powered starter liquid is the best choice. Essentially, producing a beverage for sale means making compromises that we don't need to make at home, and the cultures grown from those products are less potent.

One complication for commercial brewers is the need to control the naturally low levels of alcohol present in kombucha. Even though these low levels do not intoxicate, they can be slightly higher than the legally allowed levels for commercially sold "nonalcoholic" beverages (see page 348 for more on alcohol in kombucha). In 2010, fears about levels of alcohol in commercially sold bottled kombucha rising above the 0.5 percent limit led to a temporary and voluntary withdrawal of the product from store shelves.

Commercial producers underwent reformulation to address this issue. Some companies lost a lot of money in this process, both in sales and product, and a couple of them never recovered. In hindsight, these fears may have been unfounded, or at least greatly overblown, due to a lack of sophisticated alcohol measuring techniques. (See page 349 for more on this story.)

When the brands returned to shelves, a variety of methods had been employed for engineering the beverages or modifying the brewing process to artificially maintain lower alcohol content under any conditions so as to be in compliance with federal labeling laws. Some companies added lab-cultured probiotics; some altered the fermentation process itself; others made changes but kept their processes secret. Whatever the modification, the bottled product cannot be reliably depended upon to provide the vitality of a pure culture and starter liquid made for brewing at home rather than surviving bottling and storage in a warehouse.

Aside from questions of controlling alcohol, commercial producers of kombucha have a lot of other concerns. Shelf stability, price competition, the need to appeal to mainstream flavor preferences, and distribution for a product all over the country, let alone any factors that affect the ingredients and therefore the end product, can all contribute to a less vibrant brew.

Even if something does grow from a commercial bottle, and even if the first batch is successful, subsequent brews usually grow weaker in flavor and may not deliver the same nutritional benefit as a full-powered brew. The effect is similar to using store-bought yogurt to make homemade — the strength of the culture cannot be sustained over many batches, and the product eventually becomes runny and weak.

These are the realities of producing a commercial product, not an indictment of quality as a beverage (we love to buy and enjoy kombucha from the store, especially when traveling!). But as the kombucha boom continues, companies continue to stream into the marketplace, and while that's great news for the commercial consumer, so much market diversity coupled with fundamental changes to normal brewing techniques mean that growing a SCOBY from store-bought kombucha is no longer recommended. The good news is sourcing a full-powered SCOBY and starter liquid is easier than ever and by far the best way to get started brewing your own at home.

## Good Starter Liquid Is Key

Fresh, strong starter liquid is simply fermented kombucha tea taken from the top of the previous brew or from the top of the SCOBY Hotel. This liquid, which works closely in concert with the SCOBY, is crucial to brewing success. "Fresh" means it has not grown stagnant in an untended brew or hotel. "Strong" means it is at least two weeks old (four to six weeks is better). Using young starter liquid batch after batch can lead to a diluted brew.

Good-quality, well-aged starter provides the following functions:

- *Lowers the pH of the tea.* Kombucha has an acidic pH in the range of 3.5 to 2.5. Adding starter liquid to the sweet tea base, at a minimum of 10 percent by volume, protects the young brew from invasion by disruptive or even harmful microorganisms, such as mold or kahm yeast (see page 162).
- *Acts as an inoculant.* Starter liquid contains billions of bacteria and yeast that work in concert with their siblings in the SCOBY to get the brew moving quickly.
- *Maintains balanced symbiosis.* Strong starter liquid from the top of the brew helps maintain the party animal/planner balance (see Bacteria & Yeast: Party Planners vs. Party Animals, page 34). Using starter liquid from the bottom of the vessel leads to off flavors and smells as well as poor SCOBY growth.

## THE GOLDEN RULES OF SCOBYS

### Always
- Use a fresh, full-size kombucha SCOBY with strong starter liquid to begin brewing
- Use the right-size SCOBY for the batch (a dime-sized SCOBY can't ferment a gallon of tea)
- Store SCOBYs properly in a SCOBY Hotel (see page 106)
- Pass along healthy, fresh SCOBYs with 1 to 2 cups of mature kombucha tea and complete, clear instructions

### Never
- Use a refrigerated or dehydrated SCOBY
- Use a SCOBY without starter liquid
- Use vinegar (especially raw vinegar) as starter liquid
- Use commercial kombucha as starter liquid

## SCOBYs Are Like Snowflakes

Not all SCOBYs form perfectly smooth pancakes. The shape and color of your newly growing culture are not necessarily indicative of the quality of your brew. Odd-looking cultures can make a fantastic-tasting kombucha, and great-looking ones can fail.

Depending on many factors, SCOBY formation can be quite unusual looking yet completely normal (sort of like people). To the untrained eye these peculiar formations can seem startling, but over time they become the familiar stages of new SCOBY growth. New brewers quickly learn that many times what at first appears to be mold soon evolves into normal SCOBY and yeast growth.

## SCOBY Surfing

Many new homebrewers become concerned when they add the SCOBY to their sweet tea mix and it sinks to the bottom. Shouldn't the SCOBY float on top, creating a seal? Another concern is whether the SCOBY needs to go in "smooth side" up.

In fact, the mother SCOBY usually sinks at first. It may slowly rise over the first few days, or it may remain near the bottom of the vessel, but its position, and which side faces up, does not affect the brew. No matter where the mother is located, the new layer of SCOBY culture will always grow across the surface of the brew. The mother may attach to the underside of the baby SCOBY or they may stay separate.

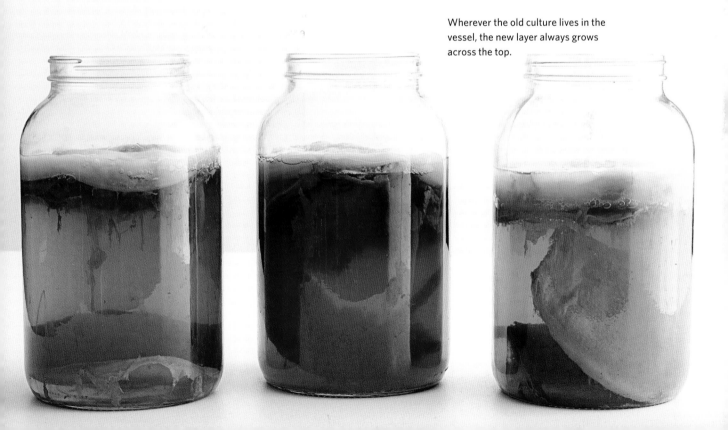

Wherever the old culture lives in the vessel, the new layer always grows across the top.

If connected, they can be easily pulled apart at harvest time.

Anytime a SCOBY layer is disturbed, as when the brew is decanted, or even just moved across the kitchen, it stops growing, but as soon as the vessel is stable again, a new layer will start to form. In the continuous brew (CB) method, this is evidenced by the development of a single, thick, multilayered culture that has to be trimmed every three to six months.

## Characteristics of a Quality Culture

### BACTERIAL MAT IS BETWEEN ¼ AND ½ INCH THICK

A SCOBY that is too thin may indicate a weak culture; one that is too thick may not allow enough oxygen to reach the brew.

### COLOR IS WHITE TO LIGHT TAN

New SCOBY growth is always white or light tan in color. As SCOBYs are reused over time, they turn darker brown and may lose potency.

### YEAST STRANDS ARE PRESENT

Yeast strands may be attached to the bottom of the culture as well as floating in the

---

*WORD NERD* **SCOBY**

SCOBY *is most commonly pronounced with a long o (as in go), but some people say "Scooby," perhaps after their favorite cartoon dog. It is also known by these names:*

- Biofilm
- Pellicle
- Zooglea
- Culture

---

starter liquid, all indicating a healthy brew. Remember, the Y in SCOBY stands for yeast, so they should be present, but in balance with the bacteria. Starter liquid that is too murky with yeast may benefit from filtering to avoid throwing off the brew's balance.

### THE STARTER LIQUID IS STRONG

The older and stronger the liquid, the more effective it will be at assisting the fermentation. A pH of 3.5 or lower is highly recommended.

### THE CULTURE REPRODUCES WITH EVERY BATCH

Healthy SCOBYs always produce new culture.

### THE BACTERIAL MAT IS HARDY

A healthy culture resists tearing when pressed tightly between thumb and forefinger.

---

**KOMBUCHA MAMMA SEZ**

### Sink or Swim

"The SCOBY can surf or dive, sink or swim, or float any which way, so just hang loose, new home-brewer, and go with the flow!"

---

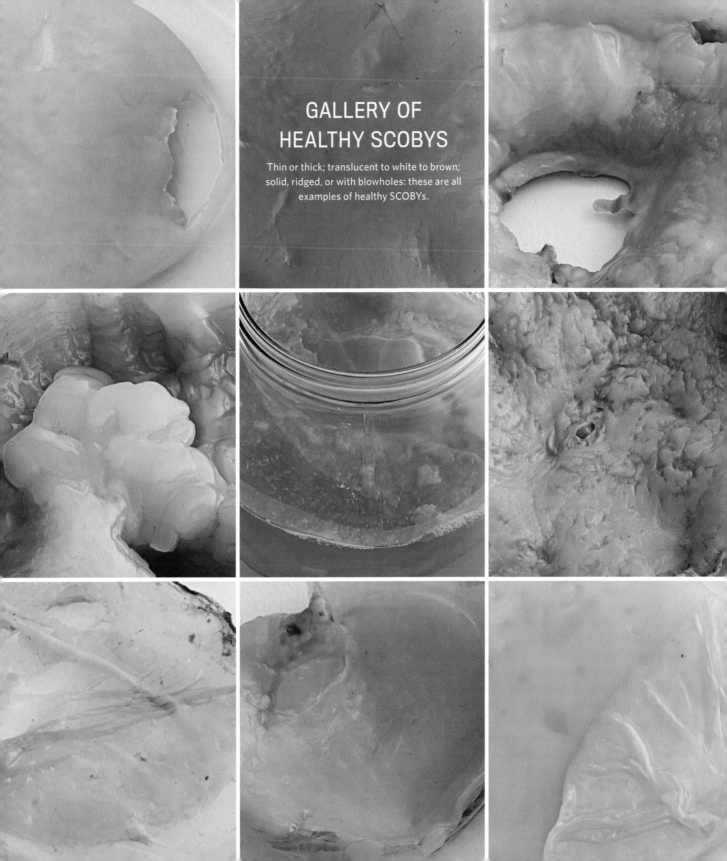

# GALLERY OF
# HEALTHY SCOBYS

Thin or thick; translucent to white to brown;
solid, ridged, or with blowholes: these are all
examples of healthy SCOBYs.

# GROWTH OF A SCOBY OVER 7 DAYS

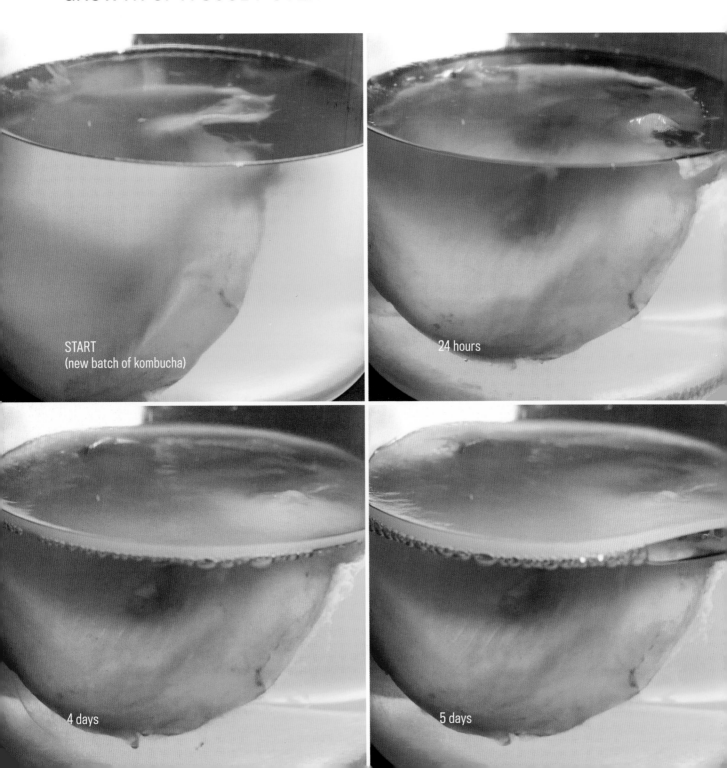

START
(new batch of kombucha)

24 hours

4 days

5 days

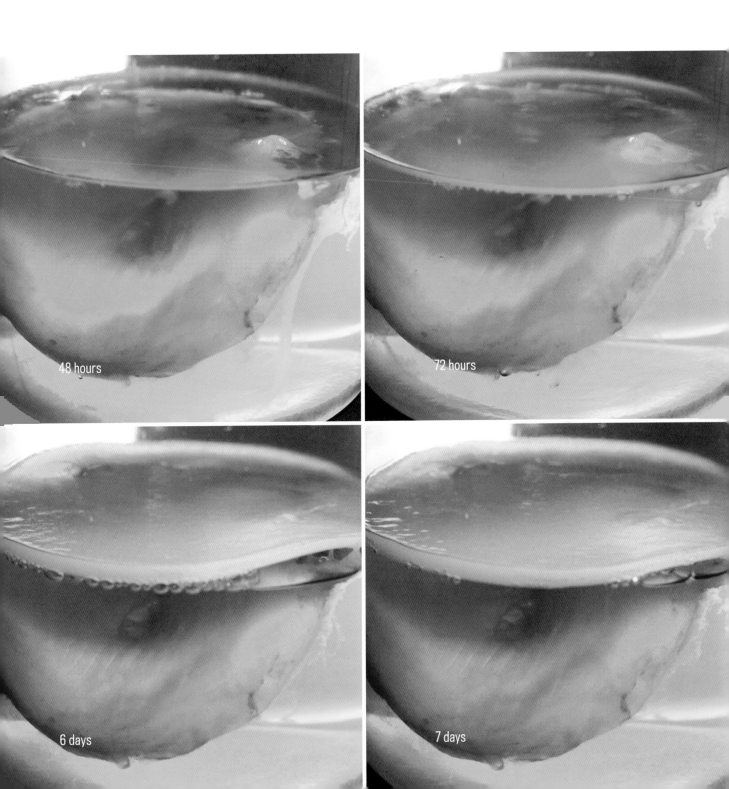

# The MANY NAMES of a KOMBUCHA SCOBY

Kombucha has accumulated numerous names throughout its long existence. Many of them either reflect how the SCOBY looks, where the culture originated, or the healthful effect of the brew. These historic and colloquial terms reflect the beliefs and benefits attributed to the culture.

**CHINESE**
Mógū
*mushroom*

**GERMAN**
Russische Blume
*Russian flower;*
Russische Mutter
*Russian mother;*
Russischer Pilz
*Russian fungus;*
Russische Qualle
*Russian jellyfish*

**DUTCH**
Theezwam komboecha
*tea sponge kombucha*

**BULGARIAN**
Meditsinski gŭbi
*medicinal mushroom*

**CHINESE**
Haipao or hǎibǎo
*sea treasure*

**DUTCH**
Thee-schimmel
*tea mold*

**FRENCH**
Champignon miracle
*miraculous mushroom*

**FRENCH**
Champignon or elixir de longue vie
*mushroom or elixir of long life*

**CHINESE**
Hóngchá jūn
*red tea bacteria*

**GERMAN**
Japanisher Schwamm
*Japanese sponge;*
Japanischer Teepilz
*Japanese tea fungus;*
Japanpilz
*Japanese fungus;*
Japanisches Mütterchen
*Japanese mother*

**GERMAN**
Heldenpilz
*hero's mushroom*

**ENGLISH**
*bacterial cellulose;*
*kombucha mushroom;*
*kombucha sponge;*
*magic mushroom;*
*Manchurian mushroom;*
*miracle mushroom;*
*pellicle;*
*SCOBY;*
*tea beast;*
*tea fungus*

**GERMAN**
Chinapilz
*Chinese fungus;*
Chinesischer Teepilz
*Chinese tea fungus*

**ROMANIAN**
Ciuperca de ceai
*tea fungus*

**LATIN**
(pharmaceutical names)
Cembuya orientalis
Fungus japonicus;

(scientific name)
Medusomyces gisevii Lindau

**FRENCH**
Petite mère japonaise
*little Japanese mother*

**SERBIAN**
Japanska gliva
*Japanese fungus*

**FRENCH**
Champignon japonais
*Japanese mushroom*

**ITALIAN**
Funko cinese/ fungo cinese
*Chinese fungus*

**GERMAN**
Wolgameduse
*Volga medusa;*
Wolgapilz
*Volga fungus;*
Wolgaqualle
*Volga jellyfish*

**FRENCH**
Champignon chinois
*Chinese mushroom*

**JAPANESE**
Kōcha kinoko
*red tea mushroom*

**SPANISH**
Hongo
*mushroom*

**ARABIC (IRAQ)**
Khubdat Humza

**GERMAN**
Kargasok Teepilz
*Kargasok tea fungus;*
Kargasok Schwamm
*Kargasok sponge*

**FRENCH**
Champignon de la charité
*charitable mushroom*

**GERMAN**
Wunderpilz
*wondrous mushroom;*
Zauberpilz
*magic mushroom*

**ITALIAN**
Alga egiziana
*Egyptian seaweed*

**RUSSIAN**
Japanskij grib
*Japanese mushroom*

**CZECH**
Zázračná houba kombucha
*kombucha wonder mushroom*

**SPANISH**
Hongo chino
*Chinese mushroom*

**RUSSIAN**
Cajnyj grib
*tea mushroom*

**LATVIAN**
Brinum-ssene
*wondrous mushroom*

**GERMAN**
Kombuchaschwamm
*kombucha sponge*

**ITALIAN**
Alga del nilo
*Nile river algae*

**GERMAN**
Gichtqualle
*gout jellyfish*

**HUNGARIAN**
Japán gomba
*Japanese mushroom*

**GERMAN**
Kombuchamost
*kombucha must*
(as in wine must)

**GERMAN**
Indischer Weinpilz
*Indian wine fungus;*
Indischer Teeschwamm/Teepilz
*Indian tea sponge/fungus;*
Indisch-japanischer Teepilz
*Indo-Japanese tea fungus*

**CZECH**
Olinka
(Nickname bestowed on SCOBYs by Bohemian and Moravian monks who wanted to keep their secret brew safe)

**GERMAN**
Mandschurischer Pilz
*Manchurian mushroom;*
Mandschurischer Schwamm
*Manchurian sponge;*
Mandschurisch-japanischer Pilz
*Manchurian-Japanese fungus*

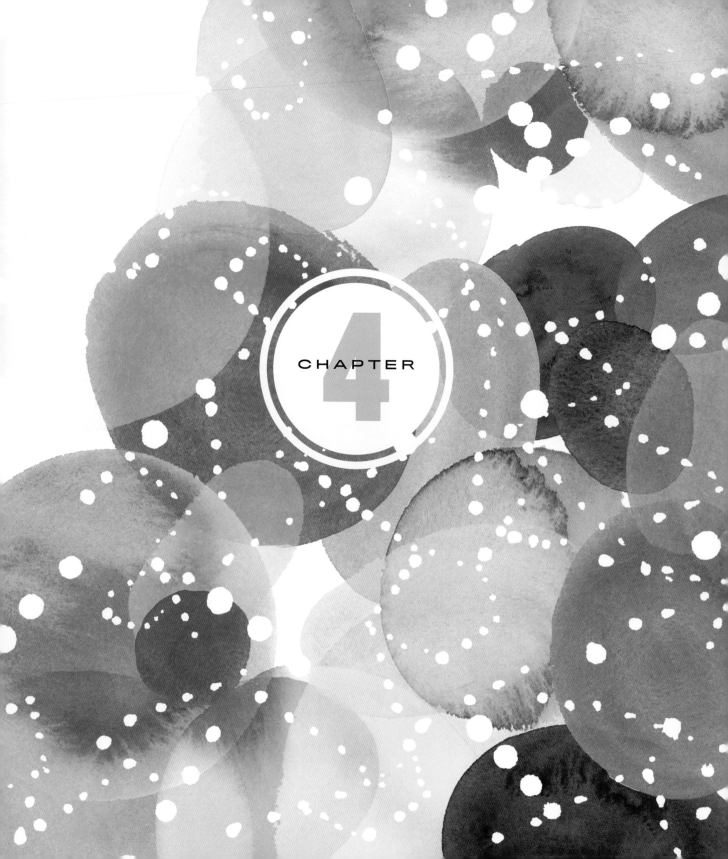

CHAPTER

4

## THE OTHER INGREDIENTS
# Tea, Sugar, Water

Kombucha is a very simple beverage, containing just four primary ingredients: tea, sugar, water, and the SCOBY with its starter liquid. As with everything in life, the higher the quality of the ingredients, the higher the quality of the final product. So use the best ingredients you can find.

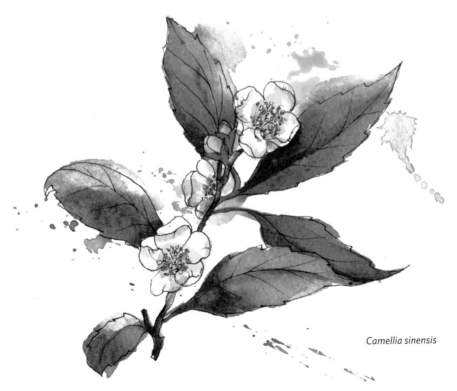

*Camellia sinensis*

# Tea

One of the healthiest and most popular beverages on the planet, tea is consumed more than all other beverages combined, including soft drinks, coffee, and alcohol. Ranging from mild to astringent and from mellow to tannic, the flavor and nutritional benefits are likely what has conferred the revered status it holds in numerous cultures from China to Europe to the Middle East and India and including the United States.

Tea is rich in polyphenols and other antioxidants, which combat free-radical damage, support long-term human health, and keep the blood clean and free from toxins. Tea also contains many alkaloids and amino acids that assist the body in metabolizing fat and controlling weight, aids in modulating blood sugar levels, helps protect the teeth and bones, and eradicates free radicals to help prevent the formation of cancer cells.

No wonder kombucha has been attributed with such a host of healing properties — it is made from a beverage that already has amazing health benefits. Utilizing nutrients like nitrogen and purines, the kombucha makes those benefits more bioavailable (that is, easier for the body to absorb) through the magic of fermentation and a little culture of special bacteria and yeast, which add vitamins and enzymes. Bonus!

When we talk about brewing kombucha from tea, we mean specifically the leaves of the *Camellia sinensis* plant. But what many people think of when they hear the word *tea* is often actually a tisane, or herbal infusion. Beverages made by steeping herbs such as chamomile and peppermint, or the leaves of rooibos and honeybush (both in the legume family), are all commonly called tea, and for day-to-day conversation there's nothing wrong with that definition. However, many herbal teas do not contain the nutrients needed to successfully brew batch after batch of kombucha. Moreover, some herbs have essential oils that may actually harm the culture and retard the reproduction of healthful bacteria. This can prevent the brew from developing important acids for flavor and other benefits and from protecting itself against invaders like mold.

When brewing kombucha with tisanes, you may initially produce a delicious, healthy fermented beverage, but over time the culture might atrophy and eventually die, or the bacterial population may simply become too weak to grow a new culture. So we don't recommend brewing kombucha solely with an herbal tisane. However, the fermentation technology of the SCOBY is incredibly flexible. By blending small amounts of herbs — ones that are free of oils or added flavors — with a majority of real tea, it is possible to create a delicious healthful brew with deep flavor and long-term vitality (see Acceptable Tisanes and Herbs for Blending, page 57).

Or, use an extra SCOBY from your hotel to brew an all-herbal batch as an experiment. (For more on this method, see Teas for Experimental Brews Only, page 60.)

## Best Types of Tea

Black, oolong, green, white, and pu-erh teas all come from the same plant, *Camellia sinensis*. The differences among them are primarily determined by the growth stage when the leaves are plucked and how they are processed.

## A KOMBUCHA LEGEND: A Long History of Tea

When hunting for the origins of kombucha, it is natural to start with the ingredients. China produces more than one billion metric tons of tea annually and has a tea history that stretches back almost five millennia. But how did humans first start drinking a steeped broth made from dried leaves of the *Camellia sinensis* bush? By accident or experimentation, of course!

Like all great histories, this one comingles with legend. Shen Nong, the "Spirit Farmer" emperor of China (also considered the father of Chinese herbalism), is commonly credited with discovering the plant around 2725 BCE. The legend may also contain an early lesson in sanitation, for it was said that he insisted water be boiled before being drunk.

When the leaves of the *Camellia sinesis* plant blew into a pot of boiling water, it was found to create a fragrant beverage that when consumed both calmed and provided a quiet, focused energy. Over the last four thousand plus years, tea has claimed a place in nearly every society on the planet, with an average of three billion cups consumed daily worldwide.

*It is better to go three days without oil and salt than to go one day without tea.*

TIBETAN PROVERB

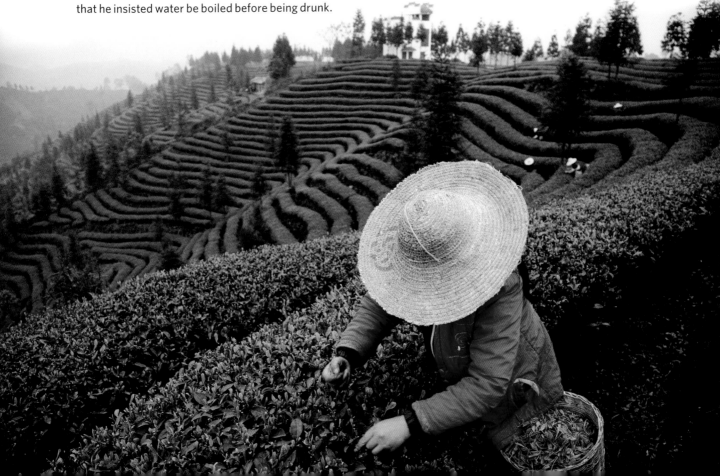

All teas are dried partially, then aged in varying ways that expose the leaves to oxygen. The oxidization of the tea leaves, also called *fermenting*, creates distinct flavors. White teas are not oxidized at all, whereas black tea is fully oxidized and green and oolong teas fall in between. Unlike traditional fermentation, bacteria (beyond what is present on the leaves) or other cultures are not used in this process (except for pu-erh — see page 54).

Though the oldest recipes call for black tea, these days all kinds of tea are used to make kombucha; usually some green and black, and even small amounts of SCOBY-safe tisanes, are blended for flavor and benefits, but the options are unlimited. Each type of tea contributes specific healing properties that kombucha's fermentation process helps unlock.

## BLACK TEA

Traditionally kombucha was brewed with black tea, which is fully oxidized to intensify the flavor and potency of the tea leaves. It produces a strong apple-cider flavor with deep earthy notes and dark golden color. For making kombucha, black teas are generally steeped at a relatively high temperature but for only a moderate length of time to maximize flavor without introducing bitterness.

Black tea has higher levels of both caffeine and purines than other types of tea. It aids blood circulation, which in turn helps to keep the body warmer. Black tea also supports beneficial intestinal microflora, helps prevent intestinal disorders, prevents tooth decay due to the presence of fluorine, and normalizes blood pressure.

## OOLONG TEA

Between fully oxidized black tea and partially oxidized green tea lies oolong (from the Chinese word for "black dragon"), which contains the benefits of both green and black teas, and is equally rich in antioxidants and detoxifying alkaloids. With its delicate, complex flavor, oolong is prized by some kombucha brewers for blending with other types of tea, offering a middle-of-the-road flavor that pleases the palate.

## GREEN TEA

Green tea leaves, which are steamed and are not fully oxidized, offer lighter flavor and color and a smoother finish than black tea. The younger the green tea, the lower the brewing temperature should be to prevent the release of excessive bitter tannins. Green tea is rich in catechin polyphenols, particularly epigallocatechin gallate (EGCG). Considered antibacterial, EGCG is also thought to inhibit the growth of cancer cells, lower LDL cholesterol levels, and boost immunity.

## WHITE TEA

White tea is made from the youngest, most delicate buds and leaves, which are covered in fine white hairs. The leaves are not oxidized but rather undergo a gentle drying process, which protects the delicate flavor and ensures the highest levels of antioxidants. White tea has been shown to reduce the risk of atherosclerotic plaques, stroke, heart failure, cancer (including tumor formation), and diabetes and to protect the skin against damage caused by UV light. It produces a milder-tasting kombucha that is high in catechins.

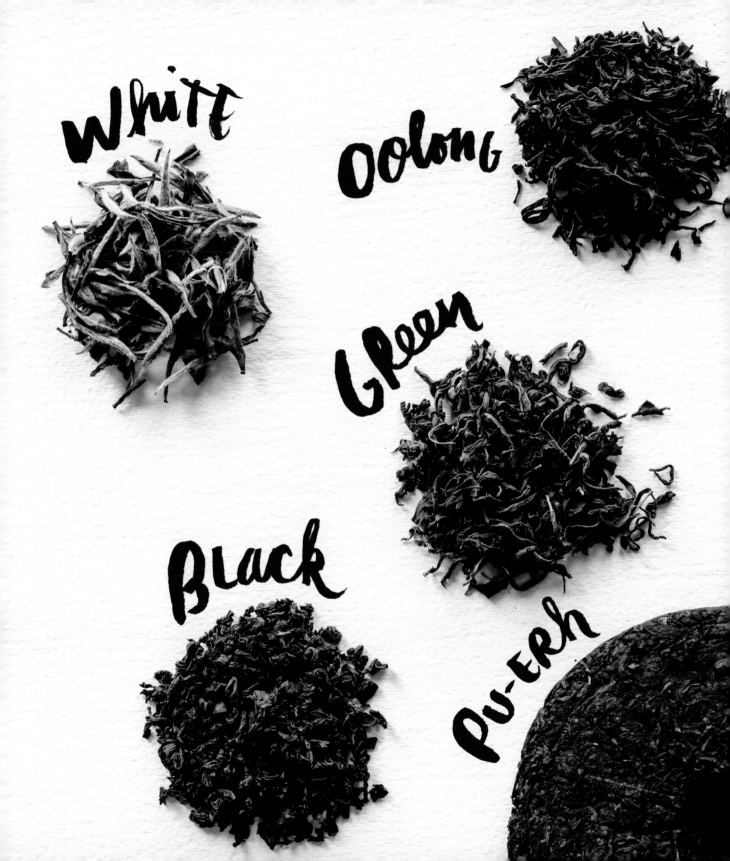

## PU-ERH TEA

Pu-erh tea is made from black tea that is pressed into bricks or balls and allowed to ferment in underground caves. Considered a "living" tea due to the natural microbial activity arising from the second fermentation, the flavor of pu-erh tea is much milder and more fragrant than its dark appearance would suggest. Many find that it harbors a pleasant sweetness.

In China, pu-erh is highly prized and considered medicinal. Just as wine collectors may pay thousands of dollars for a fine vintage, the same is true of those who collect pu-erh.

### KOMBUCHA MAMMA SEZ

## Best Choice Tea

❝As conscious consumers, we employ four criteria when purchasing tea:

- Loose leaf
- Bulk
- Organic
- Fair trade (whenever possible)

Loose-leaf and bulk teas use less packaging (more green for the earth) and are less expensive (more green for us). We choose to pay out some of those savings by purchasing organic and fair-trade teas. Organic and fair trade mean we avoid toxic pesticides (better for the earth) and the laborers were paid a living wage for their work (better for all of us)."

# The Basic Sweet Tea Recipe

Whether you're using the batch method (chapter 6) or the CB method (chapter 7), you'll start with a basic sweet tea. Use this same recipe to fill a SCOBY Hotel or to top off a CB fermenter or any other time you need sweet tea for your kombucha. This recipe makes 1 gallon, and you can scale it up or down. If you happen to make too much, it will keep in an airtight container in the fridge for up to one week.

### INGREDIENTS

4–6 tea bags or 4–6 teaspoons loose-leaf tea
1 gallon cool, chlorine-free water
1 cup sugar

### BREWING

Place the tea in a pot, bowl, or other heat-proof container.

Heat 4 cups of the water to just boiling and pour it over the tea. Let steep for 10 to 15 minutes; then remove the spent tea leaves.

Add the sugar to the hot tea and stir until completely dissolved; then add the remaining water.

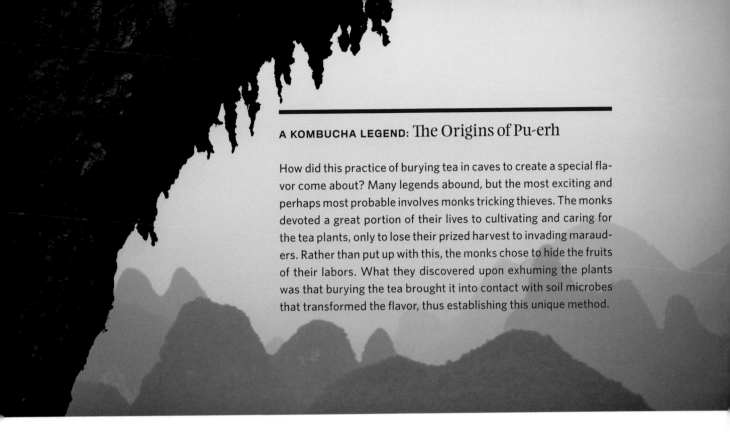

How did this practice of burying tea in caves to create a special flavor come about? Many legends abound, but the most exciting and perhaps most probable involves monks tricking thieves. The monks devoted a great portion of their lives to cultivating and caring for the tea plants, only to lose their prized harvest to invading marauders. Rather than put up with this, the monks chose to hide the fruits of their labors. What they discovered upon exhuming the plants was that burying the tea brought it into contact with soil microbes that transformed the flavor, thus establishing this unique method.

# Caffeine and Kombucha

Caffeine is a naturally occurring xanthine alkaloid found in plants like coffee, tea, and cacao. It functions as a pesticide to protect these tasty plants from hungry insect invaders. In humans, caffeine stimulates the nervous system, providing increased energy and focus. For the kombucha culture, caffeine is an important nutrient that provides nitrogen for building new cells as well as for energizing the yeast and bacteria, stimulating fermentation.

Some people are particularly sensitive to caffeine and wonder how much will be present in their kombucha. The answer is "not very much," but as with many of the questions about homebrew, the final amount will vary widely based on your brewing methods and environment. The original sweet tea base already has less caffeine than a cup of tea, and that amount of caffeine is reduced during the fermentation process by as much as two-thirds in just the first week. Moreover, caffeine from tea is paired with L-theanine (see page 58), an amino acid analogue of glutamine and glutamate (see appendix 1, page 357). L-theanine balances the caffeine to provide calm, focused energy minus the crash and burn that coffee and energy drinks are famous for.

One thing's for sure, the total amount of caffeine is much less than that in a typical serving of tea, coffee, or soda. It is little wonder that many have found they are able to consume kombucha in the evening without experiencing negative effects on their sleep patterns.

However, those sensitive to caffeine may wish to decrease or eliminate it altogether. It is possible to reduce that content to almost none without losing the benefits of brewing.

## How Much Caffeine?

While the amount will vary widely, due to the type and quality of tea, the steep time, and the fermentation cycle and temperature, a properly fermented kombucha brew contains relatively low amounts of caffeine. That amount can be further reduced, but first let's look at how much caffeine is in a serving of kombucha.

To make a cup of tea, usually 1 tea bag (1 teaspoon of loose-leaf tea) is put into 6 to 8 ounces of hot water and steeped for five or more minutes. When we brew tea for kombucha, we use just 3 to 5 tea bags for an entire gallon, which cuts the caffeine content by 70 to 80 percent before fermentation even begins. Several studies note that the caffeine levels in kombucha decrease throughout the fermentation process, by as much as one-third within 24 hours and between 50 and 65 percent after seven days (See studies cited on page 370.)

Going by our steeping recipe and these numbers, black tea, which might normally contain 40 to 80 mg of caffeine per 8 ounces, would yield kombucha with 3 to 12 mg of caffeine per 8 ounces, and green tea kombucha could contain from less than 1 mg up to 6 mg per 8 ounces. Of course it is possible to steep the tea longer or just use more of it and increase the caffeine from these levels, but it is clear that the levels can be kept low.

## Reducing Caffeine Levels

With such low levels, it may not be necessary to take additional steps, but here are a few techniques that can reduce the levels of caffeine safely:

*Use a tea blend.* Black tea contains more caffeine than green or white, and other teas, such as hōjicha (a type of green tea roasted over charcoal), contain even less. The kombucha culture prefers variety when it comes to tea, so to significantly reduce the caffeine content, use mostly green and/or white tea (up to 80 percent of the total tea blend), rather than black tea alone.

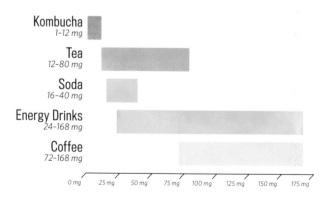

AVERAGE CAFFEINE
CONTENT OF POPULAR
BEVERAGES
(PER 8 OUNCES)

Kombucha
*1–12 mg*

Tea
*12–80 mg*

Soda
*16–40 mg*

Energy Drinks
*24–168 mg*

Coffee
*72–168 mg*

0 mg   25 mg   50 mg   75 mg   100 mg   125 mg   150 mg   175 mg

***Use an herbal tisane blend.*** As discussed earlier, we don't recommend using herbal tisanes as the sole "tea" for kombucha, as doing so may slowly degrade the health of the SCOBY and the vitality of the kombucha. However, you can use tisanes as the primary ingredient in a tea blend, contributing up to 75 percent of the total, with a *Camellia sinensis* tea making up the other 25 percent (this is the minimum — we recommend 50 to 75 percent real tea for best long-term results).

Alternatively, you can use a pure tisane and brew every fourth batch with real tea to reinvigorate the culture. Keep in mind, though, that strong oils and artificial flavorings can kill the SCOBY bacteria; experiment to find a blend that suits your flavor preferences and the microorganisms.

***Brew longer.*** Studies show that the caffeine content in kombucha decreases as the ferment continues. Brew for a longer cycle, and then dilute with juice or water to temper the sourness resulting from the longer fermentation.

***Steep-and-dump method.*** Just as it sounds, this method calls for steeping the loose tea for 30 to 60 seconds in a cup or two of very hot water, then dumping the liquid and using the steeped leaves to brew the kombucha. Though many brewers swear by this "presteeping," most studies show that there is little caffeine reduction with such short steep times. If the tea was presteeped for, say, seven to nine minutes before being used to brew the kombucha tea, the caffeine reduction might reach 50 percent, but for most teas the associated reduction in flavor wouldn't be worth it.

## USING DECAFFEINATED TEA

While using a commercial decaffeinated tea might seem like an obvious and convenient option, we do not recommend it, as most brands (even "naturally decaffeinated" ones) have been chemically treated. The culture may be able to adapt to decaffeinated tea, but if you notice poor SCOBY growth or flat flavor, consider adding some regular tea to a batch to invigorate the culture.

# Blending Teas to Make Kombucha

As long as you are brewing with real tea, any blend of types is acceptable. Once tisanes or other herbals are introduced, the long-term health of the culture and the brew must be taken into account. As mentioned, the general rule of thumb is to include a minimum of 25 percent real tea, though the best blends contain at least 50 to 75 percent *Camellia sinensis*.

By blending different teas and tisanes, anyone can achieve an endless variety of brews, each slightly different in taste, body, aroma, and nutrients. This is one of the secrets to the unique nature of each brewer's offering.

## Acceptable Tisanes and Herbs for Blending

Although kombucha thrives best in a solution of straight tea and sugar, the advanced brewer is highly encouraged to experiment by using other herbal infusions to maximize the potential health benefits from herbs that have been "predigested" through the fermentation. Basically, kombucha acts as a solvent; that is, it trades molecules with the healthful elements, breaking them down until they are in a form that is more bioavailable.

Wait to try these types of experiments until you have a stash of backup SCOBY cultures in a SCOBY Hotel (see page 37), so that it's no great loss if the SCOBY molds or fails to thrive. Some herbal infusions with high levels of volatile oils act as a bactericide and retard the culture's growth. If the SCOBY in the experimental brew shows positive growth, it may be okay to incorporate that blend into your primary fermentation regularly.

The following herbs do contain some elements that nurture the kombucha, but the exact constituents and concentrations will vary by the type and even the source, so no one can say for sure how they will brew every time. (See Caffeine and Kombucha, page 55, to learn about using these tisanes to make a less caffeinated brew.)

## CINNAMON

There is no denying the smooth, gently spiced flavor of a well-done cinnamon brew (see page 141). The addition of a few short sticks or a little ground bark likely lowers the acetic-acid production to produce the lighter flavor, but SCOBY growth and carbonation are generally robust, indicating an otherwise healthy brew.

## GINGER

All rhizomes do very well with kombucha, but ginger seems to be uniquely well suited as a partner. While a purist would never do so, adding a small amount of fresh ginger (so that it makes up 5 to 10 percent, at maximum, of the blend) to the primary ferment can inject a unique taste and complexity to the brew.

# L-THEANINE: TEA'S RELAXATION EFFECT

One unique amino acid found almost exclusively in tea is L-theanine. Structurally similar to the essential amino acids glutamine and glutamate, L-theanine crosses the blood-brain barrier and has positive psychoactive effects on the tea drinker. L-theanine plays a vital role in modulating the effect of the caffeine in tea, so that it is stimulating yet soothing; in contrast, the caffeine in coffee lacks the balancing presence of L-theanine and so delivers a jagged spike of stimulation that increases anxiety.

L-theanine acts by stimulating alpha brain waves, calming the mind similarly to meditation, while also boosting the body's production of dopamine and serotonin. This combo platter of good vibes promotes improved memory and learning ability in a relaxed state. Studies show that when taken together, L-theanine and caffeine also improve cognitive performance and mood, which is why many people turn to tea and kombucha for focused energy.

CINNAMON

ROOIBOS

HIBISCUS

GINGER

YERBA MATÉ

### HIBISCUS

Many brewers use dried hibiscus petals in the first ferment, lending a nice tartness to the brew. Use up to 20 percent hibiscus in a tea blend without affecting the health of the brew. As a visually stimulating bonus, the hibiscus turns the SCOBY a lovely pink color.

### ROOIBOS/HONEYBUSH

Rooibos (pronounced ROY-bos and meaning "red bush" in Afrikaans) is naturally caffeine-free and slightly sweet, plus it's high in flavonoids. Popular for generations in southern Africa, where it originates, it is actually a legume that is cured in a process similar to tea, creating a naturally sweet herbal tisane that goes by many names, including rooibos, red-bush, or red tea. It is purported to help calm colicky babies and soothe skin afflictions when applied topically. A cousin to rooibos is honeybush, which is similar in flavor but sweeter.

### YERBA MATÉ

Yerba maté (*Ilex paraguariensis*) is a species of holly tree native to subtropical South America. According to a study at the University of Illinois at Urbana-Champaign, yerba maté tea contains high levels of polyphenols and other antioxidants, as well as having anti-inflammatory properties and lowering low-density lipoprotein (LDL) cholesterol. (See study cited on page 370.)

Maté has as much caffeine as coffee, but its nutritional profile offsets the typical "coffee crash" experience. Instead the energy felt is often described as focused, without causing jitteriness.

### AYURVEDIC AND TRADITIONAL CHINESE MEDICINAL HERBS

Traditional medicinal herbs from Ayurvedic or Chinese medicine are often excellent choices for blending with all types of tea to infuse additional benefits into the kombucha. Some great choices for blending are angelica, ashwagandha, astragalus, ginkgo, ginseng, gotu kola, and turmeric, to name just a few. (See Flavor Inspirations: Medicinal, page 216.)

Of course, always keep a SCOBY Hotel active when experimenting with these (and any) new herbs in case a brew experiences issues and you need to toss the culture.

## Teas for Experimental Brews Only

The most important consideration when blending teas, tisanes, or herbs for brewing kombucha is to avoid essential oils or chemical flavorings that may produce a delicious beverage but harm the bacteria and therefore the culture. Nearly any type of tea or herb — even fruit juice (see Flavoring the Primary Fermentation, page 142) — can be used as a substrate for kombucha, though success and repeatability will vary on the crazier experiments.

That's part of the fun: let your imagination run wild, and try something new, using a backup SCOBY of course. If the brew looks or smells strange, it might be safest to toss it rather than risk an adverse reaction. Trust *your* gut!

# BREWING TEMPERATURES AND STEEPING TIMES FOR VARIOUS TEAS

## Best Teas for Kombucha

### BLACK TEAS

| Variety | Brewing Temperature | Steeping Time (minutes) |
|---|---|---|
| Assam | 200°F (93°C) | 4-6 |
| Ceylon | 212°F (100°C) | 3-5 |
| Darjeeling | 200°F (93°C) | 3-5 |
| Golden Monkey | 200°F (93°C) | 2-3 |
| Keemun | 195°F (90°C) | 3 |
| Yunnan | 195°F (90°C) | 2 |

### BLACK TEA BLENDS

| Variety | Brewing Temperature | Steeping Time (minutes) |
|---|---|---|
| English Breakfast | 212°F (100°C) | 4-5 |
| Irish Breakfast | 212°F (100°C) | 4-5 |

### GREEN TEAS

| Variety | Brewing Temperature | Steeping Time (minutes) |
|---|---|---|
| Bancha | 180°F (82°C) | 2-3 |
| Dragonwell | 185°F (85°C) | 3-4 |
| Gunpowder | 150-160°F (66-71°C) | 2-4 |
| Sencha | 170°F (77°C) | 3-4 |

### WHITE TEAS

| Variety | Brewing Temperature | Steeping Time (minutes) |
|---|---|---|
| Silver Needle | 180°F (82°C) | 3-5 |
| White Peony | 180°F (82°C) | 4-6 |

### OOLONG

| Brewing Temperature | Steeping Time (minutes) |
|---|---|
| 190°F (88°C) | 5-8 |

### PU-ERH

| Brewing Temperature | Steeping Time (minutes) |
|---|---|
| 212°F (100°C) | 4-6 |

## Teas, Tisanes, and Herbs for Blending

| Variety | Brewing Temperature | Steeping Time (minutes) |
|---|---|---|
| Cinnamon | Slow boil | 15-20 |
| Earl Grey | 200°F (93°C) | 4-6 |
| Ginger | 212°F (100°C) | 4-6 |
| Hibiscus | 212°F (100°C) | 4-6 |
| Rooibos and honeybush | 212°F (100°C) | 4-6 |
| Yerba maté | 170°F (77°C) | 3-5 |

# The Many Names of KOMBUCHA Tea

**ARABIC**
Al-nabtah
*the plant*

**DUTCH**
Komboecha drank
*Kombucha drink;*
Komboecha thee
*kombucha tea;*
Theebier
*tea beer*

**ARMENIAN**
Teyi saki
*tea wine*

**GERMAN**
Reimentangtee
*seaweed belt tea;*
Russische Tee-essig
*Russian tea vinegar;*
Teemost
*tea must/cider;*
Tee Kwass
*tea kvass;*
Zaubersaft
*magic juice;*
Zaubertrank
*magic potion*

**RUSSIAN**
Caj kvas
*tea kvass*

**FRENCH**
Elixir de longue vie
*elixir of long life;*
Thé kombucha
*kombucha tea*

**TURKISH**
Kombuçay
*Kombucha*

**ROMANIAN**
Ceaiul kwas
*tea kvass*

**GERMAN**
Algentee
*algae tea;*
Combuchagetrink
*kombucha drink;*
Japanische Combucha
*Japanese kombucha;*
Kargasoktee
*Kargasok tea;*
Kombuchawein
*kombucha wine;*
Medusentee
*jellyfish tea*

**CZECH**
Čajová houba kombucha
*kombucha mushroom tea;*
Čajová japonská houba
*Japanese mushroom tea*

**UNKNOWN ORIGIN**
Kongo
Spumonto
T'chai from the sea
Te-aramoana
Titania
Tschambucco
Tsche of kombu
Yaponge

**ENGLISH**
Booch
Buch
Fungus tea
Kombucha tea
Manchurian elixir/tea
Medusa tea
Mushroom tea
Tea beer/cider/wine

# Sugar

Humans have cultivated and consumed sugar for over five thousand years, but only recently has our access to it become so unfettered that we've been able to overdose on it. The excessive consumption of high-fructose corn syrup, other highly processed sugars, and chemicalized sugar substitutes has intensified the recent plague of physical ailments to afflict our society — diabetes, cancer, candidiasis, inflammation, and arthritis among them.

The reality is that sugar is a vital nutrient and nearly every organism on this planet needs some amount of it to survive. Our own DNA is held together by a sugar-phosphate backbone (the sugar is called deoxyribose). When consumed in balance, sugar gives cells the energy they need to perform vital functions. In the case of kombucha brewing, the sugar provides nutrition to the yeast and bacteria as well as the base for healthy acid formation. Without sugar, there is no kombucha. Skimping on it often leads to a weak brew that fails to replicate over time.

Many people are concerned about sugar intake, often for good reason, considering how much is needlessly added to our food supply. However, much like anything else in life, moderation trumps elimination. There is great pleasure, and even some health benefits,

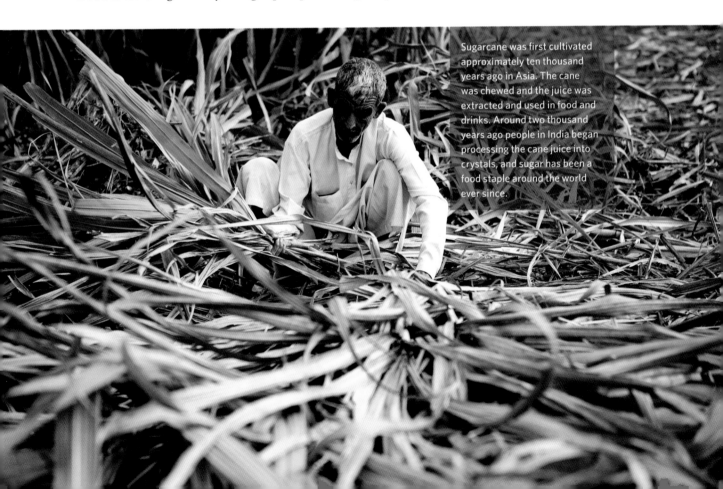

Sugarcane was first cultivated approximately ten thousand years ago in Asia. The cane was chewed and the juice was extracted and used in food and drinks. Around two thousand years ago people in India began processing the cane juice into crystals, and sugar has been a food staple around the world ever since.

in eating fresh fruit, homemade ice cream, or creamy custard, rather than sugar-laden packaged snacks. And a pinch or two of sugar enhances the flavor of many savory foods.

With kombucha, balance is also the key, as the right amount of residual fermented sugar smoothes the harsh flavor of the acids to create a pleasurable combination. Try a small sip of the sweet tea before fermentation for proof of the change; the sickly sweetness is overwhelming. How could anything delicious emerge from such a mix? Yet a beautiful alchemy occurs as the fermentation breaks down sucrose into the fructose and glucose that feed the yeast that feed the bacteria that feed us.

While it is obvious, based on taste, that the fermentation process reduces sugars in kombucha, tools traditionally used to measure fermentation, such as hydrometers and refractometers, produce inaccurately high estimates of the sugar content. This is due to a variety of complex reasons related to the presence of acids that skew readings, the symbiotic nature of the ferment, and the nature of other dissolved solids in kombucha. For a rough estimate of the actual remaining sugar, research seems to indicate that readings from these tools should be cut in half. (See Testing Tools and Protocols, page 175.)

## Remaining Sugar in Kombucha

Sugar comes in several forms. Fructose is naturally found in fruits and vegetables. Glucose, aka dextrose, is the most common energy source in the biological world. Much of the sugar that remains in the kombucha after fermentation has already been broken down from table sugar (sucrose, a disaccharide), into fructose and glucose (monosaccharides), which have a lower glycemic impact on the body. In kombucha, the bacteria then transform glucose into healthy $g$ acids such as gluconic and glucuronic acids. (Learn more about healthy acids in appendix 2, page 364.) Enzymes further break down the sugars during the brewing process, meaning even less is present in the final beverage.

A number of studies conducted since 2000 show that fermentation reduces the sugar in kombucha by varying amounts based on time, temperature, amount of starter liquid used, and likely many other factors researchers did not account for. Though the studies used varying recipes and techniques, they consistently showed that the reduction in sugar is modest at first and then quickly becomes increasingly marked from days 3 to 8, after most of the sugar has been cleaved and is waiting to be used more gradually. The reduction in sugar varied around 50 to 70 percent between 7 and 14 days and up to 80 percent after 30 days. (See studies cited on page 370.)

Using our recipe of 1 cup of sugar per gallon, that's 200 grams of sugar, which is 12.5 grams of sugar per 8 ounces of sweet tea. For an average ferment, this leaves 4 to 6 grams of sugar per 8-ounce glass of kombucha, and as low as 2.5 grams per 8 ounces in a longer brew, depending on conditions. However, when we say "sugar" we mean all residual sugars, including sucrose but also glucose and fructose, which as stated before do not have the same glycemic impact on the body.

All of this is to say: relax and enjoy the brew. Let your taste buds guide you to the sweet/tart balance that works best for you!

## Best Types of Sugar

Cane sugar is the most common fuel source used for brewing kombucha. Different processing of the cane leads to a variety of different products, the most familiar being plain white table sugar and evaporated cane juice crystals. If you are wondering if you can combine different types of sugar into one kombucha brew, the answer is absolutely! Just as with tea blends, sugar blends can add flavor and depth to your brew, so have fun experimenting.

Here is a closer look at cane and other types of sugars suitable for brewing kombucha.

### EVAPORATED CANE JUICE

This is the best choice for brewing the best-tasting Kombucha. Also known as raw sugar, it is processed enough for the kombucha microorganisms to consume it easily but retains natural vitamins and minerals, such as calcium, magnesium, potassium, and iron, that are healthful for the drinker. Evaporated cane juice crystals provide the best balance between our needs and the SCOBY's needs. Go with organic, when possible, to limit toxins and avoid GMOs.

### PLAIN WHITE SUGAR

The classic choice for brewing kombucha, ordinary table sugar puts brews into overdrive, as the yeast can quickly break down this highly refined fuel source. But how does the sugar get so white? Some people are concerned about the toxic chemicals used in the refining process, which is another reason to choose evaporated cane juice. If you choose to go with plain white, check the package for the words "cane sugar" to avoid a product that is likely derived from genetically modified sugar beets.

### OTHER CANE SUGARS

Less refined forms of cane sugar include brown sugar, turbinado, demerara, Sucanat, piloncillo, and muscovado. Each will produce a slightly different beverage. With these sugars, SCOBYs and the final brew may take on

## CAN DIABETICS DRINK KOMBUCHA?

Many diabetics enjoy kombucha without worry; some even claim it has helped their condition. Anecdotally, many have shared that not only are they able to enjoy kombucha without experiencing spikes in blood sugar levels but also that they are sometimes able to reduce or eliminate medications. A number of animal studies seem to support that possibility (Srihari, 2013; Aloulou, 2012; Shenoy, 2000). Kombucha has long been considered a potential boon to those with blood sugar issues, as far back as the early twentieth century. Of course, always consult with a primary health care provider in regard to major diet changes and medical conditions. (For more info, see Diabetes, page 367.)

darker tones and deeper flavors. Additional mineral content of less refined sugars may cause a more sour brew or even flavor issues. Most homebrewers who try these sugars tend to gravitate back to cane juice crystals or plain white sugar over time.

### PASTEURIZED HONEY

Honey can produce a delightful kombucha flavor highlighted by the bees' choice of flower. About 80 percent of a typical honey's sugar content is in the form of the monosaccharides fructose and glucose, meaning it is already broken down for the yeast to consume. This results in a shorter brew cycle and a brew more likely to grow sour after bottling unless refrigerated immediately. Substitute ⅞ cup honey per 1 cup regular sugar.

**Warning: do not use raw honey!** Raw honey's native bacteria will compete with the kombucha microorganisms, and the combination can produce a foul concoction. Stick with pasteurized honey in this case.

### MAPLE SYRUP

Maple syrup can act as a high-octane substitute for regular sugar, requiring only ½ to ⅔ cup to replace 1 cup of sugar. It has high levels of trace minerals such as zinc and manganese. Use only 100 percent pure maple syrup; common "pancake brands" are often supplemented with corn syrup.

## Sugars for Experimental Batches Only

The following types of sweeteners can produce drinkable kombucha, but they should be used with caution and only by more experienced brewers using extra SCOBYs. We do not recommend putting any of the SCOBYs from these experimental brews back in a SCOBY Hotel; if the kombucha brewed with them did not turn out as intended, dispose of them.

### MOLASSES

This thick, syrupy by-product of white sugar processing contains even higher concentrations of minerals and yields a nutrient-dense brew with a unique flavor profile. Some drinkers detect notes of caramel, whereas others find the minerals create too much tartness. Though it can be substituted for regular sugar in a 1:1 ratio, molasses-only batches typically show poor culture growth.

### COCONUT WATER

Containing 50 to 60 percent less sugar than the standard sweet tea, this refreshing beverage can work as a base for fermenting, though it sometimes results in off flavors or produces a weak brew. Use it in place of water to make the entire amount of sweet tea; rather than heating the coconut water, people often choose to cold-infuse, using the same amount of tea.

Another option is to mix coconut water into the sweet tea infusion. In this case, figure the amount of loose tea to use based on the total liquid (water plus coconut water). Brew the tea in the water; then add the coconut water. Depending on the proportion of water to coconut water, add less sugar (25 to

EVAPORATED
CANE
JUICE

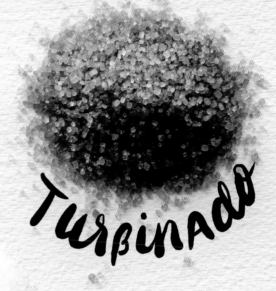

TURBINADO

MOLASSES

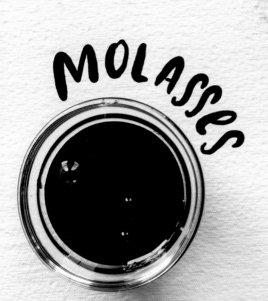

WHITE
SUGAR

MAPLE

SYRUP

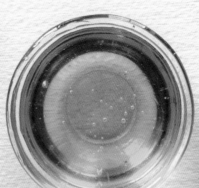

HONEY

50 percent, for example) than is normal because the coconut water will provide additional sweetness.

### COCONUT SUGAR

Due to great variations in grades and production methods, coconut sugar may or may not be a successful choice. The differing SCOBYs, with their varying yeast and bacteria combinations, likely play a part as well. Some home-brewers report mold or flavor issues, while others enjoy the result.

### LIQUID CANE JUICE

Fresh sugarcane juice is a popular beverage in many countries and may be used as a base for brewing kombucha. Because of the variable sweetness of the juice, concrete guidelines about how much to use are difficult to provide, but a good starting point is combining half fresh-pressed sugarcane juice and half tea concentrate (brewed with enough tea for the total volume of liquid, but no sugar added), which should provide about 80 percent of the sugar of a normal batch. Experiment with more or less juice as desired.

### INVERT SUGAR

Popular with some beer brewers, especially at bottling time, invert sugar, often available in syrup form, is just a fancy way of saying the sugar has already been broken down from sucrose into fructose and glucose. The name comes from the lab technique used to measure sugar solutions, not the sugar itself.

Any sugar that is broken down into smaller components is going to be easier for the kombucha culture to consume, as one less step in the digestive process has to occur. However, the yeast are perfectly capable of breaking down sucrose on their own, and invert sugar makes no difference in flavor, so there is no need to incur the extra expense or spend the time making invert sugar specifically for kombucha. However, if you have some on hand anyway, it is an appropriate choice.

## SUGAR-FREE KOMBUCHA?

People often ask if they can make kombucha without using sugar, and the short answer is no. Sugar is a necessary food for the yeast and bacteria, providing them the energy to reproduce, create a new SCOBY, and process the sweet tea into acids and vitamins and bubbles for your booch! Plus the small amounts of residual sugar in the finished kombucha make the healthful acids palatable. Properly brewed kombucha contains on average about 1 to 2 teaspoons of fermented sugar per 8 ounces, and those sugars do not interact with the body in the same way as table sugar. (See Diabetes, page 367.)

## USING SUGARS IN KOMBUCHA BREWING

| | Type of Sugar | Quantity per Gallon of Tea | Brewing Cycle (days) |
|---|---|---|---|
| **BEST** | Evaporated cane juice | 1 cup | 7–10 |
| | White sugar | 1 cup | 7–10 |
| **ACCEPTABLE** | Unrefined cane sugar/ brown sugar | 1 cup | 7–14 |
| | Pasteurized honey | ⅞ cup | 5–8 |
| | Maple syrup | ½–⅔ cup | 5–8 |
| **EXPERIMENTAL** | Molasses | 1 cup | 7–14 |
| | Coconut water | Mix with 25% usual amount of sugar | 5–8 |
| | Coconut palm sugar | ⅔–1 cup | 5–8 |
| | Liquid cane juice | Mix with 25% usual amount of sugar | 7–10 |
| | Invert sugar | ⅞ cup | 5–8 |

## Do Not Use These

Someone once asked us if they could use Mountain Dew as starter. First, gross. Second, why? And third, no, you cannot. Or you could try. But please don't. Just because something tastes sweet doesn't mean it contains real sugar. High-fructose corn syrup and other artificial sweeteners and sugar substitutes such as aspartame, sucralose, and saccharin are not suitable for fermentation. They are toxic not only to you, but also to the SCOBY.

It may be tempting to make a "low sugar" kombucha by substituting one of these alternatives, but in our experience the results range from unpalatable to mold-ridden. Here are some other sweeteners to avoid.

### AGAVE

As a primarily fructose-based sweetener, this syrup lacks the glucose that stimulates the bacteria to produce the $g$ acids, such as gluconic and glucuronic acids, that aid in the detoxification process for which kombucha is prized. Questions about its highly processed nature and health effects also give many homebrewers pause.

### BAKER'S SUGAR, BAR SUGAR, AND POWDERED SUGAR

These cane sugar derivatives are processed into smaller granules than plain white table sugar, causing caking or dissolving issues.

### BROWN RICE SYRUP

This highly processed syrup breaks down into 100 percent glucose with little mineral content. The resulting brew generally features strange yeast globs and off flavors.

### DEXTROSE

Dextrose, a form of glucose, will produce a kombucha brew with almost exclusively gluconic and glucuronic acids, the acids that support detoxification. The flavor can be weak but more problematic is the eventual degradation of the culture, which requires fructose as well to thrive over time.

### RAW HONEY

Do not use raw honey for kombucha, as it contains its own bacteria and yeast colonies that may disturb the SCOBY and throw the brew out of balance. You may use it with jun, a similar-looking yet differently balanced kombucha culture that is uniquely adapted to work with raw honey.

### SUGAR SUBSTITUTES

Products called *sugar alcohols* — stevia, xylitol, sorbitol, erythritol, and mannitol — are neither sugar nor alcohol. They are processed from other sugars, and while they contain far fewer calories than regular table sugar, they do not contain the necessary fuel for the primary fermentation process. They can be used for sweetening a brewed kombucha, but their flavor may change over time, so it's generally best to consume those brews soon after opening the bottle.

# Water

As it does in a New York City pizza crust or San Francisco sourdough bread, water has a profound impact on the flavor of kombucha and the health of the SCOBYs. Many types are suitable for brewing kombucha, but most important is that the water be free of contaminants that may harm the culture.

**KOMBUCHA MAMMA SEZ**

## Best Water Practice

"For homebrewing, your best option is to use the water that you have easiest access to and that costs the least, provided it is able to support the kombucha culture. This may mean investing in a filtration or purification system if your home water supply is less than ideal, or dechlorinating water prior to brewing with it.

Concerned about the chemicals in our water supply, we installed a whole-house filtration system with a recyclable coconut charcoal filter, as well as a separate point-of-use filter specifically to remove fluoride. This way the water we drink and bathe in does not have a negative impact. Invest in clean water, invest in health!"

## Well Water

According to the U.S. Environmental Protection Agency, about 15 percent of Americans rely on private wells for drinking water, but the quality varies. Since well water is not treated, chlorine and fluoride are rarely a concern, but it may be high in other minerals that can cause off flavors in the kombucha. Well water with a water softener added often yields better-tasting results. Check with your local health or environmental department about certified water-testing labs in your area. If your water is of good quality and produces good-tasting tea and healthy SCOBYs, keep using it!

## Spring Water

Spring water provides a wonderful option; follow standard purification practices if necessary. As with private well water, spring water may have high levels of minerals that may affect the flavor of your kombucha and the health of your cultures, so test the spring water quality as needed, monitor for changes in your kombucha over time, and adjust as necessary.

## Bottled Water

If the bottled water truly comes from a spring, as opposed to being repackaged from municipal tap supplies as many brands are, it is likely a great choice. It is possible that the water will have been properly filtered and remineralized prior to bottling, but every brand is different.

## Municipal Tap Water

Municipal tap-water supplies (where most people obtain their water) are controlled and monitored by local government agencies. Tap water nearly always contains chlorine and other additives that make it "safe" to consume. In the United States, municipal systems often also contain sodium fluoride or hexafluorosilicic acid, purportedly added for dental health but controversial in many communities.

It is critical that the water be chlorine-free. Added to kill pathogens, chlorine's antibacterial nature makes it an unwelcome element when brewing kombucha. Fortunately it can be removed easily using any of the following methods:

*Evaporation.* Fill a pot with water and leave it out, uncovered, for about 24 hours. Chlorine is a gas and will evaporate given enough time.

*Boiling.* Boil water for 15 minutes to remove the chlorine.

Though these methods will remove chlorine, we recommend filtering tap water to remove not just chlorine but other impurities. Some compounds in the water supply may be "harmless" to the brew but questionable for human health. Regular filters do not remove all contaminants, most notably chloramines or sodium fluoride, so top commercial breweries employ special filters for the cleanest water possible. Home filters fine enough to remove nearly all contaminants can be installed under a kitchen sink to help improve the flavor and purity of the kombucha, not to mention make all the water your family consumes more healthful.

## Water Filtration Methods

More and more families are turning to home filtration systems, reverse osmosis systems, and distillation as less expensive, less wasteful, and safer alternatives to bottled or tap water. There are many options.

*Pitcher filter.* Most simple pitchers use an activated charcoal filter to remove chlorine and about 30 to 60 percent of the total contaminants, though not sodium fluoride. This is a good start and should provide clean enough water for brewing in most cases.

*Countertop or under-sink cartridge systems.* Many of these filtration systems also use charcoal, but their more sophisticated design can remove 99 percent or more of contaminants. They generally do not remove fluoride.

*Gravity-fed water filter.* These units use gravity to pull the water through extremely fine filters that absorb pathogenic bacteria, viruses, and other contaminants without removing minerals. They are an excellent choice for filtration or purification.

*Reverse osmosis (RO).* RO works by forcing water through a semipermeable membrane, separating pure water from chemical-laden, which is directed down the drain. The filtered water then passes through charcoal before coming out the tap. Because of its 50 percent water loss, some consider it expensive and wasteful.

*Distillation.* It was once believed that distilled was the only appropriate water for brewing kombucha, but quite the opposite has proven to be true. Most find this "dead" water to be a source of brewing problems due to the lack of minerals. If only distilled is available, using a mineral-rich sugar, such as evaporated cane juice crystals or brown sugar, and a strong tea infusion can usually provide enough nutrition for the culture to brew properly.

## WHAT'S IN YOUR WATER?

It would be folly to deny that the drinking water supply is becoming increasingly contaminated via problems both environmental and systemic. Pharmaceutical drugs, agricultural chemicals, and other pollutants have been flooding into both municipal and groundwater supplies for decades. Just as dangerous is the aging infrastructure of many city tap-water facilities. Add fracking and oil spills to the mix, and that's a whole cocktail of yuck potentially ending up in our water and wreaking havoc on our body's internal ecosystem.

This does not even take into account the chemicals that attract plenty of controversy on their own, such as the chlorine and fluoride that municipalities add to their water. To know for certain what is in your tap water, you may consider sending a sample to a regional lab to be tested or purchasing an at-home water-quality testing kit.

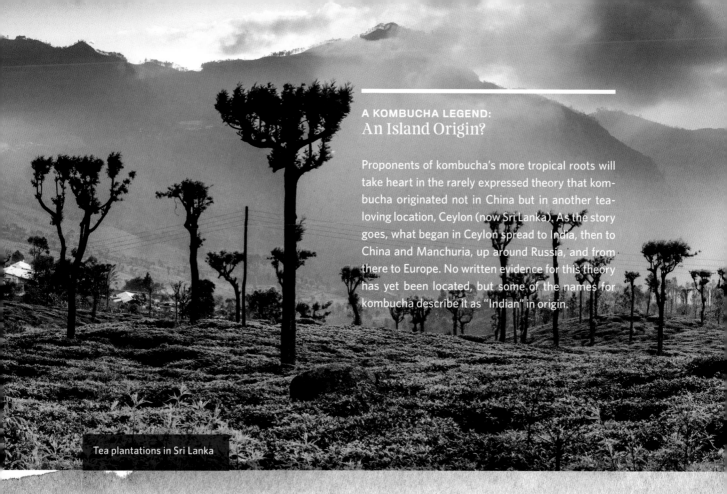

## An Island Origin?

Proponents of kombucha's more tropical roots will take heart in the rarely expressed theory that kombucha originated not in China but in another tea-loving location, Ceylon (now Sri Lanka). As the story goes, what began in Ceylon spread to India, then to China and Manchuria, up around Russia, and from there to Europe. No written evidence for this theory has yet been located, but some of the names for kombucha describe it as "Indian" in origin.

Tea plantations in Sri Lanka

# FLUORIDE IN TEA?

Occasionally concerns arise regarding the fluoride content of tea or the risk of "fluoride poisoning" from drinking too much tea over a long period of time. While these warnings are issued in good faith, they are based on a faulty understanding of the chemical constituents of tea. Tea leaves do contain naturally occurring calcium fluoride, but that form of fluoride is quite different from the types of fluoride commonly added to municipal water supplies.

Calcium fluoride is a natural substance that the body needs. You can, of course, have too much calcium fluoride in your diet, just as is possible with any other necessary vitamin or mineral. However, reports of "fluoride poisoning" from tea involve people consuming gallons of superstrong brew every day, not something that is ever recommended for tea or especially kombucha, or frankly for any food or drink.

When making kombucha, we start with relatively weak tea, containing trace amounts of naturally occurring fluoride. Once the kombucha is brewed, you won't be drinking excessive amounts of it. All of this is to say that there's no reason to be concerned about the fluoride content of tea or kombucha.

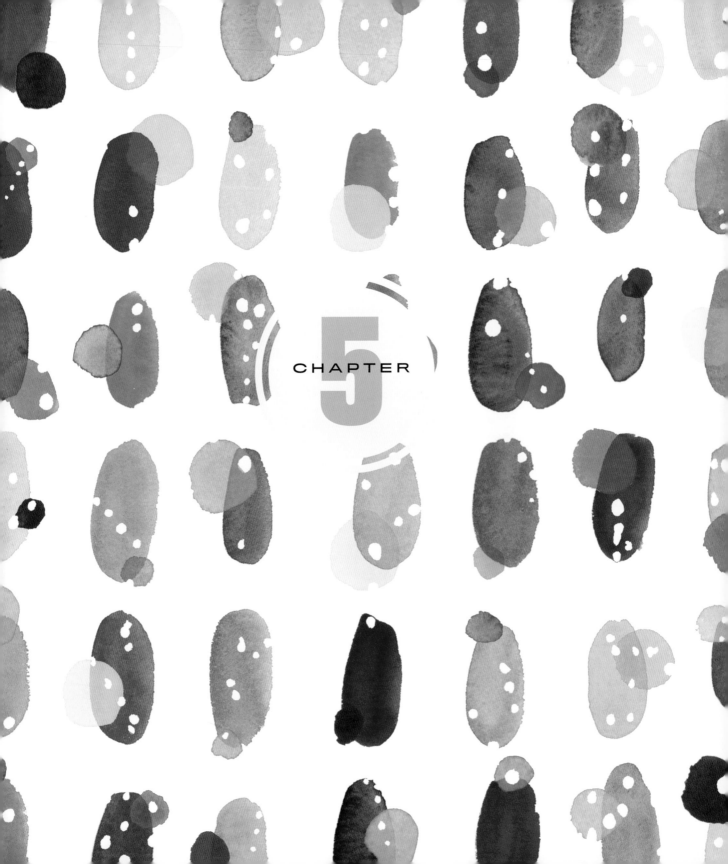

CHAPTER

5

# Brewing Equipment and Supplies

Brewing kombucha is a simple process, but many factors play a role in brewing success. Of course you'll need to have the right equipment and tools at your disposal, but you must also pay attention to the brewing environment. Kombucha is alive, and the bacteria and yeast are sensitive to all kinds of inputs — temperature, light, humidity, sounds, energy, and vibrations. Create a safe, warm kombucha nursery for a lifetime of delicious brew.

# Choosing the Right Vessel

Many begin their kombucha brewing adventure with a single batch made in a 1-gallon (or smaller) glass container. This works well for limited production, though to make a full gallon of kombucha, you need a vessel that is slightly larger to accommodate the SCOBY, the starter liquid, and the gallon of sweet tea. Ideally, the vessel will have a wide mouth for ease of access and to provide adequate surface area for optimum brewing.

For a CB system (see chapter 7), we recommend using a vessel that holds between 2½ and 5 gallons. For the homebrewer, anything larger than that can be difficult to handle and clean, let alone find room for. The serious hobbyist or budding professional brewer may decide to invest in an even larger vessel such as a brew-safe plastic bucket or tub of up to 30 gallons, or even a stainless steel fermenter, available in sizes from 50 to 500 gallons.

As tempting as it may be to brew a ton of kombucha all at once, beware! Batches larger than 5 gallons can experience issues of inconsistent flavor, extremely slow fermentation, and sometimes total failure due to problems in maintaining temperature, providing adequate oxygen to the entire brew, and other considerations.

First decide on your brewing vessel size, then investigate the options. There are many suitable choices made of various materials, as long as you follow a few guidelines.

**KOMBUCHA MAMMA SEZ**

## Recycling Rules!

"Repurposing vessels found in thrift stores or at garage sales can be an affordable way to find a home for your brew. Be aware, though, that vessels not intended for food use, such as vases or other kinds of pottery, may leach dangerous elements such as lead or aluminum into the brew. Even some 'food-safe' vessels use lower-grade plastics, paints, or glazes that were never intended for constant contact with the high acidity of kombucha. Inspect all vessels closely prior to use and if unsure, consider a simple lead-testing kit. (For more, see Selecting an Appropriate Spigot, page 80.)

## Glass

A large glass jar is perhaps the most common first brewing vessel and always a fine choice, especially for a batch brew (see chapter 6). Colored glass that is not intended for food consumption such as vases or etched glassware may contain lead. Use only food-safe glass for brewing. Clear glass jars are readily available, relatively light, and easy to clean, and they offer a view of what is happening in the brew, which many people enjoy. An old pickle jar might do the trick.

A glass vessel with a spigot is useful for continuous brewing (see chapter 7), but many commercially available beverage dispensers, the kind often used for lemonade or iced tea, are not suitable for use with kombucha due to the poor quality of the materials. (See Selecting an Appropriate Spigot, page 80.)

## Porcelain or Ceramic

Porcelain or ceramic vessels are historically the most common type of container used for fermenting, and their opaque nature protects the brew from light and offers a more discreet look, which some brewers prefer. Look for a vessel designed to be used with food, which will be best able to withstand the high acidity of the kombucha. Avoid flowerpots or containers with brightly colored glazes. Nearly all porcelain and ceramic kitchenware made in this century is lead-free. If you are unsure about a particular vessel, a simple lead test can confirm its safety.

## Stainless Steel

Most metals are not safe to use for brewing kombucha since the acidic solution will leach their compounds into the tea (see Materials to Avoid, this page). However, stainless steel (grade 304 or higher) is corrosian-resistant. It is a stalwart of the beer, wine, and, most important, the vinegar brewing industries as it can withstand the low pH and high acidity conditions of acetic-acid-producing fermentation. Vinegar can be 20 times as acidic as kombucha during production, so if they use it, we can be sure the material is safe.

## Wood Barrels

High-quality barrels can be used for brewing a unique and delicious version of kombucha, with broader flavor dimensions and mellower acetic-acid notes. The type of wood that is used imbues its own unique flavor profile into the brew. American toasted oak barrels — the traditional choice for vinegar, as well as wine and beer — are an excellent option, but a variety of other woods may also be used.

Most barrels are constructed for fermenting alcoholic beverages, and as such they lack an appropriate opening at the top for access to the brew and the SCOBYs. Suppliers familiar with the specific needs of kombucha brewing may be able to cut a barrel accordingly. (For more on barrel brewing, see page 127.)

## Plastic

Some kombucha enthusiasts prefer to brew in food-grade plastic buckets such as those found in brewing-supply stores. And there are commercial brands that choose high-density brewing-grade plastic for their vessels, as these higher-end materials are better able to withstand the acidity of kombucha. Consumer-grade plastics, however, are never recommended, and this extends to the lower-grade plastic used in manufacturing many spigots and the epoxies used to hold them together.

## Materials to Avoid

Do not use containers made with metals such as brass, cast iron, or aluminum to brew kombucha. Many beer-brewing supplies include brass fixtures or other metal pieces that cannot withstand the low pH. Kombucha will leach these metals into the brew.

Another material to avoid is crystal. Traditionally made with lead, it should not be used to ferment kombucha, as it may leach lead into your brew. A home lead test kit can confirm the safety of any vessel.

Brewing vessels are available in a range of materials and sizes to fit either method of brewing and any size batch.

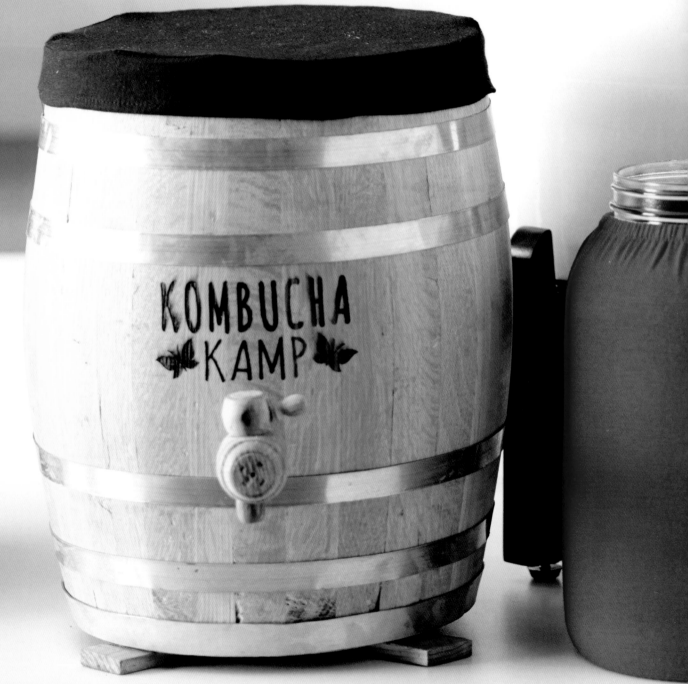

KOMBUCHA KAMP

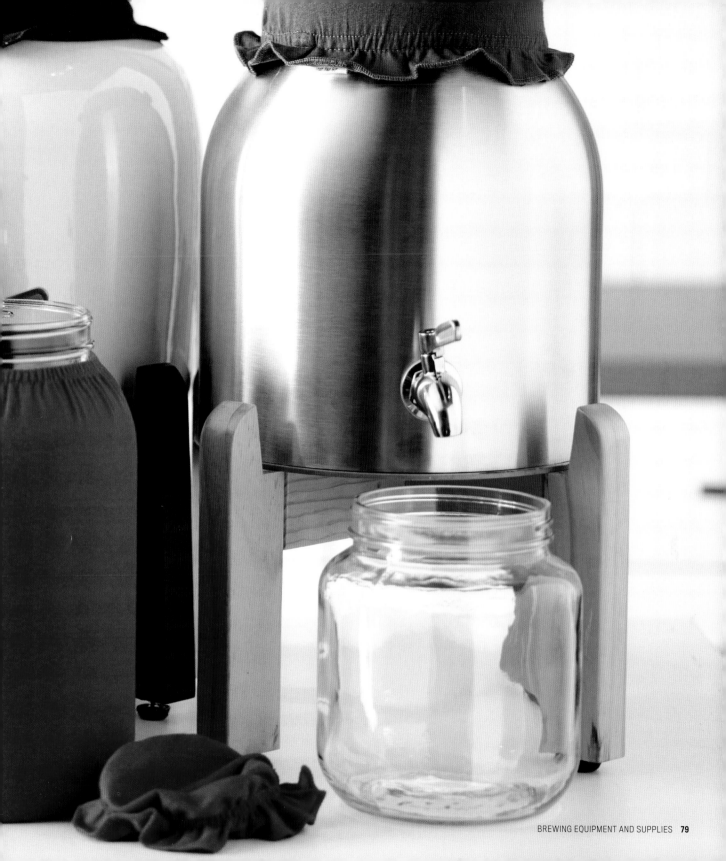

# Selecting an Appropriate Spigot

With the continuous brew method, the larger vessel size and weight of all that liquid make a spigot pretty much a requirement. There are ways to get around it (a siphon or ladle can be used to remove the brew), but adding another step defeats many of the advantages of CB, such as ease of bottling, less cleanup, and overall convenience.

Not just any spigot will do, however, and unfortunately many included on everyday beverage dispensers are unsafe for use with the high acidity of kombucha. It is common for new homebrewers to attempt to save money by choosing vessels with these spigots only to find out down the road that they've been brewing with toxins! Nearly all consumer-grade spigots and fasteners found on these jars feature one or more of the following issues: low-grade plastic (more than 95 percent have this problem), metallic-looking paints or other coating, actual metal fasteners, and epoxies/glues.

If the spigot cannot be easily removed by unscrewing the fasteners and leaving a clean hole in the vessel, it should not be used. If any part of the assembly is made of milky white, partially translucent plastic, it is a poor choice. Metal paints erode into the brew over time, and glues, as well as any real metal pieces (aluminum, brass, chrome) will result in toxins in the brew.

The best spigot options have the following qualities:

- Made from wood, stainless steel (304 grade or better), or professional-grade plastic
- Unpainted and uncoated
- Free of epoxies or glues in assembly or attachment
- Held together with corrosion-resistant nuts and washers
- Quickly and easily removed for cleaning

American-made professional-grade plastic spigots have an excellent reputation and have worked well for us for years, but stainless steel models are also very popular due to their striking appearance and high flow rate. Wood remains an appealing option for those who want only natural materials, but generally the decant takes a little longer than with plastic or stainless. Any of these options is safe for long-term use with the booch, so take your pick or try them all to find the one you prefer!

# Other Brewing Supplies

In addition to an appropriate vessel, making kombucha requires only a few tools, all of which can be found in most kitchens. It's important to make sure these tools are very clean before you use them, but remember that chlorine, and even soap, can harm your kombucha culture.

You might consider keeping a separate set of tools for your kombucha operation to avoid contamination from foods, oils, spices, and so on. Or you can thoroughly wash your tools and then "cure" them with a quick wash in mature kombucha or distilled white vinegar prior to using them for brewing.

## Kettle or Pot

You'll need a pot or kettle for heating water to make the base tea. Any vessel will suffice, as it is not being used to brew the kombucha. We use an electric teakettle, which heats water quickly and requires only a plug.

Alternatively, save some energy and brew up sun tea! Combine the loose tea with room-temperature water in a clear glass vessel. Set the vessel in a spot that gets direct sunlight. Cover loosely and let steep for 12 to 24 hours.

## Reusable Tea Bags, Tea Balls, or Strainers

For use with loose-leaf tea, cotton tea bags and tea balls are excellent choices because they can be used again and again, reducing waste and saving money. Tea bags may become stained with tannins but can be used until they fall apart. Tea balls may allow some tea particles to escape into the tea liquor, ending up in the brew and occasionally attaching to the SCOBY as small flecks of black, brown, or green. This is not an issue, though; the particles will not affect the culture or the brewing process. Whichever you choose, be sure the tea bag or ball is large enough to accommodate the leaves as they expand, to allow for optimum extraction and flavor.

Another option is to add the tea leaves directly to the water, steep, and then strain them out prior to adding the sugar.

## Long-Handled Spoon

Any spoon or other stirring implement will do as long as the handle is long enough to reach the bottom of the brewing vessel. Metal, wood, plastic — the material is not of concern, as you are using it to stir the sweet tea base before it ferments and becomes acidic.

## Cloth Cover

As an aerobic ferment, the kombucha brew needs airflow, but it also needs to be covered to protect it from dust, fruit flies, and other potential contaminants. For Kombucha Kamp (our kombucha retail business), we invented the Brewer Cap, a fitted, breathable cotton cover with elastic edging to hold it securely over any wide-mouth fermentation vessel. But you can use any tightly woven cloth (a cloth napkin or a piece of old sheet or T-shirt works fine) and secure it in place with a rubber band.

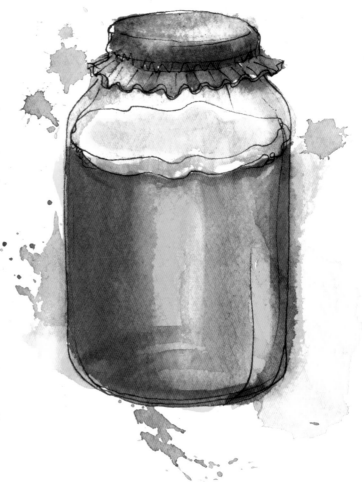

Cloth covers don't need to be replaced with every batch, but they do benefit from a cleaning now and then. Some choose to use coffee filters or paper towels; while these certainly work, we prefer to use cloth as a more sustainable option that generates less waste.

## No Cheesecloth!

"Never use cheesecloth to cover your brewing vessel! The weave is too loose, allowing fruit flies and other contaminants to colonize the brew. Folding the cheesecloth into a double layer will not help; the fruit flies will wriggle between the layers and get in anyway. Unless you enjoy a little extra protein in your booch, choose a more tightly woven cloth cover."

## Thermometer Strip

Monitoring the temperature of the brew is helpful for ensuring healthy progress, troubleshooting, and most important, maintaining consistent flavor. Adhesive strip thermometers attach to nearly any material and provide an accurate measure of the liquid temperature inside the vessel. If temperature readings are not immediately apparent on the thermometer, shining a flashlight on it can make the reading more visible.

Do not use thermometers with probes in kombucha, as the probe material may not be designed to withstand the high acidity. Another problem is that inserting a probe under the cloth cover will leave a gap for fruit flies to contaminate the brew.

## Heating Pad

Should the brew fall below the ideal temperature range, additional heat may be added via a heating pad. While homebrewers have, of course, rigged up myriad makeshift warming systems, heaters constructed specifically for kombucha that heat from the sides of the vessel give optimum results. (A heater that warms only the bottom of the vessel will encourage yeast over bacteria, pushing the brew out of balance.) (See page 86 for more on maintaining temperature.)

## Strainer/Filter

While optional, a fine-mesh strainer or filter comes in handy for filtering yeast at brewing or bottling time, removing flavoring agents prior to bottling, or collecting the loose-leaf tea after steeping. Stainless steel or plastic may be used, and even folded cheesecloth, while not a good choice for covering the fermenting brew, works fine as a strainer.

## Funnel

The batch brew method requires a funnel for the bottling stage; stainless steel and plastic are both viable options. (Incidental contact with metal and plastic does not harm the brew as it passes through.) A funnel with a detachable filter, found at brewing-supply shops, can be very useful.

## pH Strips or pH Meter

While it is not necessary to test the pH of every batch, test strips or a high-quality meter can come in handy for troubleshooting by indicating if the brew is acidifying properly or not.

Kombucha falls on the acidic end of the pH scale, so short-range test strips on the low end (0 to 6) or a pH meter would be the best choice. (For more, see page 175.)

# Types of Bottles to Use

As with any fermented beverage, kombucha should be stored in heavy-duty bottles that are designed to withstand the pressure of carbonation. Bottles intended for decoration may not be a safe choice.

While it is possible to bottle in plastic, we don't recommend it, as most are not made to withstand high acidity and may leach chemicals into the brew. With so many other options available, plastic bottles are not worth the risk. Plastic lids, on the other hand, are excellent, and they do not have more than incidental contact with the kombucha, so leaching isn't a concern. Due to the acidic nature of kombucha, never allow metal lids or any metal linings to come in contact with the brew.

Here are the best bottle choices, in order of our preference.

***Swing-top glass bottles.*** Glass bottles with swing-top closures come in many different grades of thickness, but the heaviest ones you can find are the best choice for kombucha because they are built to more effectively handle the pressure of carbonation. Of course any bottle can break, but often the bottom cracks off rather than the whole thing exploding outward. Sometimes the cap will leak, creating a mess but preventing any breakage. Round bottles tend to break less often than square ones due to more even pressure distribution.

***Recycled commercial kombucha bottles.*** Many homebrewers repurpose store-brand bottles for their own brew, and this is an excellent idea, especially at first, when homebrewers may not be ready to invest in bottles. However, these thinner glass bottles break much more easily than thicker, heavier-duty reusable bottles. Another issue is that the caps may degrade

## CLEAR OR TINTED GLASS?

Many commercial brands of kombucha come in tinted bottles. Why? Primarily because light is antibacterial, and kombucha depends on bacteria. For commercial bottlers, putting kombucha on trucks and through warehouses and finally on shelves directly under bright store lights introduces questions about how much damage the bacteria and yeast will suffer before making it to the consumer. Packaging the beverage in dark bottles reduces those impacts.

For homebrewers, who are in complete control of the brewing environment and bottling storage, there is no real need for tinted or colored glass. Clear bottles allow the often beautiful colors of the flavorings to shine through. That said, glass colors like blue or green can add personality to a bottle collection, so the choice is yours!

quickly, so that they no longer provide a tight seal, but swapping them for professional-grade caps, available from homebrew-supply shops, can extend the life of these bottles and provide better carbonation as a bonus.

**Beer bottles with capper.** While thinner beer bottles have been known to shatter, thicker ones are a popular choice for homebrewers. For safety, always keep them stored upright to prevent kombucha from degrading the metal cap. Whatever type of beer bottle you use, you'll need a cap that fits it, and possibly a capper to put on the cap; both are available from homebrew suppliers.

**Mason jars.** Many people who ferment at home have a collection of mason jars and lids. While heavy enough to handle carbonated beverages, they may leave the kombucha flat due to lack of proper seal. Oxidation of the metal lids can also be a concern as liquid condensing on the lid may drip metallic and off flavors into the brew. Plastic lids (available wherever canning supplies are sold) may be a better choice, but as long as the jars remain upright metal lids are acceptable (ditch them immediately if any rust appears).

**Recycled wine or champagne bottles.** Some people choose to recycle wine or champagne bottles because if too much carbonation builds up, the cork, acting as a safety mechanism, will pop out before the bottle shatters. This can be messy, as kombucha will go everywhere and fruit pieces may get lodged in the ceiling! We prefer to master our brewing and bottling cycle and take the small risk of manageable explosions, but as a safety-first option these bottles can be useful.

# Where to Brew

When choosing a brewing location, consider these factors:

- **Temperature.** The brew prefers a relatively warm temperature, in the range of 75 to 85°F (24–29°C), for best results.
- **Airflow.** The initial stage of fermentation, when the SCOBY is forming a new layer thrives with fresh air.
- **Exposure to sunlight.** Direct sunlight may have an antibacterial effect, so it's best to avoid it. Indirect overhead lighting will not have an adverse effect.
- **Convenience.** You'll want to taste the brew as it ferments. Most brewers prefer keeping it close to the kitchen.

For many, the kitchen counter is an ideal location for brewing. (Try to leave a few feet between the ferment and the stove, however, as grease and cooking fumes may lead to off flavors.) However, it may not always be possible to keep the brew in the kitchen. Keeping the above factors in mind, it's usually possible to find a suitable alternative location. Some people keep their brews in the garage, in a spare bedroom, on an office shelf, or on top of the fridge. Any protected nook will do.

## Conditions to Avoid

Environmental factors such as the following can have a detrimental effect on your brew:

- Cigarette smoke
- Pollen (from houseplants and outdoors)
- Grease and cooking fumes
- Toxic chemicals and harsh fumes (such as those in a closet where cleaning products are stored)
- Direct sunlight
- Excessively warm or cold temperatures (see Optimizing the Temperature, page 86)
- Stuffy or unventilated areas
- Proximity to any other ferment

Avoiding cross-contamination with other ferments is important. Kombucha yeast and bacteria are hardy, and they invisibly cling to clothes, hair, and skin or even just float around the fermenting area. If kefir, yogurt, sauerkraut, or other ferments are being made in the same area, cross-contamination is possible. Some homebrewers report a SCOBY suddenly growing in kefir, or strange yeast taking over their sauerkraut. Such is the case sometimes with the more dominant kombucha bacteria and yeast.

To prevent these issues, keep ferments well apart from each other, preferably in their own areas, and use separate covers, utensils, and vessels for the ferments. If cross-contamination does occur, it's not ideal, but it's also not dangerous unless you see mold. Move the crossed ferment to a separate area; microbiological balance should return over time. Cross-contamination is not always a bad thing, but if any of your other ferments develop a funky flavor, consider moving the kombucha to its own location.

# Optimizing the Temperature

The recommended temperature range for brewing kombucha is 75 to 85°F (24–29°C), with the ideal being 78 to 80°F (26–27°C). While the yeast perform well at a wider range, these temperatures provide the best environment for the bacteria to thrive (see Bacteria & Yeast: Party Planners vs. Party Animals , page 34).

At lower ranges, the flavor may be weak as the range of acids present is reduced. Higher temps cause the brew to become intensely sour or sharp. In both cases, yeast can overpopulate the brew, leading to diminished bacteria and SCOBY growth. That said, as long as no mold develops, kombucha brewed at any temperature is safe to consume, though maybe not as delicious.

## When It's Too Warm

In most locations at most times of year, maintaining the right temperature means heating the brew, but in rare cases too much heat can be the issue. There's nothing unsafe, unhealthy, or wrong about brewing above 85°F (29°C), and some people may prefer these temperatures. As long as the brew remains below about 100°F (38°C), the culture will survive; sustained

## TOO HOT? TOO COLD? JUST RIGHT!

### 109°F (43°C) and above

Yeast die-off begins within a few hours and the SCOBY cannot survive for more than a few days.

### 101–108°F (38–42°C)

Bacteria cease activity and yeast become hyperactive, resulting in a terrible brew.

### 86–100°F (30–38°C)

This range favors the yeast and retards bacterial development, so over time or successive batches it throws off the brew's microbial balance and flavor. It does not cause bacterial death but may eventually cause the yeast to choke out the bacteria.

### 81–85°F (27–29°C)

This is the high end of ideal brewing range, and it produces a kombucha with more full-powered flavor, higher acid levels and yeast production, and potentially stronger SCOBYs as well. This is a good range early in the fermenting process but is not recommended for a mature kombucha.

### 78–80°F (26–27°C)

This is the ideal range for kombucha, especially during the first three to seven days of fermentation; it produces the best balance of yeast and bacterial activity as well as acid production.

temperatures of over 108°F (42°C) are required to damage the bacteria.

**Note:** This also means that if your kombucha heater accidentally raises the temperature above optimum range overnight or for a day, it's no big deal.

When brewing at higher temperatures, the flavor will turn sour more quickly and the brew will be done faster. If brewing conditions are normally above 85°F (29°C), the first and best possibility is to find the least-warm spot in the house, perhaps on the bottom shelf of a shaded pantry or in a breezy hallway or wherever there might be a pocket of cooler air.

Other ways to reduce the effects of high temperature brewing include the following:

- Taste frequently, harvest sooner — the warmer it is, the faster it will be done; check several times a day when it's close to ready.
- Harvest when it's sweeter than you like — we do this anyway to allow for extended bottle-aging, but in warm conditions we consider even sweeter kombucha potentially ready for bottling.
- Make smaller batches. Since they will complete faster anyway, it doesn't hurt

## 71–77°F (22–25°C)

At the low end of ideal brewing range, the result is a smoother beverage with good flavor but less bite. It works with close-to-mature CB setups to slow development.

## 65–70°F (18–21°C)

This range permits slow but acceptable fermentation; the kombucha may achieve the desired flavor over a longer brewing cycle. It may result in weaker SCOBY growth and more yeast. It is an acceptable temperature range for SCOBY Hotel storage or second fermentation.

## 50–64°F (10–18°C)

For brewing kombucha, this range causes very slow fermentation with weak or yeasty flavors and the possibility of mold. However, 60°F (16°C) is the ideal temperature for long-term SCOBY Hotel storage.

## 50°F (10°C) and below

Too cold for bacterial activity, temperatures this low lead to mold in both SCOBY Hotels and kombucha brews. This temperature range — which can be found in refrigerators — is *never* recommended.

to make less, and it will be easier to finish the bottles on hand before they go sour.

- Flavor, then move directly to the fridge; the flavors will still infuse, though carbonation may be weak. Pull the bottles from the fridge and leave at room temperature for 4 to 24 hours to reawaken the yeast and develop some effervescence.
- Use 25 percent less sugar and/or tea; giving less fuel for creating acids means a smoother brew.

## When It's Too Cool

One of the most common issues new homebrewers confront is low temperature, resulting in a weaker brew with potential for mold. Brewing in the 68 to 75°F (20-24°C) range should still yield a drinkable brew, especially at the higher end, but it will take longer and may lack the appley sour bite produced by

### One Exception

"Every rule needs an exception, and this is the *only* exception to our refrigerator rule: Under extreme conditions, where the brew itself (not just the weather outside, but the liquid) could reach close to 100 degrees, it is okay to put the whole brew in the fridge for a few hours during the hottest part of day, but *do not leave it overnight*. Remember, this is only a brief and temporary exception, and it need not be done every hot day."

proper temps. Attempting to ferment below this range, especially under 64°F (18°C), usually results in a flat, "dirty" taste or a batch that goes to mold, as the bacteria become sluggish and often have a difficult time acidifying the brew in time to protect it from contamination.

## SEASONAL CHANGES IN BREWING CYCLE

The seasons affect the speed and flavor of kombucha brews. Adjusting to the needs of the brew will ensure delicious kombucha year-round.

*Spring* — Cooler temperatures prevail as winter slowly melts away. Use a heating element to keep the brew between 78 and 80°F (26 and 27°C).

*Summer* — As temperatures rise outside, the fermentation cycle shortens significantly, so taste your brew more often. Staying on top of it will prevent lost batches. To slow the brew, take a break before starting the next batch or topping off a CB vessel. Some overly sour liquid may need to be drained in order to achieve the right brewing cycle. Don't worry — there are lots of uses for it (see page 256 and page 309).

*Fall* — Brewing cycles lengthen but flavors remain robust. When temperatures drop at night, use a heating element to maintain the right temperature, but monitor during warm days to prevent overheating.

*Winter* — When it is cold out, kombucha gets sluggish and wants to hibernate. Even when heated to the correct temperature, the brew may take longer than usual.

If no proper heating solution is available, look for the naturally warmest spot in the kitchen. If that's not enough to boost the temperature, try setting the fermentation vessel next to a working appliance, like a refrigerator or slow cooker. Sometimes wrapping the jar in a towel or blanket helps. Keeping the vessel off cold kitchen countertops by setting it on a wooden cutting board, for example, can keep the brew a few degrees warmer.

Some also place their vessel in a closed cupboard, closet, or oven with the light on. In general, we don't recommend using light bulbs or heat lamps at close proximity to warm kombucha because light is antibacterial, plus the vessel and brew will experience hot spots rather than even heat.

Airflow is also important, so find a spot that has a good balance between the temperature and air circulation. And yes, people have forgotten and turned on the oven, baking their entire SCOBY Hotel in the process, so use your best judgment when selecting a location!

## Best Practices

In the end, most people choose to heat their kombucha in some way to achieve the desired brew. Even in the summer, people in coastal areas or northern climates, as well as those using air-conditioning, find that maintaining the vessel at SCOBY-friendly temps requires a heat source.

A highly efficient mat specifically designed to heat kombucha will always be the best option, but seedling mats or belts may provide enough heat in a pinch if the temperature needs to be raised only a few degrees. That said, where the heat is delivered — from the sides rather than the bottom — is critical for flavor and brew balance. The reason, as it often is with the booch, is to keep those yeast in check.

When the yeast complete respiration a few days into the brew, they descend to the bottom of the fermentation vessel, and the bacteria, which have been working quietly to this point, ramp up their activity at the top of the brew near the newly growing SCOBY. Placing a heat source below the vessel, as many new homebrewers unwittingly do, prevents the yeast from resting, which disturbs the balance.

A proper heater works from the sides of the vessel, which assists the bacteria's efforts to acidify the environment, build SCOBY, and protect the brew by delivering the warmth right where they do their best work. For the most consistent results batch after batch, but especially with continuous brew, maintaining temperature with the right heat source makes all the difference.

# Kombucha to Go

Sometimes it's necessary to take your brewing operation on the road. Here's how to handle traveling with a SCOBY and even a full batch of kombucha tea.

## By Plane

Current airline regulations require that amounts of liquid over 3 ounces be stored in checked luggage. Package SCOBYs with starter liquid in a ziplock bag; then wrap that bag in a small towel and seal it in a larger ziplock bag. The towel will absorb liquid and help protect the contents of the suitcase should the bags leak.

For even more protection, pack the SCOBY with just enough liquid to keep it wet during

# HOW MUCH BOOCH TO BREW

**1.**

Estimate how much kombucha each drinker in the household consumes per day (don't forget to include the neighbor, babysitter, and dog!) Use the chart at right to calculate weekly consumption for each drinker.

**2.**

Once everyone is accounted for, add up the total household consumption per week.

**3.**

Use that total in the chart below to find the household category — **Samplers, Sippers, Regulars, Lovers,** or **Pros** — that fits your needs and estimate how much kombucha to keep on hand. This chart assumes a 1-gallon (4 L) batch brew and

2.5-gallon (10 L) continuous brew. Because people drink more some days and less others, these numbers are just estimates — you can always add extra vessels as your demand increases.

| Kombucha per Day | × | Days per Week | = | Weekly Consumption |
|---|---|---|---|---|
| 4 ounces (125 mL) | | 4 | | 16 ounces (.5 L) |
| 4 ounces | | 7 | | 1 quart (1 L) |
| 8 ounces (250 mL) | | 4 | | 1 quart (1 L) |
| 8 ounces | | 7 | | ½ gallon (2 L) |
| 16 ounces (500 mL) | | 4 | | ½ gallon (2 L) |
| 16 ounces | | 7 | | 1 gallon (4 L) |
| 1 quart (1 L) | | 7 | | 2 gallons (7.5 L) |
| More than 1 quart | | 7 | | Start a company! |

| If your household consumes this much kombucha per week | Your household category is | Consider brewing this much kombucha |
|---|---|---|
| Up to ½ gallon (2 L) | **Samplers:** You may prefer to purchase kombucha commercially or to make half-size batches at home, spaced out as needed. | 1 batch brew (or just buy it) |
| ½ to 1 gallon (2–4 L) | **Sippers:** Brew a standard gallon batch brew for your needs, or make life easier with one standard CB. | 1–2 batch brews or 1 regular CB |
| Up to 2 gallons (7.5 L) | **Regulars:** As a regular consumer with serious kombucha needs, rotate a number of batch brews or set up at least one CB to meet demand. | 2–4 batch brews or 1–2 regular CBs or 1 large CB |
| Up to 4 gallons (15 L) | **Lovers:** Keep that love flowing with a number of batch brew jars or a few CBs pumping the booch every day. | 4–8 batch brews or 2–3 regular CBs or 1–2 large CBs |
| 4+ gallons (15+ L) | **Pros:** You are one step away from starting your own kombucha company! Rotating as many as four CBs is the easiest way to keep a steady supply on hand. | 2–4 regular CBs or 2 large CBs |

travel. Pour the starter liquid into a separate plastic or glass bottle, close tightly and apply packing or duct tape around the edges of the lid to minimize leaking, and then wrap in plastic bags and a towel as described above.

If you don't pack bottles without these precautions, they will almost certainly leak.

## By Vehicle

Move the SCOBYs and kombucha to glass jars with screw-on lids, preferably plastic lids to prevent rusting. To protect the bacteria from sunlight and keep them at hospitable temperatures, store the jars in a box with a lid or, better yet, in a cooler.

If stopping for an extended period on a sunny day, you may need to take the brew inside to keep it from overheating in the vehicle. The culture can tolerate brief periods of exposure to colder temperatures, but extended exposure to temperatures of 108°F (42°C) and above may harm the culture.

Kombucha may slosh out from under the jar's lid even when it is screwed on tightly, as it is more mobile than water. One trick to prevent leaking is to place a piece of plastic wrap over the mouth of the jar before screwing on the lid. Even so, consider wrapping the jar in a towel to absorb any leakage. Keep the jar(s) or brewer upright, or leakage is guaranteed.

With a continuous brew vessel, you can leave the cultures and brew inside the vessel, provided it isn't full to the brim (remove some of the liquid if necessary). Pack the entire vessel in a box, and wedge it into a secure spot in the vehicle. To ship bottles or bring them on a driving trip, look for wine shippers, which are often molded from packing materials to create a safe slot for each bottle. Keep in mind that shipping full bottles can be expensive.

## Brewing on the Go

If you're not just transporting kombucha but actually brewing in a vehicle that's constantly on the go, like an RV or houseboat, you shouldn't experience any specific problems unless the ride is particularly bumpy. SCOBY growth can be affected by the constant disturbance of liquid, and you may see strange-looking SCOBYs forming in strands or in many thin layers that start anew each time the culture is dislodged. The constant agitation of the brew may also cause it to mature more quickly, as it is exposed to more oxygen, leading to faster ferment times.

## Moving

If you're moving to a new home and bringing your kombucha cultures with you, they may need a bit of time to adjust to their new environment. The first batch or two that you brew in your new home may not turn out exactly right, but eventually the cultures will adapt and you'll be back in business.

---

**KOMBUCHA MAMMA SEZ**

### Kombucha Tourism!

"Can't travel with your booch? Look up local brands wherever you are, grab a few different bottles, and have a sampling party with whoever is adventurous enough to try. Some kombucha breweries now offer tours and tastings. Call ahead to find out!"

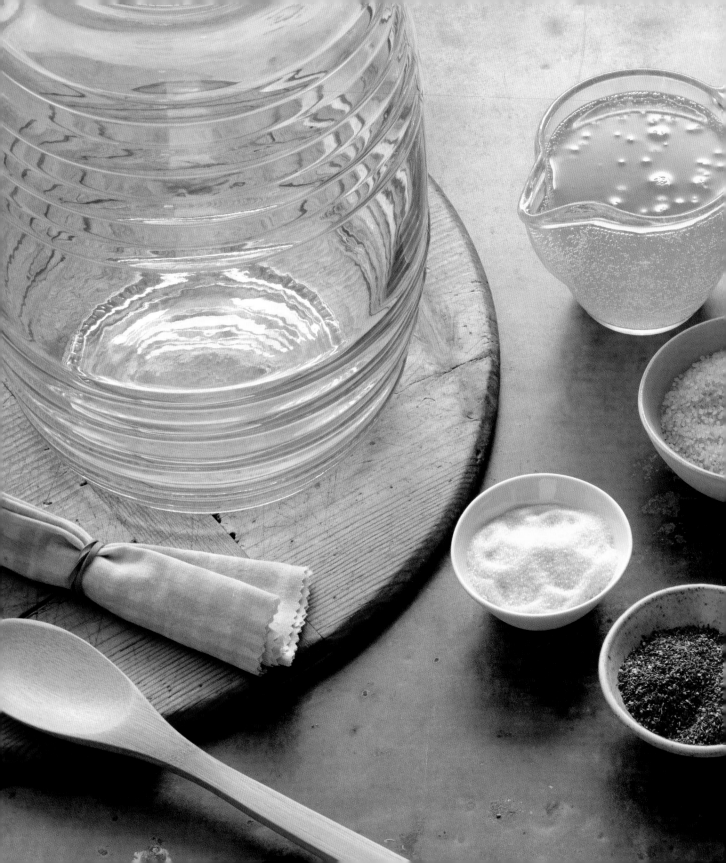

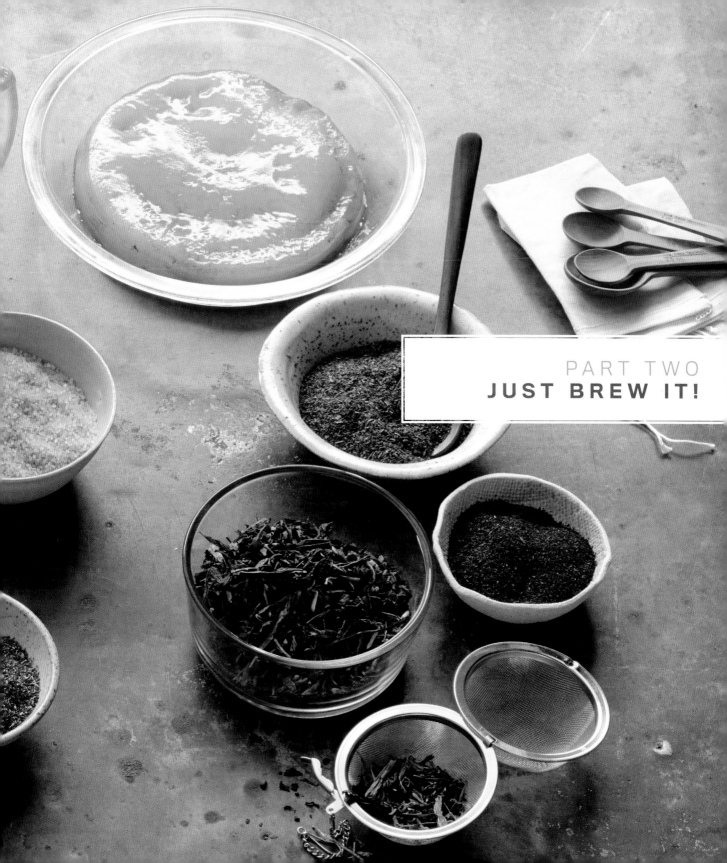

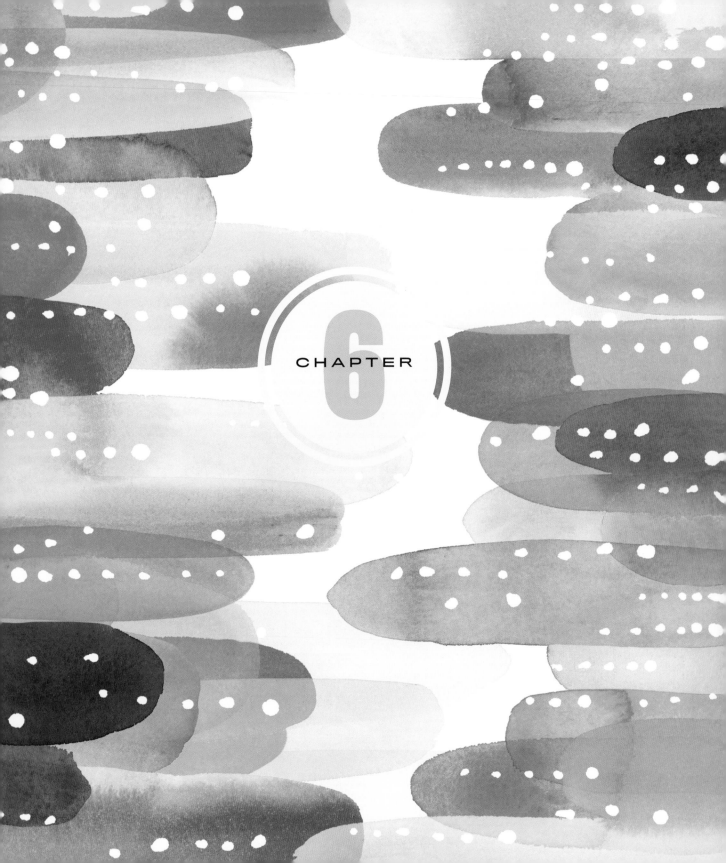

CHAPTER

6

# The Batch Brew Method

**M**ost people use the batch brew method to start their kombucha adventure. It is the most basic of procedures: make a nutrient solution (that is, sweet tea), add the culture and starter liquid, and let the brew ferment. When it's ready, harvest and repeat. Batch brewing is ideal for those wishing to make small quantities of kombucha, from ½ to 5 gallons, and is an excellent choice for those wishing to finely control the flavor of the kombucha, especially those who prefer their brew very young and on the sweet side. It also lends itself well to experimentation.

Because you start with a SCOBY and 1 to 2 cups of starter liquid per gallon of sweet tea each time, the choices you make — the type of tea or sugar, the length of the brewing cycle, and so on — will be fully expressed in the flavor right away, as opposed to continuous brewing (see chapter 7), where the large amount of kombucha that remains in the vessel guides the developing flavor of the brew.

The flexibility of the batch brewing method appeals to newbie and veteran homebrewers alike, and many people experiment with batch brews on the side even if they choose continuous brewing for their main supply of kombucha.

Most commercial producers brew in large batches, rather than with a CB system, because they can more easily control the process from batch to batch, using an exact recipe and producing a more consistent product. That said, different batches of kombucha are likely to turn out differently no matter how diligently the brewer attempts to reproduce conditions. Place two identically prepared batches next to each other, and in almost every case, they will develop differently — there may be great SCOBY growth on one batch but not the other, or one may remain sweeter for longer, despite identical ingredients, starter liquid, SCOBY weight, and so on. This is the joy of living things.

The larger the batch of kombucha, the greater the likelihood of variation in the brewing process. Batches larger than 5 gallons can experience issues with incomplete fermentation and uneven or weak flavors, to name just a couple of potential problems. The culture's bacteria and yeast utilize oxygen to ferment the sweet tea, but in a deep vessel the sweet tea at the bottom may not receive the same vigorous attention from the bacteria and yeast as the sweet tea nearer the top of the vessel, where the SCOBY develops.

This issue can be mitigated by brewing in a shallower, wider vessel that allows oxygen to penetrate more evenly into the brew. But in general, homebrewers work in batches of 1 to 5 gallons, which are of a manageable size, ferment evenly, mature in 2 to 4 weeks, and can be consumed within a relatively short period.

## A KOMBUCHA LEGEND:
## Emperor Qin Shi Huang

The most famous legend of kombucha's origin dates it to the Qin dynasty (221 to 206 BCE), during which time many claim it was referred to as the "Tea of Immortality" or "Divine Tsche." The emperor Qin Shi Huang is said to have sought to lengthen his life by any means available, and this Tea of Immortality was purportedly delivered by alchemists at his request.

However, specifics of this tale do not bear out, as the term *Divine Tsche*, or *lingzhi* in Chinese, refers to reishi mushrooms, and while the kombucha culture has been called a mushroom, it seems unlikely that *lingzhi* would ever have referred to the kombucha.

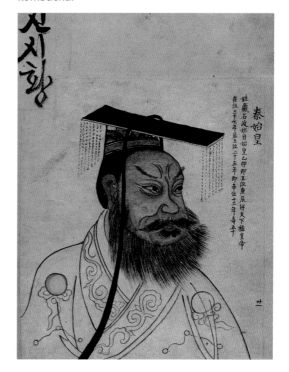

# How to Brew 1 Gallon of Kombucha

Recipes for batch brewing most commonly provide measurements and directions for a 1-gallon batch, which happens to be a size that works well for homebrewers. Unlike some ferments that are ready in just a couple of days, kombucha requires time to mature. So making at least a gallon at a time ensures there is enough (maybe!) to drink while waiting for the next batch.

When prepping the vessel, utensils, and counter, avoid antibacterial soaps, which may have a negative effect on the culture. Instead, opt for very hot water or a 1:1 dilution of distilled/pasteurized vinegar (*never* use raw vinegar, as it will alter and potentially contaminate the brew). You may also choose to "cure" the inside of the vessel by rinsing with distilled vinegar or kombucha vinegar immediately prior to adding the sweet tea, but this is optional.

Brewing a full gallon of kombucha requires a fermenting vessel that holds at least 1.25 gallons to accommodate the SCOBY and starter liquid and give adequate headroom for air circulation. If all that is available is a 1-gallon vessel, never fear — simply reduce the tea, sugar, and water by 25 percent. (See Measurements, Brew Times, and Methods on page 113 for more details.)

This basic recipe reflects centuries of consensus developed through experiments and research by brewers of all types from around the world. In addition to the equipment discussed in chapter 5, you'll need the following ingredients:

1 gallon cool, chlorine-free water
4–6 tea bags or 1–2 tablespoons loose-leaf tea
1 cup sugar
1 full-size kombucha SCOBY (4–5 ounces)
1–2 cups mature kombucha for starter liquid

We usually prepare a 1-gallon batch right in the glass vessel. However, one must use caution when doing so because pouring hot liquid into a cold jar could cause the glass to crack, creating a dangerous mess. Most of the time this is not an issue and precautions can be taken to prevent an accident from happening.

One way to avoid the issue altogether is to prepare the quart of hot sweet tea concentrate in a separate container than the fermentation vessel; it could even be the pot used to heat the water. (It doesn't matter what material that container is made out of because there's no acid content to worry about.)

A benefit to adding the cool water to the brewing vessel first, then adding the hot sweet tea concentrate is that it evenly distributes the heat and prevents the bottom of the vessel from warming up. This means the temperature of the liquid will drop faster and you can brew sooner. In fact, waiting is usually unnecessary as the temperature is already under 100°F (38°C) with this technique.

However, there's nothing wrong with preparing the sweet tea in the brew vessel and adding the water afterward. Just make sure the glass is not so cold as to crack when hot water is added.

# How to Brew 1 Gallon of Kombucha, *continued*

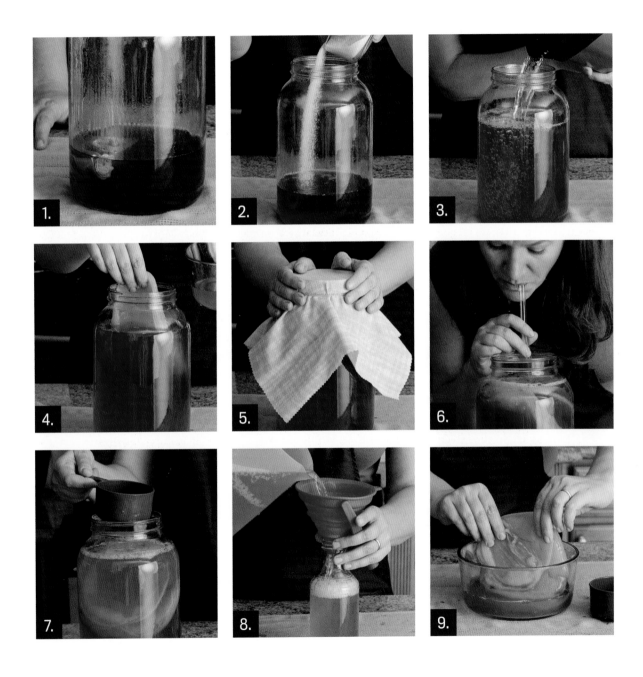

1 Heat 1 quart of the water to just below boiling. Combine the tea and hot water in the pot, a separate bowl, or in the brewing vessel. Let steep for 5 to 15 minutes, then remove the tea leaves.

2 Add the sugar to the hot tea, and stir until completely dissolved.

3 Pour the remaining 3 quarts of cool water into the brewing vessel. If prepared separately, add the sweet tea. Dip a clean finger into the mixture to gauge its temperature. If warmer than body temperature (about 100°F [38°C]), cover with a clean cloth and set aside until lukewarm.

4 With clean hands, place the SCOBY in the sweet tea solution. Pour the starter liquid on top of the SCOBY; this acidifies the pH of the tea near the top of the vessel, where the culture is most vulnerable, offering a layer of protection from potential pathogens.

5 Cover the vessel with breathable cloth, secured with a rubber band if necessary. Set it in a warm location (ideally 75–85°F [24–29°C]), out of direct sunlight, unless brewing in an opaque vessel. (At this stage you have the option to say a prayer, send good vibes, or otherwise commune with your new brew. It is a culture of living organisms and responds to energy — positive and negative.)

6 Allow the sweet tea to ferment for 7 to 21 days. After 5 days (or sooner, if you're curious), it's okay to begin tasting once a day. To taste, remove the cloth cover, gently insert a straw beneath the SCOBY, and take a sip. Or dip a shot glass or other small cup past the new layer of SCOBY into the brew.

7 Once the brew reaches the flavor you prefer, it is ready to harvest. Before bottling or flavoring, collect at least 1 cup of starter liquid for the next batch from the top of the brew (2 cups if you can spare it or if the brew is young) and pour it into a clean bowl. Then remove the SCOBYs to the bowl, cover with a clean towel, and set aside. (We take the liquid first because removing the cultures can kick the yeast off the bottom, which is fine for drinking but not for starter liquid.)

8 The rest of the kombucha is now available for drinking, either straight from the vessel or, more commonly, after bottling with or without flavors. For tips on flavoring, filtering, bottle-aging (to further develop the flavor and carbonation), and other advanced techniques, see chapter 8.

9 To start the next batch, use one or both of the SCOBYs, either the original and/or the new one from the previous batch, with the starter liquid. The extra culture may be used to start another batch or placed in a SCOBY Hotel. Enjoy the first batch while the second brew is in progress!

# DOING the KOMBU-CHA-CHA

## The Next Steps

One of the beauties of brewing kombucha is the way it carries forward. At the end of each cycle you bottle your supply, saving enough of the current brew to start the next batch, and on it goes! When we're finishing up one batch and ready to start another, we find it most efficient to work in a "brewing dance" wherein we start the water boiling for the next brew, then rotate to flavoring and filling the bottles while the tea brews, and finish by setting the SCOBY into the fresh sweet tea. Of course this is just what we've found works best for us — each person will find his or her own flow. Here's how we do our kombu-cha-cha:

**2.** Start water boiling.

**1.** Assemble all equipment and supplies.

**START HERE**

**3.** Cut up any fruit/flavorings and place in the bottles. (See chapter 8.)

**4.** Remove SCOBYs & starter liquid for next batch to separate bowl. Decant kombucha into the bottles.

**5.** Rinse the brewing vessel with filtered water to remove excess yeast.

**6.** Put tea bags in a pot or pitcher. Pour the just-below-boiling water over the tea and set a timer for the desired steeping time.

**10.** Enjoy the finished kombucha!

**7.** While the tea brews, finish capping, labeling, and storing the bottles of kombucha.

**8.** When the timer goes off, remove the tea bags and stir in the sugar.

**9.** Pour cold water into the brewing vessel, then add the sweet tea, the SCOBY, and the starter liquid. Cover with a cloth and return to the brewing location.

# The Brewing Cycle

Typical brewing cycles can differ in length based on, among other things, the temperature in the fermentation space and your personal taste preference. You may need to brew a couple of batches to discover the best timing; patience is rewarded.

The Brew Minder Logs (page 371) can help determine your preferred kombucha brewing rhythm. Each successive batch will offer new insight into the symbiosis. (See Seasonal Changes in Brewing Cycle, page 88).

| Batch Size | Fermentation Time |
|---|---|
| ½ gallon | 3–7 days |
| 1 gallon | 7–21 days |
| 2½ gallons | 10–28 days |
| 5 gallons | 18–42 days |

### KOMBUCHA MAMMA SEZ

## Handling SCOBYs

"I love handling my SCOBYs — they are soft and smooth, yet have a firm texture like squid. I believe that as a collection of living organisms, the SCOBY appreciates personal contact and bacterial exchange. Just wash your hands first (avoid antibacterial soap). But if you are uncomfortable with the feel of the culture, it's okay to opt for rubber gloves or tongs, which will also prevent the culture or tea from staining your fingers, an occasional and temporary effect."

# Signs of a Healthy Kombucha Brew

Once you've brewed a few batches of the booch, the process will become familiar, but at first it pays to know what signs to look for that indicate the kombucha is progressing safely. The good news is that as long as there is no mold, which would appear as blue, black, or white fuzz on the SCOBY, there is no risk in tasting the brew to see how it is coming along. (Kombucha mold is not really dangerous, though it might make you sick if you are allergic, and a moldy culture should absolutely be thrown away; see page 170.)

While it is common for the mix of yeast and bacteria to evolve and adapt to its new environment over the first few cycles, most people experience a delicious beverage from the very first batch. Though the flavor may change over time due to this gradual evolution of the culture, it rarely causes issues. Kombucha has been passed around the world for centuries and has survived by rebalancing as required in new environments. Here are some signs of a healthy brew to keep an eye (and nose) on:

*Slightly vinegary aroma.* Kombucha has its own special smell that longtime brewers will immediately recognize. The signature sweet-sour waft from the vessel is a particular delight. Sometimes described as fermented, cidery, or beerlike, those notes of vinegar and that slightly sour pungency indicate a healthy brew.

*SCOBY growth.* One of the most obvious signs of a healthy kombucha brew is the formation of a new SCOBY. SCOBYs do not appear all

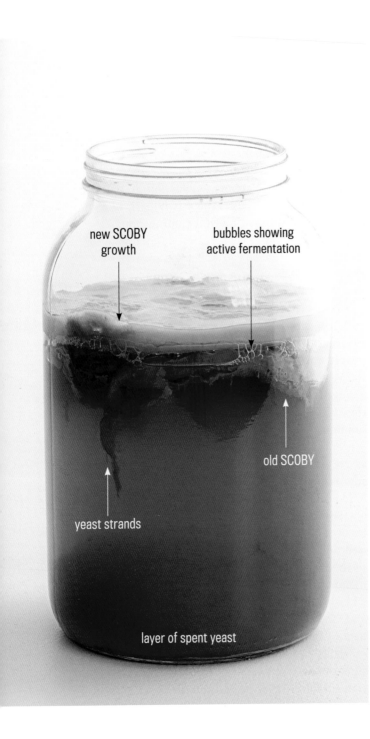

new SCOBY growth

bubbles showing active fermentation

old SCOBY

yeast strands

layer of spent yeast

at once, fully formed, but grow gradually until they cover the entire surface area of the brew, creating a seal that slows evaporation and allows for anaerobic fermentation to occur. When it's warm, kombucha ferments quickly and SCOBY growth is rapid. In cooler conditions, SCOBY growth is often slower and thinner, and batches may take longer to ferment.

*Yeast activity.* The formation of yeast strands or tendrils suspended from the culture is not only normal but desirable. In the early stages of fermentation, before the baby SCOBY has fully formed, yeast globs congregate at the top of the brew. These brown strands or clumps eventually attach themselves to the underside of the culture or fall to the bottom of the brewing vessel. New brewers may confuse these yeast blooms with mold because beneath the newly forming culture they may look bluish or black. (For more information on identifying mold, see page 170.)

*Protective pH.* One of the kombucha culture's most important defenses against pathogenic organisms is its low pH, which generally drops below 3.5 within three to five days of beginning the ferment. This acidic environment favors the particular bacteria and yeast of the SCOBY yet prevents other potentially harmful microorganisms from colonizing. The pH will not indicate that the brew is ready to drink; only your taste buds can determine that. Often a brew will reach the desired pH while it is still much too sweet to enjoy. Still, that pH lets you know the brew is progressing safely.

*Lightening in color.* A freshly brewed batch of starter tea can be quite dark, depending on the type of tea used and how long it steeps. As the culture goes about its business of converting sugar into healthy acids, it also breaks down the tannins, which lend the tea its color. The result is transformation from a dark brown to light tan or even golden color, depending on the original tea.

## Tasting and Perfecting Your Brew

Taste is king with kombucha. After the culture has had some time to consume the sweet tea, start tasting the brew to see how it's coming along. If you are new to homebrewing, we recommend that you start tasting a 1-gallon batch at five days and sample the flavor daily after that to teach your taste buds how the brew develops over time and to recognize when it's ready to harvest.

As kombucha fans know, though it's made from tea, kombucha does not taste like tea. Rather, because of the acetic acid, it has a sweet-tart, apple-cidery flavor. Adjectives commonly used to describe kombucha include *tangy, tart, smooth, crisp, dry, refreshing, thirst quenching, satisfying, alive.*

The taste may seem strange to a first-timer, but by even just the second or third sip your perception of the flavor will evolve. Those consuming lots of sugar in their day-to-day diet often have more trouble enjoying kombucha at first, but as the body shifts and rebalances, every sip becomes more satisfying. If the sourness is too intense, dilute with water or juice.

The batch brewing method makes it easy to adjust each batch to your personal tastes by shortening the fermentation cycle to make kombucha that is a little bit on the "younger"

side, hence sweeter, or lengthening the cycle to build stronger flavor.

Matching your tea and sugar recipe with your preferred brewing cycle and temperature, experimenting with flavorings, and then determining the length and condition of the second ferment to build carbonation and infuse flavor are the true art and joy of this wonderful homemade beverage. Science gives us the understanding and the parameters, but our instincts must take over. What's important is that you brew a kombucha that you like. Trust *your* gut! (See chapter 8 for details on flavorings, bottle-aging, and carbonation.)

## Playing with the Basic Recipe

Of course, our basic 1-gallon recipe is only a beginning point and can be modified to suit individual tastes. Every change will affect the final brew; for example, changing the amount of tea used or the length of steeping time will change not only the flavor but influence the culture and fermentation process. The minimum amount of tea to sustain continued culture growth is 3 tea bags, or about 3 teaspoons of loose-leaf tea, per gallon of water.

At the upper limit, 12 tea bags or around ¼ cup of loose-leaf tea is close to the maximum that can be used batch after batch without harming the culture. Overly strong tea may adversely affect the brew's balance by overstimulating the yeast and creating off flavors. Mixing lighter teas such as green and white into the blend may reduce the impact. Experiment with different teas and different steep times to produce a variety of kombucha flavors.

There is less wiggle room with the amount of sugar. The prescribed ratio of 1 cup of sugar per gallon of tea produces consistent results batch after batch. Experiment with a range from ½ cup to no more than 2 cups, if desired, but even that may be pushing it. Too little sugar

## CATCHING THE RIGHT FLAVOR

We like to share our kombucha, so we make large batches, flavor them, and then bottle-age in a cool location for a few days, weeks, or months. When we flavored and bottled kombucha that tasted just right at harvest, it would often end up too tart after bottle-aging. So we started harvesting and bottling when the kombucha was still just a little on the sweet side for our personal taste, and it works very well for us. The results are a lighter and drier drink with more carbonation and a flavor that holds longer before turning sour in the bottle. Here are some guidelines for capturing just the right flavor:

### Too sweet

Taste daily until optimum flavor is achieved, or bottle and move to refrigerator immediately to preserve flavor.

### Sweet-tart

For dry, crisp kombucha, flavor now and bottle-age at 74 to 78°F (23–25°C) for 1 to 7 days, or continue brewing if full-flavored booch is preferred.

### Just right!

Flavor now and bottle-age for 1 to 3 days, monitoring closely to prevent too much sourness from developing, or bottle and move to refrigerator immediately to preserve flavor.

### Too tart

Shorten brewing cycle and/or reduce temperature for next batch; try mixing this batch with water or juice to cut the sourness or try a fining agent (see page 136). If the kombucha is too sour to salvage, use as starter liquid, a booster for a SCOBY Hotel, or household and beauty products (see chapter 17).

inhibits the brew's normal healthy development: no SCOBY and no acetic acid. Too much sugar causes the yeast to either "flush" and overrun the bacteria or fall completely asleep and do nothing.

If you reduce or increase the sugar in successive batches and the kombucha's flavor or SCOBY growth show signs of failing, return to the original ratio of 1 cup of sugar per gallon. A culture may need to undergo one to three rounds of fermentation to recover from an experiment gone wrong.

## SCOBY Growth and the Next Brew

Kombucha SCOBYs are infinitely abundant, as the "mother" produces a "baby" with each batch. That new culture forms gradually and always grows across the top of the liquid. It may first appear as little dots or patches, eventually creating a thin skin that thickens the longer it is left undisturbed. (See pages 44–45 for photos of a SCOBY growing.)

As it takes shape, it may grow in a layer on top of the mother SCOBY, like a stack of pancakes, or it may develop around the mother and become one, as we often see in CB. SCOBYs in a CB or SCOBY Hotel often fuse into a solid pad of dozens of thin layers.

The mother may also float below the surface of the brew and remain unconnected to the new SCOBY growth. These are normal manifestations and vary with each batch.

Note that once a SCOBY is disturbed, from moving either the vessel or the layer itself, it no longer continues to grow. If added to another batch, it may float to the top and connect with

the new culture growth, appearing to thicken by combining with the new SCOBY. But SCOBYs floating below the surface of the brew do not grow thicker on their own.

Sometimes SCOBYs that have grown together can be easily peeled apart. If the cultures have truly fused, there's no harm in leaving them connected, but eventually you will want to separate some of them, either to brew more than one batch of kombucha at a time or to start a SCOBY Hotel (see page 106) or to find other uses for them (see chapter 17). Pulling them apart or cutting them is a simple process. (See Thinning and Trimming SCOBYs, page 108, and CB Maintenance, page 124.)

If your original culture came from a quality supplier, it is likely thicker than what would typically grow during a single batch brew of 7 to 10 days. The cultures produced by your brews may be noticeably thinner. For this reason, keep the new baby together with the mother for at least the second batch. Once a third SCOBY grows, consider starting a SCOBY Hotel with one and keeping the other two together to brew, and then rotate SCOBYs as desired, always using two if they are thin.

## How Much SCOBY Do You Need?

Maintaining the correct balance of starter liquid and culture is important to making a tasty brew batch after batch, but much like the quantities of tea and sugar, the amounts can be varied within reason. We recommend 4 to 5 ounces of SCOBY plus 1 to 2 cups of strong starter liquid per gallon of sweet tea; you could add more culture and liquid, which might shorten the brewing cycle slightly, but for best results we wouldn't recommend adding less. If a culture has grown too large or thick to be used, just trim it to size (see Thinning and Trimming SCOBYs, page 108).

New SCOBY growth will vary in thickness, but remember that the goal is to produce a delicious beverage, not to grow a culture of a given size. Some batches develop thicker SCOBYs than others, and while it is important to see some culture growth, it is possible to have a thick, healthy culture on a batch that is still too sweet to enjoy or to have a thin, measly culture on a perfectly flavored batch.

With batch brewing, there is no way to tell when the batch is complete simply by looking at SCOBY growth. You have to taste the kombucha. When it tastes right, remove whatever SCOBY is there and go ahead with the next steps. That particular SCOBY might be awesome and rubbery and beautiful, or it might be very thin and fragile, but if the flavor of the brew is good, that's all that matters.

## The SCOBY Hotel

Unlike other, more delicate cultures such as kefir grains, which will disintegrate and disappear if not fed regularly, the kombucha SCOBY is a hardy organism and can remain in stasis for extended periods. After a few brewing cycles, with the SCOBY producing a baby in each batch, you will have extra SCOBYs. That's the perfect time to start a SCOBY Hotel, which is simply a place to safely store cultures with some strong starter liquid so that you'll always have backups for a lifetime supply of kombucha. The SCOBY Hotel is one of the most important tools in the homebrewer's arsenal.

To house extra SCOBYS, the best option is a large, clean glass jar (a ½- or 1-gallon jar works well), a tightly woven cloth cover to fit over the jar, some mature kombucha, and sweet tea (see The Basic Sweet Tea Recipe, page 54). From there you're just three steps away from a proper hotel:

1. Rinse the jar with hot, nonchlorinated water or clean it with nonantibacterial soap and cure with pasteurized vinegar or kombucha vinegar.

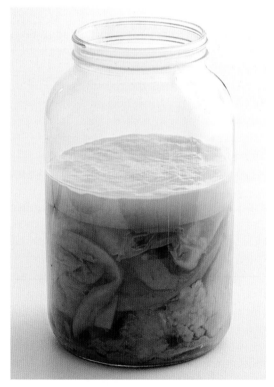

Left undisturbed, a SCOBY Hotel will grow a thick layer of new culture.

2. Place the SCOBY(s) in the jar and add 2 to 4 cups mature kombucha. If necessary, top off with enough sweet tea to fully submerge all the SCOBYs. Add mature kombucha or sweet tea anytime the level dips low or starter liquid is removed for another purpose.

3. Cover the jar with the cloth cover and set in a relatively dark location at room temperature. **Do not refrigerate.** That's it!

If a small amount of sweet tea is added and the hotel is left undisturbed for at least a few weeks, a thick layer of SCOBY can grow across the top. This new SCOBY layer will act as a lid to slow the evaporation process. If left undisturbed for an extended period of time, that layer can become several inches thick! We prefer to use a tightly woven cloth cover on our hotels and allow a new SCOBY to form to create the "lid," but you can also use a plastic lid.

## Hotel Maintenance

The SCOBY Hotel does need a bit of attention from time to time to ensure that the cultures remain viable. Generally all we do is feed the bacteria and yeast every once in a while, trim

### Livin' It Up at the Hotel SCOBY-fornia

"I invented the term SCOBY Hotel to refer to the jar of extras I kept on hand in case someone asked for one. Then I tried to come up with a parody of Hotel California, but could never quite work out the lyrics — give it a try and send me your version!"

the top SCOBY as needed to allow oxygen to penetrate to the lower layers, and keep the yeast in check.

### FEEDING THE SCOBYS

The bacteria and yeast living in the SCOBYs and the liquid in the hotel will remain viable indefinitely, provided they remain at room temperature and get a little food every few months. And the liquid will slowly evaporate over time, so check the hotel every couple of months and top off the container with sweet tea as needed. Anytime you add a dose of sweet

## VACATION TIPS FOR A BATCH BREW

Heading out of town but don't have a SCOBY-sitter? Need to take a break? Here are a few options for suspending activity.

- Start a fresh batch right before you leave so the kombucha will be ready when you return.

- Let the current batch go to kombucha vinegar (see page 256).
- Store the cultures in a SCOBY Hotel.
- Teach a friend how to tend the brew.

tea, use a cloth cover for the next couple of weeks so it can ferment the new fuel normally, then switch back to a lid if preferred.

## THINNING AND TRIMMING SCOBYS

If the SCOBY that forms on top of the hotel grows to more than an inch in thickness, fresh oxygen may not reach the liquid below, causing bacteria and yeast to stagnate or die off over time. One option to prevent this is to push the SCOBY down under the liquid before it grows too thick, but even then multiple SCOBYs may float to the top and create a very thick culture by fusing together with the new growth.

However it happens, eventually you will want to pull apart and thin or trim the extra SCOBYs (this process also applies to CB, when the culture from inside the CB must be cut down to rebalance the brew).

To complete this task, gather a large container (stainless, glass, ceramic, or wood), a cutting board or cookie sheet with a rim, a clean towel, and a pair of sharp scissors or a serrated knife.

1. Remove the thick top SCOBY from the hotel, and place in the container, covered with the clean towel to prevent fruit flies or contamination. As it rests, some of the liquid will drain from the culture, making it easier to handle.

2. Remove other SCOBYs that require maintenance one at a time. Trim off any soft, gelatinous edges or dark bits; compost those pieces or set aside for other uses (see chapter 17). If any SCOBY looks ready for retirement, dispose of it. As each SCOBY is cleaned, return it to the hotel. (With the cultures out of the hotel, this is a good

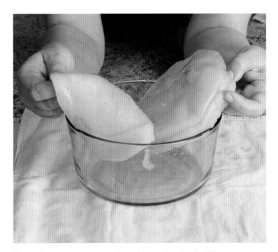

Some layers may seem fused together but will easily tear apart.

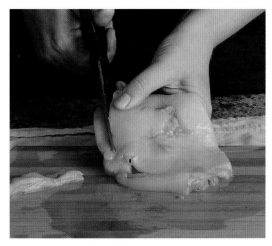

Trim thick layers into smaller SCOBYs. Don't worry, cutting them won't harm the culture.

time to filter the yeast if necessary — see Removing Excess Yeast, below).

3. After the largest SCOBY has drained for a while, try to simply pull it apart while holding it over the container; the layers may peel easily, and if they rip, it won't make the SCOBY any less viable.

4. If you cannot pull the SCOBY apart, use the scissors or the knife to trim the culture as desired. You may place one hand on top to hold the SCOBY steady, then slice horizontally through the thick culture like a bread roll (see photo, page 124). Or cut it like a pizza in halves or quarters. Or just trim off the biggest parts.

### REMOVING EXCESS YEAST

Yeast create carbonation and provide nutrition for the bacteria (and humans!). Although the bacteria and yeast live in symbiosis, they also compete with one another, and the yeast will tend to win unless you, as the homebrewer, intervene to maintain balance. As the yeast enter the dormant phase of their life cycle, they drop to the bottom of the vessel. Over time the liquid may become dark or cloudy.

---

**KOMBUCHA MAMMA SEZ**

### Yummy Yeast!

"Save the yeast you filter out of the hotel liquid to make kombucha sourdough starter! Learn how on page 261."

---

This is a signal that it's time to remove excess yeast; expect to do it every two to six months. Gather the following supplies:

- Clean towel
- Two containers, one large enough to hold all the SCOBYs in the hotel, the other large enough to hold all the liquid
- Fine-mesh strainer, sieve, or cheesecloth
- 2 cups sweet tea (1 tea bag/teaspoon tea, 2 tablespoons sugar)
- Optional: cutting board and knife/ scissors to trim the SCOBYs

1. Remove the SCOBYs from the hotel into the first container. Cover with the towel to prevent contamination.

2. Filter the liquid from the hotel through the strainer into the second bowl or jar. The large yeast strands will not pass through the filter, but plenty of yeast will remain in the liquid.

3. If the vessel now holding the liquid is appropriate, it can become the SCOBY Hotel. If it isn't, rinse the hotel vessel with hot water to remove all traces of yeast from the bottom and sides. It isn't necessary to use soap, but a good scrubbing might be required. Pull off any large globs of yeast, but do not rinse the SCOBYs.

4. Now is a great time to trim the SCOBYs as needed before placing them into whichever vessel is now the hotel. Add the filtered liquid, extra kombucha from your brews to boost levels if necessary, plus 2 cups sweet tea (more if desired) to the hotel, cover it, and return it to storage.

Overfiltering the yeast can lead to issues as well, so don't be too zealous. Leave some of those friendly guys in there to help maintain balance, build carbonation, and help with flavor.

## A Potent Source of Starter Liquid

With so many cultures in such a small space, the liquid in the hotel will become super-sour over time. Go on, take a sip or a whiff — Kombucha Face guaranteed! It smells powerful because it is liquid gold for fermentation. You can pour off some of this potent brew for use as starter liquid for a new batch.

You don't need to replenish the hotel with sweet tea each time you harvest some starter liquid from it, but after a few batches you should top it off with a few cups (use a cloth cover for a few weeks after adding sweet tea) and give it a chance to convert that sugar, which it will do quickly.

People who prefer a shorter brew cycle get particular benefit from using a SCOBY Hotel because using starter liquid that is only five or six days old — as they would if they collect it from each batch they brew — is fine once, but doing that for multiple batches in a row dilutes the strength of the bacteria, resulting in dominant yeast and off flavors. The super-sour liquid from a hotel gives shorter brews a full-powered starter.

Best of all, using the hotel for starter liquid means that 100 percent of the batch is available for drinking, rather than using some for the next batch. More kombucha to drink plus backup SCOBYs swimming in a constantly regenerating pool of healthy bacteria and yeast, ready to go at a moment's notice — that's a win-win!

## SCOBY Rotation

Some brewers prefer to rotate SCOBYs through their batches and hotel, taking both the starter liquid and a SCOBY from the hotel for a new batch and returning the previously used SCOBY (and maybe also the new baby) to the hotel until they're needed. This creates a dynamic hotel environment that keeps more SCOBYs vibrant and active while also providing them with rest periods.

Other brewers prefer to keep one SCOBY going from batch to batch once they have found a balance and flavor they like. Each brewer must find their own rhythm and discover what works best in their environment and with their SCOBYs.

A single SCOBY might last for 10 or more brewing cycles, though we've heard of people using the same one for years. We prefer to use younger ones in our brewing vessels, reserving older ones for experimental batches or recipes (see chapter 16).

## Don't Toss That SCOBY!

"Freshly trimmed pieces of healthy SCOBY make excellent bandages for cuts or burns, or you can toss them into a blender to make SCOBY face cream. If you have a small burn and no bits of SCOBY available, haul a culture out of a container, cut off a piece, and toss it back in, or keep a small jar with some starter liquid on hand for storing small bits and pieces of SCOBY. (Learn more in chapter 17.)"

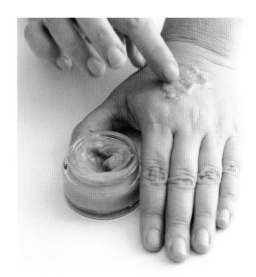

# SHARING SCOBYS WITH FRIENDS

There is a long tradition of sharing fermentation cultures of all kinds with friends. If you want to share a culture with friends, it's best to pass along a large SCOBY (measuring approximately 6 inches across and ¼ to ½ inch thick and weighing 4 to 6 ounces) with at least 1 cup of strong starter liquid (2 cups is even better) for each gallon of kombucha the recipient intends to make. Always include complete brewing instructions from a reputable source.

To mail a kombucha SCOBY to a friend, double- or even triple-bag it and its liquid in plastic ziplock or vacuum-sealed bags. Kombucha will often leak even if the culture is well packed, so wrap the plastic bags in paper towels or newspaper to absorb any seepage in transit.

Read Obtaining Your First SCOBY, page 36. If you are unable to meet those standards in starter liquid, shipping, and support, consider recommending a quality supplier instead for the best experience.

# Brewing Dos

| Brewing Dos | Brewing Don'ts |
|---|---|
| Wash the prep area, vessel, utensils, and your hands with chlorine-free hot water. If needed, use small amounts of nonantibacterial soap, and then rinse well with hot water and cure with pasteurized vinegar or kombucha vinegar. | Don't use antibacterial soaps or chlorinated water, which harm the bacteria in SCOBYs. Other soaps may leave a potentially harmful residue as well. |
| Select a glass, food-grade ceramic, stainless steel (grade 304 or higher), wood barrel, or food-grade plastic vessel for brewing. | Don't select a crystal, low-grade plastic, metal (aside from stainless steel), or decorative or antique ceramic vessel for brewing. |
| Brew with filtered, distilled, spring, or bottled water. | Don't brew with chlorinated or unfiltered tap water. |
| Brew with real sugar and real tea (*Camellia sinensis*). Organic is preferred but not required. | Don't brew with decaffeinated tea or herbal tea or with artificial sweeteners or sugar substitutes. |
| Use a tightly woven, breathable cloth cover over your fermentation vessel to prevent contamination. | Don't use cheesecloth (the weave is too loose) or a solid lid (the kombucha needs oxygen). |
| Let the tea ferment in a relatively warm location with good airflow. | Don't let the tea ferment in direct sunlight, in a closed cupboard, or in a cool location. |
| Allow the brew time to develop before tasting it. | Don't disturb the fermentation vessel in the first five days. Too much movement prevents the new SCOBY from forming properly. |
| Take starter liquid from the top of the previous batch. | Don't take starter liquid from the bottom of the previous batch. |
| Make a SCOBY Hotel for extra cultures and as a source of potent starter liquid. | Don't store all SCOBYs in one brewing vessel — you won't have any backups if that vessel is compromised. |
| Throw away any batch, both the liquid and the SCOBYs, that exhibits mold. | Don't try to salvage a moldy batch of kombucha. |

# Measurements, Brew Times, and Methods

Always brew in a vessel that is slightly larger than the desired amount of kombucha. For example, a 1-gallon vessel holds about ¾ gallon of sweet tea plus the SCOBY and starter liquid. Small batches can be brewed in large vessels if desired; the extra space is not an issue. The amount of sweet tea roughly equals the batch size, as the starter liquid plus a little more usually evaporates during the process.

| Vessel Size | Max Batch Size (sweet tea) | Tea Bags (loose leaf) | Sugar | SCOBYs | Starter Liquid | Brew Cycle (days) | Recommended Method |
|---|---|---|---|---|---|---|---|
| ½ gallon | 6 cups | 2–3 (1 tablespoon) | 6 table-spoons | 1 small | ½–1 cup | 3–7 | Batch only — too small for CB |
| 1 gallon | ¾ gallon | 3–5 (1–2 tablespoons) | ¾ cup | 1 large* | 1 cup | 7–14 | Batch only — too small for CB |
| 1½ gallons | 1 gallon | 4–6 (1–2 tablespoons) | 1 cup | 1 large | 1–2 cups | 7–21 | Batch only — too small for CB |
| 2 gallons | 1½ gallons | 6–9 (2–3 tablespoons) | 1½ cups | 2 large | 2 cups | 10–24 | Ideal for serious batch brewers; works for CB |
| 2½ gallons | 2 gallons | 8–12 (3–4 tablespoons) | 2 cups | 2 large | 2–4 cups | 10–28 | Ideal for CB |
| 5 gallons | 4 gallons | 16–24 (5–8 tablespoons) | 4 cups | 4 large | 4–8 cups | 18–42 | For serious hobbyists and homebrewers |

*A large SCOBY = approximately 6 inches across, ¼ to ½ inch thick, 4–6 ounces.

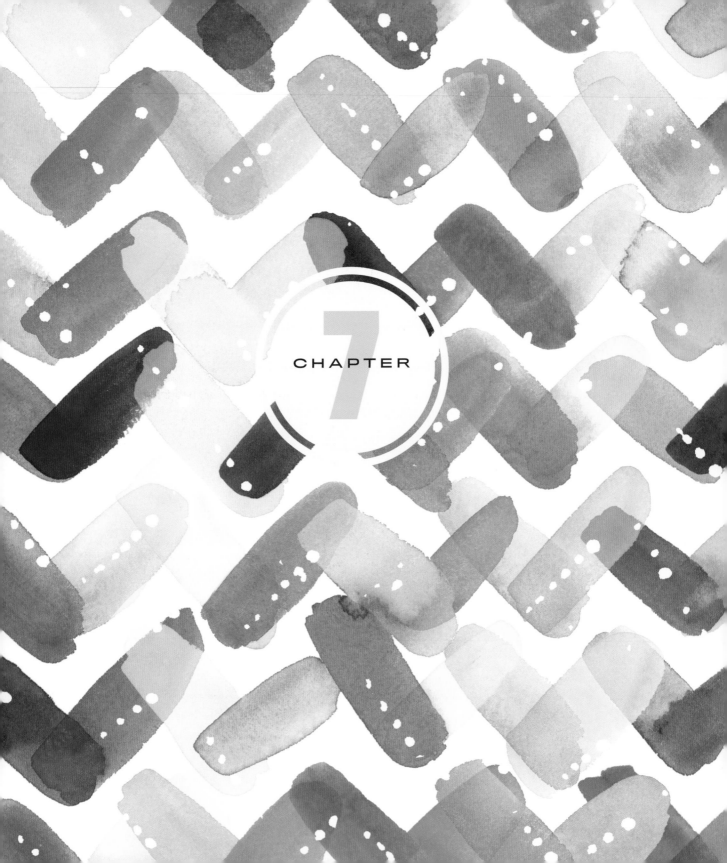

CHAPTER

7

# The Continuous Brew Method

**C**ontinuous brew (CB) is the most versatile method for making kombucha. It significantly reduces the amount of time, effort, and cleanup involved in batch brewing, and it works for individual homebrewers making a couple of gallons a month as well as for commercial breweries producing large batches. Brewers select for themselves the CB cycle and rhythm that fits their needs in terms of taste and volume.

CB is simple: make a large batch of kombucha — usually 2 to 5 gallons — in a vessel with a spigot, ferment to the preferred flavor, and then remove between one-third and two-thirds of the brew through the spigot. Add more sweet tea right away to keep the process going or wait until your supply has dwindled to refill the brewer to slow the process a little. This added sweet tea is often referred to as nutrient solution, substrate, or top-off tea. With the large amount of mature kombucha left in the vessel as starter liquid, the SCOBY converts the sugar in the top-off tea quickly enough that another portion of brew may be drawn off in two to five days.

That's the whole process in a nutshell, but because each brewer's needs differ, not to mention brewing conditions and personal tastes, there is no one right way for CB. It doesn't take long, though, for new brewers to discover a rhythm that works for them. Here we cover the basic process, with a variety of techniques for harvesting and replenishing.

# Why Choose CB?

Simply put, continuous brew is the easiest, tastiest, safest, healthiest, and most versatile method for making kombucha. It may appeal to those who wish to make a lot of kombucha as well as to those who simply wish to reduce their time commitment to the process, even if they're brewing for one.

Anyone looking to make a lot of kombucha in less brewing time should definitely give this method a try. The minimum recommended size for CB is 2 gallons, which is just large enough to allow you to harvest regularly while leaving enough mature kombucha in the vessel to maintain a balanced brew. Vessels of up to 5 gallons are popular choices for CB homebrew setups. Whatever the volume, a vessel with a spigot is essential to the ease of CB, greatly reducing the mess and effort associated with a typical batch brew.

Once the initial brew has reached the preferred flavor, one-third can be harvested straight from the spigot. Once the CB as a whole has matured (after three or four batches), even more can be removed, up to two-thirds per harvest. In most cases, we do not recommend taking more than 50 percent at a time in order to maintain the appropriate balance between the bacteria and yeast, but experienced homebrewers may adopt more aggressive decanting schedules to keep up with demand.

Homebrewers add top-off tea based on their particular brewing rhythm. They may choose to follow the "drink a cup, add a cup" method, serving themselves straight from the spigot and topping off with sweet tea as they go. Or they may choose to harvest several bottles of kombucha at a time, replenishing the CB with sweet tea either right away or once the supply has dwindled.

Because the CB setup retains a large amount of mature kombucha as starter liquid, the brewing cycle is greatly shortened. A fermentation that would normally take 7 to 14 days with the batch brewing method takes just 2 to 5 days with continuous brewing. This method also eliminates the need to handle the SCOBY between batches, minimizing the risk of contamination.

One of the best benefits of CB kombucha is that during the fermentation of tea, higher levels of healthful acids, such as gluconic and glucuronic acid, are expressed later in the process, between 15 and 30 days, when the kombucha will likely be too sour to enjoy. With the CB method, acids can develop fully while the flavor is tempered with younger kombucha.

## CB for One Person?

Since the minimum size for a CB setup (2 gallons) is larger than that for a standard 1-gallon batch brew, those making kombucha for one may wonder if CB is still a good choice. The answer is a resounding yes!

First, many people find they consume more kombucha once they have it available on tap (and it doesn't cost $3 to $5 a bottle!). Also, single brewers often bottle up their brew when it's ready and then just let the SCOBY and liquid hang out in the brewer at about the half-full level. When they are a few days from running out of bottled kombucha, they top off the brewer with a fresh batch of sweet tea, so that it delivers a new harvest in just a few days.

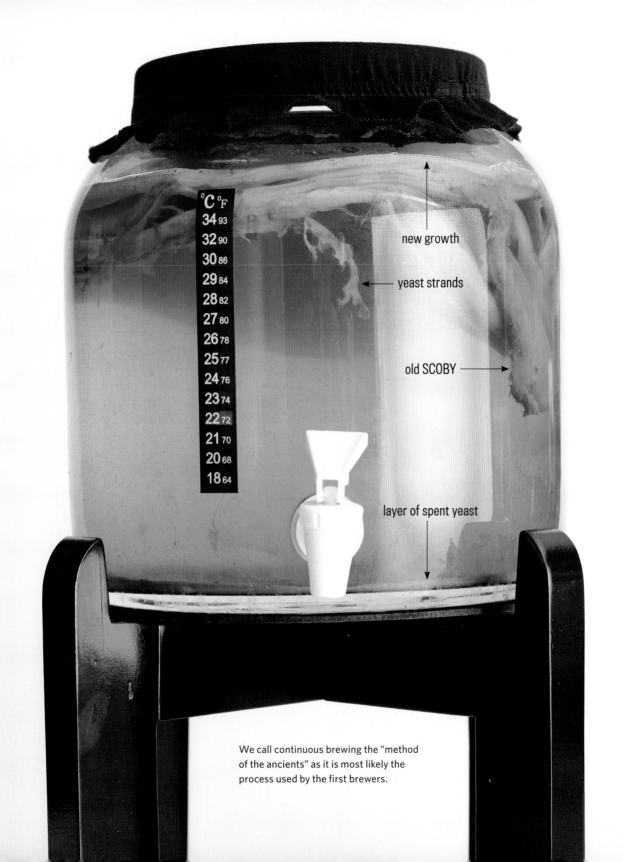

°C °F
34 93
32 90
30 86
29 84
28 82
27 80
26 78
25 77
24 76
23 74
22 72
21 70
20 68
18 64

new growth

yeast strands

old SCOBY

layer of spent yeast

We call continuous brewing the "method of the ancients" as it is most likely the process used by the first brewers.

No matter how much time passes between bottling one brew and starting the next, as long as the SCOBYs remain covered in mature kombucha, the low pH will keep them ready to brew as soon as fresh sweet tea is provided, so the CB acts as a self-contained SCOBY Hotel, meaning everyone can find their own rhythm and flow.

## Preparing the Brewing Vessel

Prior to beginning your first batch, double-check to make sure the spigot is removable and made of corrosion-resistant materials (see Selecting an Appropriate Spigot, page 80). The next step is to test the spigot for leaks.

To do this, fill the brewing vessel with enough water to completely cover the spigot and leave it for a few hours. If water seeps through the spigot seal, unscrew it, adjust the washers, and tighten. (Sometimes the washers need to be reversed in order to create a tight seal.) Test again. Wood or cork spigots may require additional soaking time to resolve the issue.

Once the seal is established, test the flow. Spigots made of wood or other natural materials may experience some initial friction; turn the spigot several times to loosen prior to inserting into the vessel (for more on spigots, see page 80). With the spigot in place, rinse with hot water and cure the inside of the vessel to set the proper pH for the brewing environment. Pour about a cup of pasteurized vinegar or kombucha vinegar into the brewer, swish it around to coat every part of the vessel, and then dump out the remaining liquid. Oak barrels have a unique preparation protocol. (See Barrel Brewing, page 127, for a discussion of how to properly seal a barrel.)

## Starting a Continuous Brew

We'll assume that you're using a 2½-gallon vessel, the most popular size for CB homebrewers, which calls for 2 gallons of sweet tea. (If you have a different-size vessel, see the chart on page 113 for the proper ratios of ingredients.) The rest of the equipment and the ingredients are the same as for batch brewing. Here are the amounts called for:

8–12 tea bags or 3–4 tablespoons loose-leaf tea
2 gallons cool chlorine-free water
2 cups sugar
2 full-size kombucha SCOBYs
   (4–5 ounces each)
2–4 cups mature kombucha for starter liquid

The initial process is basically the same as for batch brewing. We usually prepare the sweet tea concentrate in a separate bowl or vessel, or even right in the pot used to heat the water (see page 80). However, there's nothing wrong with preparing the sweet tea in the vessel for the first batch. Just make sure it is not so cold as to crack when hot water is added.

1 Heat 2 quarts of water to just below boiling. Combine the tea and hot water in the pot, a separate bowl, or in the brewing vessel. Let steep for 5 to 15 minutes; then remove the tea bags or leaves.

2 Add the sugar to the hot tea and stir until completely dissolved.

3 Pour the remaining 6 quarts (1½ gallons) of cool water into the brewing vessel. If prepared separately, add the sweet tea. Dip a clean finger into the mixture to gauge its temperature. If it seems warmer than body temperature (about 100°F [38°C]), cover with a clean cloth and set aside until lukewarm.

4 With clean hands, place the SCOBYs in the sweet tea solution. Pour the starter liquid on top of the SCOBYs; this acidifies the pH of the tea near the top of the vessel, offering a layer of protection from potential pathogens.

5 Cover the vessel with a breathable cloth cover, secured with a rubber band if necessary. Set it in a warm location (ideally 75–85°F [24–29°C]), out of direct sunlight, if not using an opaque vessel. (At this stage you have the option to say a prayer, send good vibes, or otherwise commune with your new brew. It is a culture of living organisms and responds to energy — positive and negative.)

6 Allow this first batch to ferment for 10 to 28 days. After 7 days (or sooner, if you're curious), begin tasting once a day or every few days from the spigot to determine when the kombucha reaches the flavor balance you are seeking.

7 Once it reaches the flavor balance you are seeking, decant some of the fermented kombucha into bottles (take no more than one-third of the total volume from this initial batch). Flavor as desired, and store at room temperature (to build flavor and carbonation) or in the fridge (to preserve the current flavor for as long as possible); see chapter 8 for details.

8 Refill the brewer with sweet tea, or wait and refill later, depending on your personal schedule.

**Tip:** Let the kombucha remaining in the brewing vessel continue to mature, even if the flavor gets a little tart. The CB performs best with the power of well-fermented kombucha as the base to offer the proper flavor. When your supply of bottled kombucha begins to run low, refresh the vessel with sweet tea. We'll talk timing specifics next.

# Establishing a CB Rhythm

Two of the great advantages of continuous brewing over batch brewing are (1) a flexible schedule for brewing and drawing off each batch and (2) the quick turnaround made possible by the larger proportion of starter liquid. However, that versatility means that it may take a few brewing cycles to discover exactly what works best for you.

## The First Few Cycles

When starting a CB, it is important not to draw off too much kombucha too soon. Early on in the process, the brew is not yet fully matured. If too much kombucha is decanted, the weak kombucha remaining in the brewer is excessively diluted when top-off tea is added, and it won't have the opportunity to build to full strength to support an ongoing fermentation.

For the first few batches we recommend decanting no more than one-third of the vessel (for example, about ¾ gallon from a 2½-gallon vessel), leaving the brewer about two-thirds full. While you are enjoying the first batch of bottled kombucha, let the brew ferment without adding sweet tea, as this helps build the "Sour Power" of the brew. Continue tasting from the spigot daily to monitor the progress and learn how to identify the stages of fermentation.

When your bottled supply is a few days from running out, add up to 1 gallon of sweet tea (depending on the vessel size and how much tasting has been happening from the spigot) and wait two to five days for the next decant, tasting until it is ready. Again, remove just one-third of the brew, and continue this pattern for at least the first four brews.

If the kombucha in the vessel ever turns so sour that you are concerned it will instantly become undrinkable even after adding the sweet tea, drain some mature kombucha into a jar and set it aside to add to a SCOBY Hotel or use in other ways. Then add the full gallon of sweet tea and taste until it's ready.

There are many other ways to adapt CB to your own rhythm, so be creative. Kombucha is forgiving and has many uses beyond drinking, so it never goes to waste!

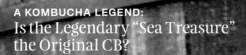

## A KOMBUCHA LEGEND:
### Is the Legendary "Sea Treasure" the Original CB?

*(This legend was passed directly to Hannah in Mandarin from a Chinese brewer; she has translated it for the first time into English.)*

This origin story, offered to us by a Chinese kombucha brewer, may reflect the beginnings of CB and kombucha itself. Like most good legends, there are various iterations, but it begins fourteen hundred years ago along the Bohai Sea coast, not far from Beijing, in a grocery and sundries shop. A shop assistant rinsing out a honey jar sloshed some of the rinse water into a nearby earthen crock of wine. Being lazy, when he noticed his mistake, he simply covered the crock with a cloth to hide the liquid inside.

Over the next few days, a strange fragrance began to waft through the shop. Everyone was curious to discover its source, but they could not locate it. Eventually it came time to sell some wine, and the shop assistant lifted the cloth and then cried out, "That sweet-sour smell is coming from here!" When the people rushed over to have a look, they saw a rubbery milky-white film sealing the mouth of the vessel. They fell into solemn praise of this wonderful curiosity, believing the earthen jar had given birth to a treasure.

It was midsummer, the hottest days of the year, and the thirsty assistant couldn't resist trying the nectar in the jar. Each person in the store drank half a dipper, and they all exclaimed over its delicious sweet-tart flavor.

Remembering the spilled honey water, the assistant used the same technique to make another batch of "sweet-tart vinegar," and then another and another, and so on. The shopkeeper, who not only drank kombucha but also ate the milk-white culture prepared cold with dressing, became a local celebrity known as the "Long Life Expert." After he died at a ripe old age, his mysterious treasure was shared with the world, and since that time, it has been handed down for all to use. To this day, families in the Bohai region use this ancient technique to ferment their own longevity "vinegar" using their beloved "sea treasure."

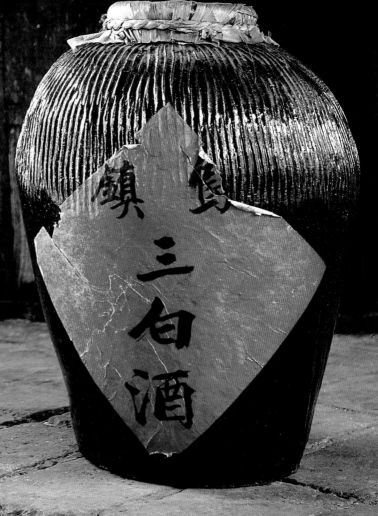

# The Mature Continuous Brew

As the bacteria and yeast fully inhabit their CB home, fermentation time becomes shorter. Taste is king, but balancing flavor/tartness with the production demands of all those greedy guts that suddenly need the booch can sometimes be a challenge. Once the CB has been through three to five cycles, it's possible to remove up to two-thirds of the vessel per harvest, though we recommend 50 percent in most cases.

At some point you may decide to add a second CB system. We like to keep five going at all times so we can share our brew with friends and have plenty of kombucha vinegar on hand for cooking. Experiment to find out what works for your household. Mix and match the following techniques as needed to develop your own brewing rhythm.

### DRINK A CUP, ADD A CUP

Keeping a container of sweet tea in the fridge makes this process easy. When you decant the daily allotment of kombucha, refresh the brewer immediately with the same amount of sweet tea (no need to warm it up). If your household is only consuming a couple of cups a day, this may be the best option.

### DRINK FROM THE TAP, ADD MORE

You may prefer to drink straight from the vessel, taking what you want when you want it. In this case, consume up to one-third of a young brew or half to two-thirds of a mature brew before topping off. This typically results in a four- to seven-day cycle.

### BOTTLE AND TOP OFF

Perhaps the most popular option for busy households is to decant a portion of kombucha into bottles and immediately top off the brewer with sweet tea in order to maintain a steady supply. This method makes it easier to gauge how much kombucha will be available to keep up with the needs of several drinkers. If you remove one-third (as for a young brew), the next batch may be ready in two to five days. If you remove half to two-thirds (as for a mature brew), the next batch could be ready in four to seven days, or maybe sooner depending on your environment.

### BOTTLE AND WAIT

If you've decanted enough kombucha to last a while, slow the cycle by simply letting the SCOBYs and liquid rest in the brewer, without topping off. As long as the vessel remains at least one-third full and the SCOBYs are fully submerged, the resting bacteria and yeast will be ready to brew when called upon. SCOBYs can live in mature kombucha for many weeks or months without being fed, just like in a SCOBY Hotel.

When your supply of kombucha begins to dwindle, add top-off tea and the next batch will be ready in a few days. If it's been a while, give the brew a taste, and if you're concerned the flavor is too acidic and will instantly turn sour when sweet tea is added, drain off more mature kombucha first for better balance. This method works very well for those with inconsistent needs or those who simply want to make booch on demand.

## SCOBY Growth in Continuous Brew

Whenever a SCOBY is disturbed, including when you dip into the vessel for a tasting sip, that culture stops growing and a new layer of SCOBY begins to form. In a batch brew, that disturbance mainly comes at harvest time when the culture is physically removed. With a CB, the kombucha is harvested straight through the spigot, leaving the SCOBY untouched until it's time to add sweet tea.

The newly formed upper layer of SCOBY is often dislodged at least partially when the top-off tea is poured in, though it may float back to the top. When a new layer begins to form, it may form only in the places where the surface of the liquid is exposed to oxygen. At first glance the SCOBY appears to change very little over time, but as the brew is topped off with tea many times during the CB process, layers of culture may fuse together like a stack of thin

pancakes, or a single, very thick culture may form. To see how thick a SCOBY is, depress it gently with a spoon at one edge until the opposite side lifts above the liquid.

Eventually the mother SCOBY becomes so thick that it impedes the fermentation process. Before that happens, it's best to do a little brewer maintenance.

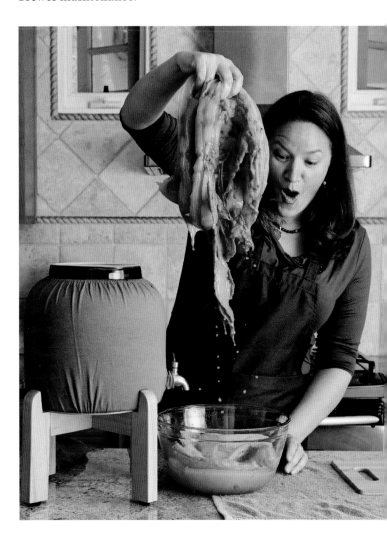

# Continuous Brewer Maintenance

With a CB, "maintenance" involves trimming the SCOBY, decanting the kombucha, cleaning the brewer, and restarting the CB. When to reset is determined primarily by flavor: if the brew is becoming too sour too quickly or if the kombucha appears overrun by yeast, it is likely time for maintenance. On average, you'll reset the CB only once or twice a year, though some brewers prefer more frequent upkeep and others go years before starting over.

While the size of the SCOBY may be intimidating at first, the entire process is very easy and takes only about 30 minutes or less from start to finish, even for first-timers.

## Removing and Trimming the SCOBY

You'll need a serrated knife and scissors for trimming, a large bowl or a rimmed cookie sheet lined with wax paper or plastic wrap for holding the SCOBY. You'll probably also want a few clean kitchen towels to catch drips. Follow all normal cleaning and curing protocols prior to beginning.

Depending on how long it has been since the last maintenance, the SCOBY may be heavy and difficult to handle. Use both hands to lift it from the brewer, holding it above the vessel for a moment to allow all the liquid to fully drain, and then move it to the bowl or cookie sheet.

For best results, reduce the SCOBY down to about three-quarters of the diameter of vessel and no more than ½ inch thick. Or you can

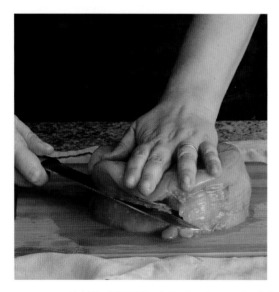
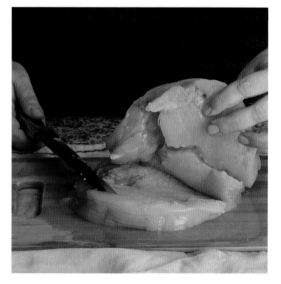

Hold the SCOBY firmly in place by pressing it down with your hand while you work the serrated knife through the cellulose.

return the SCOBY to the CB in smaller pieces that equal about that amount; the shape won't affect the brew and the new SCOBY always starts growing across the top.

Start by pulling off or slicing away the oldest layers, which are found on the bottom of the SCOBY. They will be darker in color due to prolonged exposure to the tannins in the tea, and they may peel easily or even rip apart. Next trim away any gelatinous pieces from the edges, so that only healthy solid white or tan SCOBY remains.

Then use the serrated knife to break down the culture. You may choose to place one hand on top to hold the SCOBY steady and then slice horizontally through the thick culture like a bread roll. Or cut it like a pizza in halves or quarters. Or just trim off the biggest parts.

Once done, place the trimmed-down SCOBY in the bowl, and return the extra pieces of culture you wish to keep to a SCOBY Hotel (see page 37) for backups, experiments, gifts, and other uses (see part 4).

## Starter Liquid for Restarting

Remove 5 or more cups of the kombucha from the brewer to use as starter liquid for the new CB. The more starter liquid used, the faster the next batch ferments; we commonly use a half gallon or more. If the liquid seems cloudy, filter it through a strainer, sieve, or cheesecloth to remove excess yeast. Then pour it over the trimmed-down SCOBY in the bowl and cover it with a towel.

Decant the remaining liquid from the brewer into bottles, the SCOBY Hotel, or a storage vessel for other uses (see chapter 17), or pour it down the drain.

## Cleaning the Brewer and Spigot

Now the brewer is empty and you're ready to clean it, which will help remove excess yeast and keep the spigot free of obstructions. To begin, remove and disassemble the spigot. Run all the pieces under hot water to dislodge any bits of SCOBY that may have grown inside them. Use a toothpick or similar implement if necessary.

Rinse out the brewing vessel with hot water, and then cure it with pasteurized vinegar or kombucha vinegar. Replace the spigot securely. Test for leaks.

Finally, add the SCOBY and starter liquid to the brewer, and begin a new batch of CB, following the instructions on page 118.

### UNCLOGGING A SPIGOT

A clogged spigot, while commonplace, can be frustrating. The SCOBY serves many functions, one of which is to seal off all potential places where evaporation might occur. This includes growing tiny plugs of culture inside the spigot. During regular maintenance, when the spigot is removed from the brewing vessel, it is simple to remove the SCOBY plug. But it can be trickier to unclog a spigot that is still attached to the brewer. To solve the issue, try any of the following:

*Use gravity.* Sometimes you can just open the spigot and let gravity do the work. Place a bowl or jar beneath the spigot and open it. Wait five minutes. If no flow occurs, try something else.

*Blow.* If the plug has formed inside the spigot assembly, it is possible that blowing into the spigot will push the material out of the way. Blow quickly, then get out of the way so that the kombucha doesn't flow into your face!

**Check the inside.** It is possible that the obstruction is caused by SCOBY or yeast growing over the spigot inflow on the inside of the brewing vessel. This is especially likely if the level of liquid in the vessel is low and the SCOBY is thick. Wash your hands; then reach inside to sweep a finger over the inflow.

**Sweep.** Find a hook of some sort — a pipe cleaner, toothpick, straightened-out paper clip, or the like. (An unused mascara brush happens to fit nicely inside a spigot.) Place a large bowl or jar beneath the spigot. Open the spigot and insert the hook into the spigot. Fish around with it, pulling to release any material that may be clogging the spigot. Don't be afraid to dig or tug a little. It may take a few tries, but the blockage should pull loose, allowing liquid to flow freely through the spigot.

If none of these options work, you may need to remove the spigot and clean it by hand. Drain the vessel, disassemble the spigot, and then hold it under a stream of hot water to flush away yeast and SCOBY. Use a toothpick or similar tool to pick out any remaining SCOBY pieces.

# Taking a Break

Whether you take a break on purpose or by accident, the CB process keeps the cultures and liquid protected in a low-pH environment, making it easy to start up again whenever the time comes. For a short break (up to six months), it's as easy as almost doing nothing. As long as enough liquid remains in the

## VACATION TIPS FOR A CONTINUOUS BREW

When you leave town for a bit, you have a few choices for dealing with your CB.

### If the CB vessel is full:

- Leave it alone. Harvest a batch of kombucha vinegar upon returning, and then add sweet tea and be ready to bottle in a few days.
- Bottle up what's in the brewer, leaving it one-half to one-third full, and then add sweet tea upon returning and be ready to bottle in a few days.

Bottle up what's on hand, add sweet tea right away, and taste upon returning.

### If the CB vessel is low:

- Leave it alone. Add sweet tea upon returning and be ready to bottle in a few days.
- Add sweet tea before leaving, and allow it to ferment into drinking kombucha or kombucha vinegar, depending on how long you are gone.

brewer to cover the cultures, they will be ready to brew whenever you are. Should the level of liquid dip too low, simply add sweet tea to replenish.

When the time comes to revive the booch, how to proceed depends on the status of the SCOBYs and liquid inside the brewer. If the brewer is still three-quarters or more full, drain it to about half full or slightly less and refill with sweet tea; then see how it tastes after a few days. If the brew remaining in the vessel is very low, or if it is too sour or yeasty to make delicious kombucha, follow the directions for resetting the brew (page 166).

For a longer break (more than six months), consider warehousing the SCOBYs in hotels, topping off the hotels with extra sweet tea so that they last longer.

# Barrel Brewing

Brewing in wood offers a unique flavor profile but also comes with unique challenges. Wood is an ancient material and is still used in many traditional fermentation and brewing operations. A wood barrel is the only "living" vessel, in that the wood is porous and provides a safe harbor for bacteria and yeast within the grain. It may take a little more patience to work with a barrel, but the resulting "oakiness" and smooth flavor are worth it.

## Sealing the Barrel

Every barrel is different, and they all require more attention, at least initially, until they are fully sealed. We avoid using models with chemical glues or sealants that could contaminate the brew.

A barrel without sealants must be soaked in order to swell the staves. As the wood expands, it is held together by the metal bands to create a tight seal. Once sealed, the wood must remain saturated in order to stay watertight. For this reason, always keep the barrel at least three-quarters full.

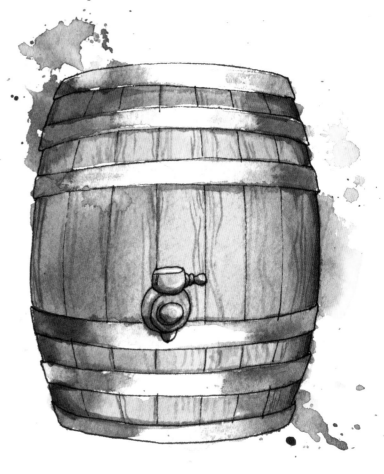

To start, fill the barrel halfway with warm water. Add 1 crushed Campden tablet (sodium metabisulfite, used for sanitizing) per gallon capacity of the barrel (for example, 2 to 3 tablets for a 2½-gallon barrel or 5 tablets for a 5-gallon barrel). Then fill the barrel the rest of the way. Let it sit for 24 hours. At this stage, some water may continue to seep through the staves as they haven't fully swelled; some of the ash of the char may also have leaked onto the exterior, creating an aged look. Don't worry if the sealing process hasn't completed; the barrel will continue to seal over the first week.

After 24 hours, empty the barrel and rinse it out three times with clean hot water to remove all traces of the sanitizer and any remaining loose char. It is important to lower the pH quickly, so it's best to brew right away, using a minimum of 1 large SCOBY (5 ounces) and 1 cup starter liquid per gallon. The staves at the top of the barrel may shift a bit during this cycle, which is normal, as is some leakage as the wood continues to completely saturate.

## Dealing with a Leaky Barrel

It is not uncommon for a barrel to experience a small leak due to slight shifts in the wood, especially as the seasons change. When this occurs, the wood normally continues to expand and eventually the leak stops. If the leak doesn't go away, apply barrel wax or beeswax to the area to reduce or eliminate any seepage.

If a leak persists for five days or more or if the wood develops a large wet patch on the outside, there may be a structural issue. As long as mold does not develop, the barrel is safe to use and may repair itself through expansion. If the area grows larger and begins to leak liquid, the barrel may need to be repaired or replaced.

## Dealing with a Moldy Barrel

Mold is a bit more common in barrels than in other vessels due to the porous nature of the wood and the potential for mold spores to exist in the wood itself. While purchasing the barrel from reliable sources considerably reduces the risk, sometimes the contamination comes from the environment.

If mold occurs, drain the barrel completely and scrub the inside with a clean soft-bristled brush to remove yeast or other particulates, and then rinse with hot water. Fill the barrel half full of hot water, add 2 cups distilled vinegar and 1 Campden tablet per gallon capacity of the barrel, and fill to the rim with more hot water. Let soak for 24 hours to allow the tablets to decontaminate the barrel.

Once the soaking is completed, rinse out the barrel three times with clean hot water to remove all traces, and immediately brew a

---

**KOMBUCHA MAMMA SEZ**

### Flavor and Alcohol Twist

"Some brewers may want to make a kombucha with a unique flavor profile and a potentially higher alcohol content. Using barrels from the wine or whiskey industry provides an opportunity to create hybrid kombucha brews."

new batch using more healthy SCOBYs than you normally would and at least 2 cups (more if available) of strong starter liquid per gallon of sweet tea as extra insurance.

## Detaching a SCOBY from the Barrel

As the kombucha brews, bacteria and yeast from the SCOBY take up residence within the wood itself. Some of the thin strings of bacterial cellulose reach right into the crevices of the wood, forming a tight seal with the sides of the barrel. As the liquid is drained via the spigot, the SCOBY may remain attached to the sides of the barrel, held in place by those cellulose strings, and may lose contact with the brew below, potentially drying out if left alone.

This is normal and easy to fix. Just use your fingers or a wooden spoon to push the SCOBY gently all around its edges until it dislodges and falls back into contact with the liquid. Once it is unstuck from the sides, the SCOBY may float or sink — either is normal — and a new layer will begin to form on top.

## Storing the Barrel

To take a break from using the barrel, a few precautions are in order. The best option, if you intend to start your brew again fairly soon, is to simply leave the SCOBY and liquid in the barrel and top off with sweet tea so that it is at least three-quarters full. When you are ready to brew again, simply drain off the sour stuff or empty the barrel completely and start a fresh batch.

If you'd like to place the barrel in storage, you can fill it with water. If the barrel has already been used for brewing kombucha, when you come back to empty it you may discover a SCOBY growing across the top. This is because the bacteria and yeast take up residence in the wood and the tannins in the oak provide enough nutrition for them to rebuild. Simply remove everything from the barrel and clean it thoroughly when you're ready to start a new batch.

Dry storage is also possible, but you may need to reposition the staves and hoops, as they can shift when the wood shrinks, and you'll need to soak the barrel to seal it, as described above. When restarting a barrel, unless it already contained kombucha, it is best to follow the instructions from the beginning.

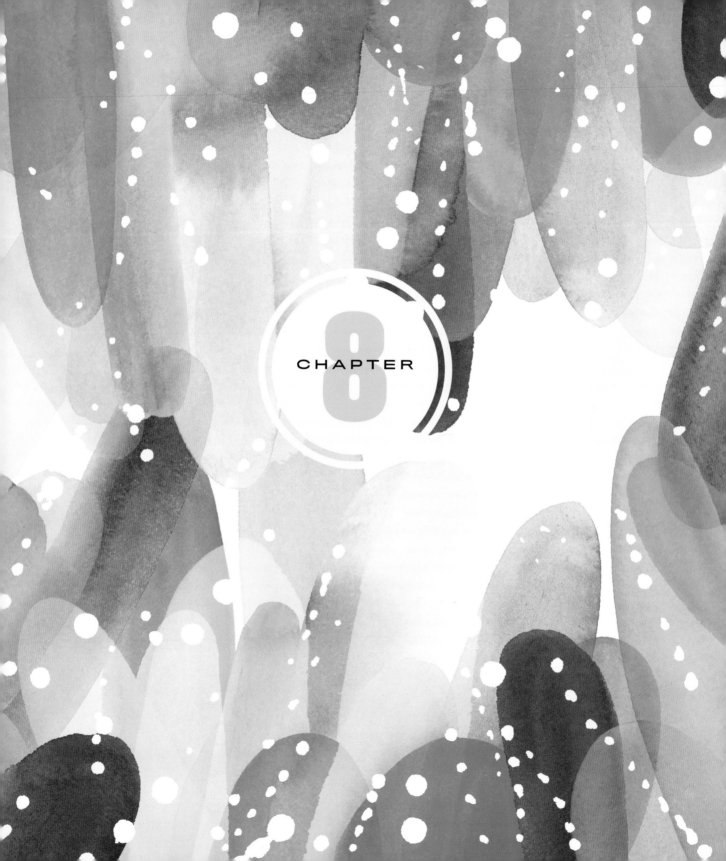

CHAPTER

8

# In the Bottle

## CONDITIONING, FILTERING, AND FLAVORING YOUR TEA

Kombucha tastes great straight from the fermentation vessel, especially over ice. But when the brew has reached the desired flavor, the best way to maintain that flavor over the long term is to bottle it and store it in the refrigerator (aka the "fermentation-slowing device" — with a tip of the hat to Sandor Katz). Bottling also allows the homebrewer to start a new batch while still enjoying the previous one, ensuring a constant supply. And, of course, bottles make transporting the booch much easier than lugging around a gallon jar or a continuous brewer!

Bottling is fun, too, as that's when you can add flavors and increase carbonation. One of kombucha's secret superpowers is that it adapts well to many flavors, both savory and sweet. The possibilities are endless — you can add fruit, veggies, mushrooms, herbs, roots, or nearly anything else your imagination can conjure. Bacon booch? Why, yes! (See chapter 11, page 211.) Even better, any beneficial elements present in the flavorings — nutrients, minerals, antioxidants, and the like — will be absorbed into the kombucha and broken down into forms that are easier for the body to assimilate.

# Flavoring Kombucha in the Bottle

Flavoring kombucha is perhaps the most creative stage and, for many brewers, the most fun. Fresh fruit, ginger, or fresh herbs are common choices. When good-quality fruit is scarce, dried fruit, jam, or juice can achieve excellent fruity flavors. High-quality dried herbs and spices may be used at any time. Creative choices for flavoring include herbal decoctions, floral tisanes, and syrups. People enjoy the flexibility of flavor experiences from sweet to tangy to spicy to savory, and kombucha has a flavor for everyone!

Remember that many flavoring agents — and most definitely ones with any type of sugar — will reawaken the latent yeast in the brew, causing a secondary fermentation that will change the flavor profile and most likely boost carbonation. Experiment with varying amounts of different flavorings to find the balance you prefer for any particular combination. (See chapter 11 for dozens of ideas to engage your imagination and start your flavor adventures.)

If you have a batch of kombucha that is too tart to drink, flavor it with garlic or spices to create delicious and healthy vinegar for marinades, salad dressings, and cooking.

### Customized Flavor

"We like to bottle our brew when it is still just a little too sweet for our taste, and then store it at room temperature for three to seven days or longer before refrigerating. For us, this yields maximum flavor and carbonation. In the cooler months, it's often unnecessary to refrigerate the bottles at all. Some may find that they enjoy the flavor of the kombucha after it has been in the bottle for longer. Balance the different factors to discover the best bottle-conditioning cycle for your palate."

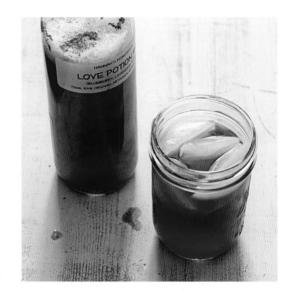

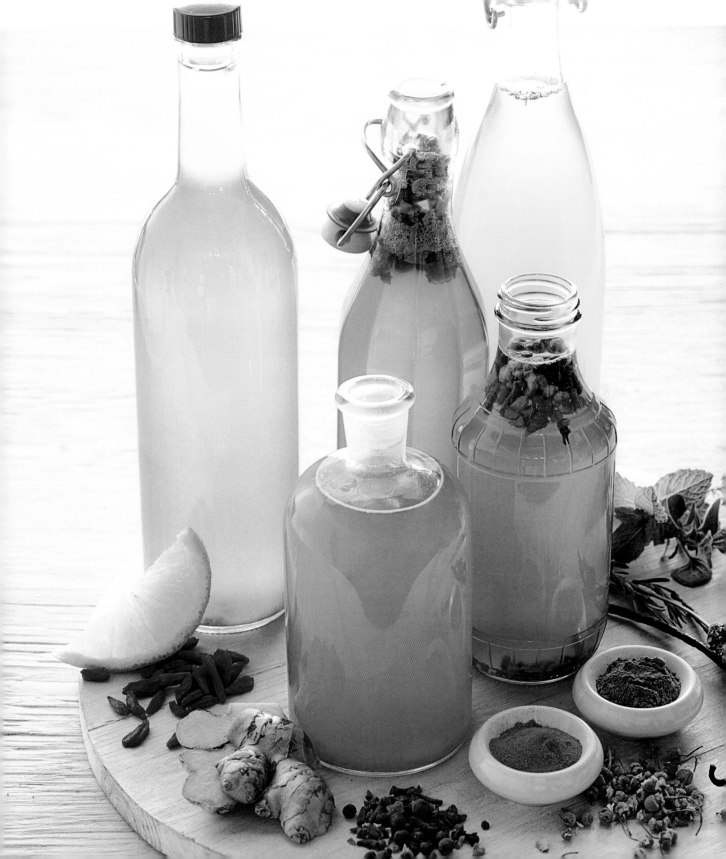

# How to Bottle Kombucha

Bottling kombucha is pretty simple. Here's what you do:

1 If you're adding a flavoring agent, put it in the bottle.

2 Carefully pour the fermented kombucha into the bottle and cap it. Fill bottles nearly to the top to preserve as much fizz as possible. Use a funnel if you're pouring from a batch-fermenting vessel; if you have a continuous brewer, simply fill the bottle straight from the spigot, keeping an eye out for overflowing foam. Repeat with remaining kombucha.

3 If you like, condition the bottles by leaving them at room temperature for one to four days, or longer, to build carbonation and flavor. Move them to the fridge when the kombucha attains the flavor and carbonation level you desire.

4 Enjoy!

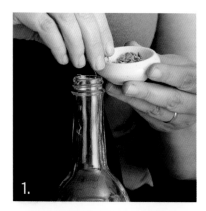

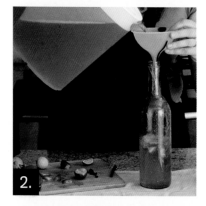

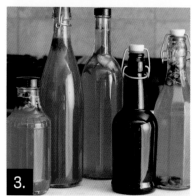

# Bottle-Conditioning

Bottle-conditioning is a continuation of the fermentation that takes place, as you might guess from the name, in the bottle. If sugar is added to the kombucha at bottling time, whether in the form of priming sugar, an herbal syrup, or some form of fruit, the yeast reawaken and initiate a secondary fermentation, during which they begin creating more of everything, especially carbon dioxide. Because the kombucha is now in a closed and anaerobic environment, those bubbles become trapped in the liquid, creating additional carbonation.

Even without the addition of sugar and other flavorings, the kombucha will continue to ferment in the bottle. This continued fermentation alters the flavor profile and balance of a brew over time and must be taken into account when deciding the appropriate time to bottle your brew.

Once you've finished bottling, leave the bottles out at room temperature for one to four days to condition. Or, if you like the flavor and balance of the brew as it decants from the fermentation vessel, refrigerate immediately after bottling to slow the ongoing fermentation, thereby preserving it longer.

Experienced homebrewers may experiment with flavorings and sugars to stimulate an in-bottle secondary fermentation, especially to boost carbonation levels; see page 148.

## WARNING: CONTENTS UNDER PRESSURE!

Sometimes kombucha becomes so fizzy that opening a bottle causes the brew to gush like Old Faithful! Although somewhat entertaining, this is messy and a waste of good booch. Moving room-temperature bottles to the refrigerator for just 30 minutes slows down the action of the yeast, making a mess less likely.

Another method for retaining overly fizzy booch is to place the bottle in a large bowl with a plastic baggie over the top, and then open the bottle, holding the baggie down tight. The liquid that spills into the bowl can then be poured into a glass.

To prevent these issues in the first place, use less flavoring or filter the yeast prior to bottling. While geysers are inconvenient, there is also cause for caution when creating carbonation as too much pressure can lead to a bottle explosion. Storing bottles at room temperature can be fine, but if there are concerns, place them in a box or cooler to reduce the risk of mess or injury.

Burping bottles during second ferment — slowly unscrewing the cap, allowing the carbon dioxide to escape, and then tightly recapping — also mitigates this risk. Use a towel over the top of the bottle to cushion fingers if the pressure is very high or there are worries of breaking glass. The more bubbles collecting at the top of the brew, the more pressure is building up, but overburping will lead to a loss of fizz, so experienced brewers will have to use their best judgment as to how much maintenance is needed for specific conditions.

# Filtering and Fining

There are many reasons why you may choose to filter or fine your brew. For some, the sight of strands of yeast and bacteria in the bottle is unattractive, while others prefer a reduction in carbonation or the already low levels of alcohol. Filtering is the most common way to remove excess particulate from the brew, but if you desire a kombucha with more clarity and a slightly softer flavor profile, then fining might be a better option.

If excess yeast populates the brew at bottling time, it may be wise to filter. Keep in mind that removing too much yeast could reduce the overall activity of the bottled beverage, eliminating carbonation entirely and flattening out the flavor.

Many people drink the yeast, as they are a great source of B vitamins (think brewer's yeast). We choose not to filter our brew to maintain maximum beverage activity. However, we also sometimes skip the last bit of brown dregs from the bottom of the fermentation vessel at bottling time and from the bottle at drinking time.

Here are some of the methods for reducing the particulates floating in the brew.

## Physical Filters

Although cheesecloth should never be used to cover a brew vessel (it lets in fruit flies), it is an excellent filter, especially when paired with a colander or strainer. Or choose a funnel with a built-in filter. Leftover captured yeast can be composted or used to inoculate a kombucha sourdough starter (see page 261).

## Fining

While we prefer to simply strain the visible yeast out with a filter, people who homebrew other ferments may have fining agents on hand. Fining makes further changes to the flavor of the brew by, as the name suggests, refining or softening any astringent or bitter notes, plus it will bring a clarity to the kombucha that cannot be achieved with mere filtering.

## OOGLIES (LITTLE BABY SCOBYS)

Kombucha continues to reproduce even without oxygen. Storing bottles in the fridge will slow the growth of new culture but won't completely prevent it from occurring. It's just part of the miracle of kombucha — it is always making more of itself! These little collections of new SCOBYs are informally called *ooglies*.

If you prefer, you can pour your booch through a strainer to filter out these little clumps, or you can simply dump the dregs down the drain or into the compost pile. Brave "Kombucheros" swallow the ooglies; many people assert that the culture contains the most concentrated forms of healthful acids. One option is to treat ooglies like oyster shooters: open wide and swallow whole. Gulp!

Fining agents are typically used to clarify wine and remove sediments from solution. Some, like gelatin, have a positive or negative electrical charge, as do many solids suspended in solution. When the fining agent is added to the solution, the positive and negative ions are attracted and bind to one another, causing the particles to increase in mass and precipitate to the bottom of the vessel. Other fining agents, such as bentonite clay, work through absorption rather than attraction, "soaking up" particles that then settle on the bottom.

All sorts of strange things from powdered blood to fish bladders (isinglass) have been used as fining agents, but we'll just discuss a couple of the most common choices here.

### BENTONITE CLAY

Bentonite clay, made from volcanic ash, works as a fining agent via both absorption and electrical charge. It is highly absorptive, able to expand to 20 times its size, and it carries a negative charge, which attracts positively charged particulate matter and weighs it down to the bottom of the bottle. Its rich mineral content also reduces some of the sourness of the brew by making the pH slightly higher.

To use with kombucha, first add 1 tablespoon bentonite clay to 2 cups water, and stir vigorously. Let the mixture stand for an hour to allow the particles to thoroughly hydrate. When you're ready to use it, add 1 to 2 tablespoons of the clay slurry for each gallon of kombucha. (Don't use any more than this, as too much fining agent can remove flavor components as well.) Give the kombucha a few days in the fridge to allow the clarifying process to complete. Then filter the brew through cheesecloth or a fine-mesh strainer to remove the denser particles.

### GELATIN

Gelatin is the collagen-rich substance extracted from the tissues and bones of animals. It holds a positive charge that helps reduce tannins, thus lightening the color and astringency of the brew. A little bit goes a long way, so start with a small amount (1 teaspoon per gallon). After the kombucha clarifies, usually within 48 hours, strain to remove excess particulate.

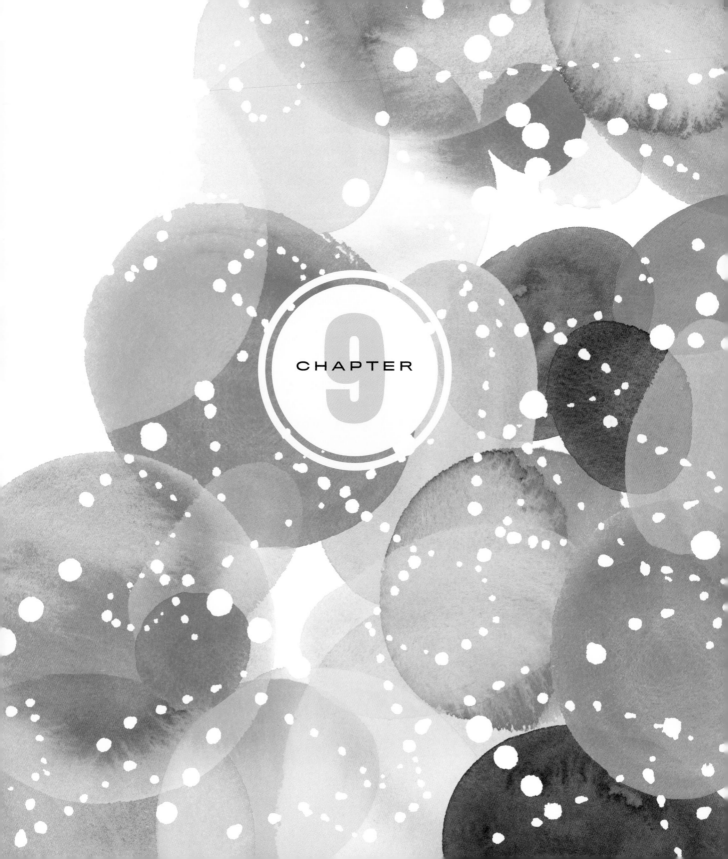

CHAPTER

9

# Advanced Techniques

## FOR FLAVORING, BREWING, AND CARBONATION

Once you've mastered the basics, you can expand the brewing experience in a variety of fun ways. Try adding flavoring agents during the primary fermentation stage instead of at bottling, or making batches with substrates other than tea, or kicking off the fermentation with a fruit purée instead of sugar, or priming the bottle with sugar or other ingredients to boost carbonation — the possibilities are endless.

It is best to keep the SCOBYs that you use for experimental batches separate from the rest of your SCOBYs, in their own hotels, to prevent cross-contamination. Over the course of sequential batches, watch SCOBY growth carefully to determine whether your experiment has the potential to maintain itself. Weak SCOBY growth or overabundant yeast means that an experiment is failing to support the culture. Then again, you may have enough SCOBYs that you don't need a particular type of brew to support itself; in some cases, such as when you're fermenting kombucha with coffee or herbs that have high concentrations of volatile oils, which will degrade the SCOBY, you can use a SCOBY once or twice and then dispose of it.

Now that we've covered the basic rules, let's have some fun figuring out ways to break them!

## Was There a Dr. Kombu?

One of the most popular kombucha origin stories, second only to the tale of Emperor Qin Shi Huang (page 96), is perhaps the origin of this brew's strange moniker. It is the story of Dr. Kombu, a Korean doctor summoned to heal the Japanese emperor In-giyō in 415 CE. The history checks out, though the connection to kombucha is tenuous.

While it is true that the Japanese emperor of that time was a sickly man named In-giyō, and that the eighth-century *Kojiki* (Records of Ancient Matters) recounts that a medically trained ambassador accompanied the yearly tribute from the Kingdom of Silla (Korea), no evidence exists that kombucha was involved.

Instead of identifying this ambassador as the Dr. Kombu of the popular legend, the Japanese texts refer to him as Komu-ha-chimu-kamu-ki-mu. This may offer a glimmer of hope, as *Komu-ha* is somewhat akin to *kombucha,* but the *Kojiki* does not describe how the emperor was cured, and there are no references to kombucha in it or in any other Japanese histories we could locate.

# Adding Flavoring Agents to the Fermentation Vessel

Many homebrewers add flavoring agents to their kombucha as they bottle it, which imbues the brew with a somewhat delicate flavor or zest. Adding flavoring agents directly to the fermentation vessel, on the other hand, whether at the outset, so that they play a role in the primary fermentation, or afterward, as a secondary fermentation, brings more intensity to the kombucha, imparting complex notes and undertones of flavor and aroma.

Popular herbs to experiment with include basil, bay leaf, chamomile, clove, lavender, rosemary, rose petal, sage, and thyme. Some herbs — peppermint and sage, for example — contain volatile oils that may adversely affect the kombucha culture, which is why we use them in experimental batches only. Of course, people have used kombucha to ferment all variety of herbs, flowers, berries, fruits, and spices, many to great success.

Try any flavoring you desire and see how it goes, then make adjustments from there. Make notes in the Brew Minder Logs (page 371) to determine which can be incorporated into primary fermentation on a regular basis. Follow The 10 Generations Rule (see page 144) to make a final determination on any flavoring agent's long-term viability. That's one of the beautiful things about kombucha: experimentation!

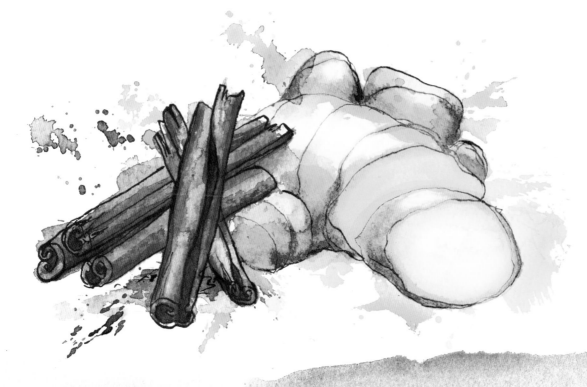

# A COUPLE OF CLASSIC FLAVOR BOOSTERS

Here are a couple of tried-and-true ideas for punching up your booch right from the start. Try adding them to your next batch at the beginning of the primary fermentation. The amounts given are for 1 gallon of brew.

## Cinnamon Brew

Cinnamon Brew has a mellow flavor that imparts gentle warmth. The oils in the cinnamon mellow the acetic bite yet complement the naturally appley flavor of the kombucha. We love to use Cinnamon Brew to make Warm Kombucha Cider (page 231).

- 2 cinnamon sticks, 2 teaspoons chopped cinnamon bark, or 1 teaspoon powdered cinnamon

## Ginger Punch

Ginger stimulates carbonation, and hibiscus in small amounts is a nice natural match for the kombucha flavor, lending an undertone of sweetness. This brew can be consumed on the young side to satisfy the kids or fermented fully for your puckering pleasure!

- 1 tablespoon chopped fresh or dried ginger

- 1 teaspoon dried hibiscus

# Flavoring the Primary Fermentation

One common way to flavor kombucha is to add an herbal tisane, fruit pieces, or juice to the traditional black/green tea mix before the primary fermentation begins, thereby brewing and infusing flavor in one step. Keep in mind that any flavoring agent added at the beginning of the process will ferment for much longer than if added at bottling and is therefore likely bring more intense flavor to the kombucha. It doesn't take much flavoring agent to affect the brew — see chapter 11 for specific suggestions. Here is the general process:

1 Make the sweet tea as normal (see page 54) and pour it into the brewing vessel.

2 Add the fruit, tisane, juice, or other flavoring agent to the tea.

3 Add the SCOBY(s).

4 Use very sour kombucha as starter liquid. The normal ratio is 1 cup of starter per gallon of sweet tea, but with this method we recommend using 3 to 4 cups of starter per gallon to prevent mold, which is more likely to develop due to the additional sugar, yeast, and other constituents in the flavorings.

5 Cover and let ferment as usual. Check the brew for flavor after just five days, as it may turn sour more quickly, and fruit sugar in particular can create a stronger brew.

Remember that in the bottle kombucha will continue to ferment, becoming stronger or slightly alcoholic, so refrigerate your flavored kombucha when it reaches the desired flavor.

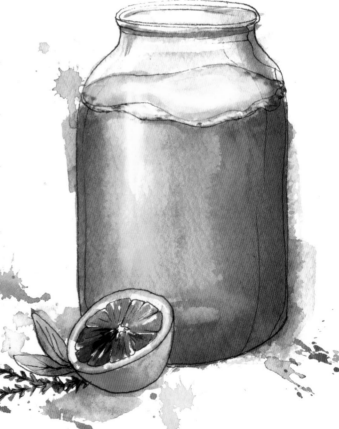

# Flavoring the Secondary Fermentation

Adding flavoring agents to the primary fermentation is an excellent experiment, but another option is to add those flavorings to the brewing vessel afterward, for a secondary fermentation. With this option, there is no risk of contaminating the SCOBY, since it has been removed prior to adding the flavoring agents. Also, because the flavorings spend less time in the brew (1 to 4 days with this method versus 7 to 14 days with the primary fermentation), and because the brew has already developed and acidified under normal conditions without additional flavors to slow the process, there is less chance (really no chance) of mold or other issues arising.

Of course you can add flavoring agents directly to your bottles and have the secondary fermentation take place there, but if you plan to store the bottled kombucha for more than a few weeks, flavoring in the brewing vessel and then straining before bottling is often the best option, as those flavoring elements may disintegrate over time, causing off flavors.

Your brew will also look cleaner and more professional without flowers, bark, berries, or bits of fruit floating around in the bottle. Finally, flavorings left in the bottle often stick to the bottom and make cleaning a challenge; flavoring in the brewing vessel avoids that potential pitfall.

1 Ferment the kombucha as usual.

2 Remove the SCOBYs and enough mature kombucha to start the next batch.

3 Add the flavoring agents.

4 Replace the cloth cover and let the brew ferment for one to four days. As with unflavored kombucha, carbonation may be unimpressive in the fermentation vessel, though bubbles should begin to appear once the brew has been bottled for a couple of days.

5 Strain the flavored booch to remove excess yeast and flavoring agents. Then bottle it. Let the bottles sit at room temperature for one to four days or longer to build bubbles, or move them to the fridge to preserve the existing flavor.

# Creating Flavoring Tisanes, Decoctions, and Syrups

Both tisanes and decoctions are herbal "teas" — tisanes are made from leaves and flowers, and decoctions from roots and woody parts. Syrups are made by boiling a tisane or decoction, usually an extra strong one, with sugar.

## Tisanes

Herbs and other plants were mankind's first medicines. Steeping the plant matter in hot water (tisanes are also called infusions) aids in the extraction of the active elements of many plants. Nearly any type of plant can be utilized provided it is recommended for human consumption. Examples of some popular tisanes for flavoring kombucha include hibiscus, elderflower, gotu kola, and mint. While any of these might also be added directly to the booch, using them in tisane form gives the brewer more control over the intensity of flavor.

The longer the herbs steep, the more intense the flavor of the tisane. Add it to the kombucha based on the level of flavor desired. Store extra tisane in the fridge (or just drink it up!) and use within a week.

## Decoctions

Decoctions are similar to tisanes in that nutrition is extracted through water, but time and temperature also play an important role in maximizing their benefit. They work best for releasing flavor and nutrition from fibrous or woody parts of plants, such as bark and roots. The typical ratio is 1 teaspoon of powdered herb or 2 teaspoons of fresh herb per 8 ounces of water. Experiment with small batches of decoctions to find the recipe and ratio that produce the flavor you desire, and then scale up or down. We recommend approximately 2 ounces of decoction to flavor 1 gallon of kombucha. Store any extra decoction in the fridge, where it will keep for up to one week.

## THE 10 GENERATIONS RULE

How do we determine if an herb, spice, or other flavoring agent is suitable for use during primary fermentation? A good rule of thumb is to brew with it for 10 generations. If the SCOBY reproduces and appears to be vibrant and healthy after 10 successive batches with the flavoring agent, then that flavoring agent can be considered safe to use in primary fermentation.

Vibrant culture is creamy white and dense. Weak culture is easily penetrated by fingers. Without DNA analysis, there is no way to know what changes the culture may undergo due to adaptation when brewing with alternative substrates. We recommend always storing experimental cultures in a separate hotel and keeping a traditional SCOBY Hotel with real tea for backups.

## Syrups

Syrups are thickened liquids that can add a quick jolt of flavor, and the extra sugar content ensures plenty of fizz. Use syrups sparingly; too much sugar can have the opposite effect and may turn the kombucha sour or create so much fizz that half the bottle is lost bubbling over when it is opened. Making syrups from tisanes or decoctions is easy. Simply steep the flavoring agent for a longer time to create a more intense flavor; then boil it down with an equal amount of sugar (1 cup:1 cup) for about 30 minutes until it is concentrated into a syrup. Add 1 ounce of syrup to each gallon of kombucha. Syrups will keep a long time due to the natural preserving quality of the sugar.

# *Root Beer Syrup*

Root beer is a traditional medicinal beverage that gained popularity during the soda fountain boom of the early twentieth century. All of the herbs in this decoction have great health benefits. Prepare this strong, delicious syrup in advance for easy kombucha flavoring. This makes enough to flavor about 12 gallons of kombucha, depending on taste preference.

*Yield: 3 cups*

### INGREDIENTS

    2 quarts water
    1 cup sassafras bark
    ½ cup sarsaparilla bark
    ¼ cup dried wintergreen leaf
    1 whole vanilla bean, cut in pieces
    1 tablespoon lemon zest or dried lemon peel
    1 tablespoon licorice root
    3 cups sugar

### INSTRUCTIONS

1. Combine the water with the sassafras, sarsaparilla, wintergreen, vanilla bean, lemon zest, and licorice root in a large pot. Bring just to a boil, then reduce the heat and let simmer, covered, for 2 hours. Strain to remove the herbs.

2. Pour the liquid back into the pot and bring to a boil. Add the sugar and cook over medium heat until the liquid is reduced to about 3 cups. Let cool, then store in the fridge.

## Rootbucha

To make root-beer-flavored kombucha, combine 1 teaspoon root beer syrup with 2 cups kombucha. Cap tightly and store in a dark, warm place for 1 to 3 days. Check daily. If bubbles are visible, turn the cap to release carbonation pressure, and then immediately retighten. Move to the fridge when the kombucha has reached the desired flavor.

For another way to make Rootbucha, see page 203.

# Using Fruit as a Primary Sugar

Sugar comes in many forms, including fruit sugar, or fructose. While we've already mentioned that valuable acids are created when we use cane sugar to brew kombucha, in some fermentation traditions, we do find the direct fermentation of fruit in place of sugar. So, if you want to avoid any kind of processed sugar or just like to experiment with different fermentation techniques, you can use concentrated fruit juice instead of sugar to brew kombucha.

Fruit can be utilized in a couple of different ways with this technique. Cut up whole pieces of fruit, and add it directly to the tea (we recommend substituting 2 cups of fruit for 1 cup of sugar as a starting point), or use a fruit-juice concentrate. In either instance, because the concentration of fruit sugar will vary, it is difficult to provide an exact recipe, but in general, about 1 cup of concentrated fruit juice provides the necessary sugar to support the fermentation. Brew the tea about 50 percent stronger than normal to maintain the balance of flavor.

SCOBY development may be weak with this method, so as always, the maintenance of a traditional tea and sugar SCOBY Hotel is recommended to provide a backup supply. As with all experiments, do not store SCOBYs used in or developed by this method in your traditional SCOBY Hotel.

## PASTEURIZATION

Pasteurization kills off microorganisms, but it is indiscriminate, killing off not only undesirable elements but also the very yeast and bacteria that are essential to kombucha fermentation. The benefit is a shelf-stable product with no "ooglies" in the bottle and a more consistent flavor, especially over time.

But isn't pasteurization of a living product antithetical to fermentation? Perhaps, but when we consider that most beers and wines are pasteurized rather than wild living ferments, it doesn't seem so strange. Many people believe that kombucha's healthy acids survive pasteurization intact. Of course, fans of the brew's probiotic benefits would do best to leave it raw.

There are two methods of pasteurization commonly employed: chemical and heat. With chemical pasteurization, sulfites are added to kill microorganisms. In heat pasteurization, the liquid is raised to and held at a certain temperature for a specific amount of time.

Most homebrewers forgo these techniques in favor of a wild fermentation process that continues to evolve in the bottle. Commercial-scale operations, however, may proudly offer a pasteurized product or, in some cases, may pasteurize and then add lab-cultured probiotics to create various offerings intended to appeal to different markets. The legitimacy of those beverages as "fermented" is always up to the consumer, though brands are under no obligation to disclose on the label whether their product is pasteurized.

# "Kom-pache"
## (Mexican Pineapple Kombucha)

Some claim that kombucha has been fermenting in Mexico since the 1500s. This adaptation of *tepache*, a traditional ferment of Mexico, utilizes the natural sugar present in pineapple concentrate in place of cane sugar in the primary fermentation. If you're substituting fresh pineapple, use 2 cups of chopped fruit for every cup of sugar.

*Yield: 1 gallon*

### INGREDIENTS

> 1 quart extrastrong tea
> 1 (12-ounce) can frozen pineapple concentrate, defrosted, or 2 cups diced fresh pineapple
> 3 quarts water
> 1 SCOBY
> 1 cup starter liquid

### INSTRUCTIONS

Combine the brewed tea with the pineapple juice concentrate and stir until completely dissolved. Pour the water into the brewing vessel. Add the tea mixture. If the mixture is warm, let cool to body temperature. Then add the SCOBY and starter liquid. Cover and set aside to ferment.

This brew may develop quickly, so begin tasting at 5 days to prevent a mouth-puckering batch!

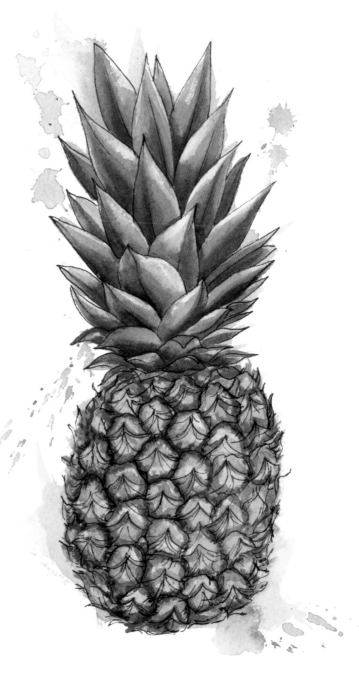

# Carbonation Tips and Techniques

One of the most common questions home-brewers have is how to get more carbonation in their kombucha. Bubbles are fun, and there is something inherently exciting about seeing a fizzy serving of iced kombucha froth over the edge of the glass. However, kombucha is naturally effervescent rather than carbonated — the difference, while subtle, should moderate your expectations. Some commercial kombucha brands add carbonation, so what you buy at the store may not be reflected in the home-brew bottle.

## What Causes Carbonation?

Carbonation is a solution of carbon dioxide ($CO_2$) dissolved in a liquid. So long as the liquid is kept under some form of pressure, the $CO_2$ remains trapped. When the pressure is released, so is the gas — as bubbles. As with many processes, there are natural and man-made versions. Forced carbonation involves adding $CO_2$ to a liquid under mechanical pressure. Natural carbonation requires only the magic of fermentation and a tightly capped container.

Kombucha is fermented in an open container with a cloth cover and requires air circulation. How can $CO_2$ build up? The SCOBY! As the new layer grows across the top, it creates an airtight seal, trapping gases beneath it. Oftentimes the bubbles are visible just below the new layer. Holey SCOBYs are the result of blowholes that form as the $CO_2$ escapes.

## Boosting Carbonation

When some homebrewers complain about their kombucha not being fizzy enough, it may just be a matter of perspective. A little carbonation can go a long way, especially if you don't expect your kombucha to look like a soda when it's poured. Pay close attention to the bubbles in your brew, and you may find that the kombucha is plenty carbonated as is. But if you like a lot of fizz, here are some ways to bump up the bubbles.

### GIVE YOUR BREW A SECONDARY FERMENTATION

Whether you are batch brewing or continuous brewing, a secondary fermentation increases effervescence. This is usually the point at which flavorings are added, many of which also lead to increased carbonation. There are two basic requirements for success here: tight-fitting caps on the bottles and the presence of yeast strands inside (yeast create carbon dioxide when fed sugar). So the easiest way to create carbonation via a second fermentation is to add yeast, feed it sugar, and keep the lid on tight! (See page 143 for more details.)

### STIR A CB BREW BEFORE BOTTLING

In batch brewing, the process of pouring the finished brew from the fermentation vessel into bottles stirs up the yeast from the bottom of the vessel, so they get distributed into the individual bottles. With the CB system, you simply drain the kombucha from the spigot, so the yeast that have collected on the bottom of the fermentation vessel stay there. Lack of yeast in the bottle can lead to weak flavors and poor carbonation.

The easy way around this is to slide a clean spoon gently past the SCOBY to the bottom of the vessel and give it a few quick stirs to agitate the yeast resting there. Immediately decant the kombucha into your bottles. Stir again as necessary to continue dispensing sufficient yeast into each bottle. The additional benefit to stirring up the yeast is that it reduces the yeast population in the vessel, thus maintaining a balanced flavor longer and increasing the amount of time one can go between cleanings.

### FILL BOTTLES COMPLETELY

In most homebrews, like beer and wine, headspace is left at the top of the bottle to allow for the formation of froth at the top. By reducing the amount of oxygen present in the bottle, more $CO_2$ remains dissolved in the liquid, which means more bubbles for you.

### LEAVE BOTTLES OUT OF THE FRIDGE

Once the kombucha is bottled up tight with very little air, set the bottles in a dark, warm location (74-78°F [23-26°C]). Now that you are no longer concerned with airflow, a cupboard

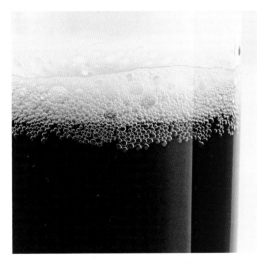

Artificial bubbles are typically more uniform, stick to the side of the glass, and tend not to interlace with each other. They also dissipate more quickly and are more aggressive in the mouth, with a much harder feel to them.

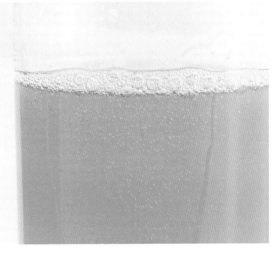

Natural carbonation, even when it causes kombucha to explode out of the bottle upon opening, delivers softer bubbles that tickle rather than burn and look a little more soaplike, with a variety of shapes, sizes, and popping speeds.

or any other enclosed space works fine. The more flavoring you've added to the bottles, the more closely you should monitor the bottles; they may need to be "burped" to prevent accidents (see page 135). Give them one to four days (or longer in winter or at cooler temperatures) to build bubbles.

### ADD A LITTLE SOMETHING

An easy way to increase carbonation in the bottle is to add some extra fuel for the bubbles. Here are a few options.

*Sugar.* A common carbonation booster is priming sugar, which is added just before you cap the bottles. This sugar reactivates the yeast, which create $CO_2$. Add ½ teaspoon of sugar per 16-ounce bottle. Sugar in the form of fruit pieces will also increase carbonation. (See chapter 11, starting on page 182.)

*Ginger.* Be it from natural sugars or from bacteria that live on its skin, ginger also increases carbonation. Add anywhere from a quarter to a full teaspoon of chopped or grated ginger per 16-ounce bottle, depending on how much fizz and flavor you want.

*Carbonation drops.* If the kombucha is not building bubbles as desired, you might try glucose and sucrose drops, which help add consistent carbonation. They look like throat lozenges. They can be particularly helpful if you're bottling your kombucha with flavorings that don't have any natural sugars to activate the yeast. They can be found at homebrew-supply shops; follow the manufacturer's instructions for using them.

*Mineral booster.* Effervescence occurs when a weak acid interacts with a base and creates carbon dioxide. Kombucha is naturally acidic,

so when you add a trace mineral booster, which serves as a base, both carbonation and mineral content are increased, making for a bubblier brew. Since this chemical reaction utilizes some of the acetic acid created by the kombucha fermentation, it also minimizes the sourness. Mineral boosters are great to use with kombucha that is slightly too sour. They are available from homebrew-supply shops; follow the manufacturer's instructions.

*Eggshells.* Because they have high levels of calcium and trace minerals, eggshells not only increase the fizz and decrease sourness but also boost the nutritional value of the final brew. Use eggshells from organic, pastured chickens for the best nutritional value.

Clean them thoroughly. Dehydrate them by baking in a 200°F (95°C) oven for 10 minutes prior to use. You might want to crush the shells, because the greater the surface area, the more calcium can be extracted. Then again, shells left in larger pieces are easier to remove. If you are concerned about the potential for salmonella, the low pH of kombucha has been shown time and again to kill those types of pathogenic bacteria on contact.

Eggshells will affect the flavor of the kombucha, so start by using a quarter of a shell for every 16-ounce bottle, and thereafter increase or decrease the dose based on taste and fizz.

*Calcium carbonate.* If quality eggshells are not available, you can substitute calcium carbonate pills. Crush them to gain maximum surface area, and add to the brew according to the manufacturer's instructions.

# Reducing Alcohol Levels

Here are some strategies to reduce the small amounts of alcohol, usually around 1% ABV or less, naturally present in properly fermented kombucha.

*Filter out the yeast.* Yeast in an anaerobic environment produce ethanol and $CO_2$, so removing the yeast strands from the brew will drastically cut down on the amount of alcohol produced. However, the yeast also provide nutrition, flavor, and carbonation, and these factors will also be reduced with this technique.

*Avoid fruit and other sugary flavorings.* Herbs, flowers, most green tea blends, and a variety of roots and rhizomes let you add flavor without sugar, thereby depriving the yeast of the fuel they require for ethanol creation. Some of the carbonation may also be sacrificed, except in the case of the rhizomes, which add fizz without adding sugar. (See chapter 11, starting on page 196.)

*Refrigerate quickly.* Keep the brew cold until you're ready to drink it. Cold temperatures quell the activity of the yeast, which cuts down on alcohol, though it may also reduce carbonation. Allowing the bottles to return to room temperature before serving should reactivate the yeast and initiate some bubbles.

*Leave more headspace in the bottle.* This tip is in direct opposition to the usual advice of filling the bottle to the top (see page 149). If you plan on consuming your kombucha within one or two weeks, leaving more oxygen in the bottle creates an environment more favorable to respiration than to fermentation, which will decrease alcohol production without reducing carbonation too much. Adding oxygen to the brew — pouring it through a filter or strainer as you bottle it, for example — may also limit alcohol levels.

*Allow an extended second ferment.* To bottle-age a batch for one month or more, fill the bottles to the very top. Eliminating as much oxygen as possible not only preserves the maximum amount of carbonation but also creates a favorable environment for fermentation, which leads to more alcohol. Giving the bacteria more time to convert the ethanol into healthy acids lowers the alcohol level and develops the flavor (it will be drier and perhaps much tarter), and the resulting brew will have lovely bubbles.

With an extended aging process, we recommend bottling the kombucha when it is on the sweeter side — just as wine starts as sweet grape juice that gradually develops a drier flavor over time, so too will the brew have a smoother flavor the longer it ages. If the brew is just right or a little on the tart side going into the bottles, aging it will produce overly tart flavors that may not be well received.

*Dilute individual servings.* Diluting kombucha by half with water or juice not only cuts the alcohol but also reduces the pH and acidity, smoothing a tart brew while maintaining hydration and flushing toxins.

# Raising Alcohol Levels

Although kombucha naturally tops out around 2 percent alcohol (and usually much less), it is possible to add other yeast and traditional beer ingredients to increase the alcohol and bring additional layers of flavor to the brew with anywhere from 3 to 14% ABV. Some companies produce kombucha beers; look for those at your local store or try these higher alcohol brew suggestions.

## "Beer"

Hybrid kombucha beers, with a taste profile similar to that of lambics (spontaneously fermented beers) and other wild-yeast beers, are garnering positive attention on the craft beer scene. Using beer yeast in the secondary fermentation builds more alcohol than a traditional kombucha would have. The hops add a bitter note, so use them sparingly, as the kombucha powerfully extracts the flavor.

Kombucha beers can be brewed in two ways: by adding a beer wort to the primary fermentation or by adding beer yeast and hop flowers as a flavoring in the secondary fermentation. Each method will produce different flavor profiles. Beer yeast typically yields alcohol levels between 4 and 9 percent.

## "Wine and Champagne"

Wine and champagne production is essentially grape juice inoculated (like kombucha) with yeast and bacteria, fermented, and bottle-aged for a fruity to dry flavor. Wine yeast drive alcohol levels to 9 to 16% ABV, while champagne yeast go even further, yielding alcohol levels of 15 to 20% ABV. Using younger kombucha with these yeast produces a dry, crisp flavor, whereas older kombucha makes tarter wine.

For a fruitier flavor, do a secondary fermentation with any fruit you desire for two days prior to adding the yeast.

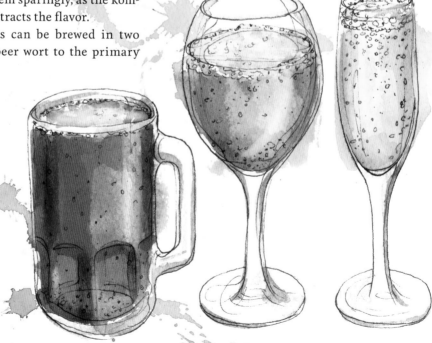

# Making Beer, Wine, and Champagne from Kombucha

To make about 1 gallon of beer, wine, or champagne, you'll need a brewing vessel that holds at least 1¼ gallons and has a lid with an airlock.

## INGREDIENTS

- 2 teaspoons of ale, wine, or champagne yeast
- 1 cup lukewarm water
- 1 cup sugar
- 1 gallon slightly sweet (young) fermented kombucha
- 1 tablespoon dried hops (for beer only)
- 1 ounce vodka

## FERMENTATION

1. Activate the yeast by combining 2 teaspoons with the lukewarm water and sugar. Stir well; the mixture should form a slurry. Let the mixture sit for 30 minutes to 1 hour and up to 2 days, until it is foaming. (Store leftover yeast in the freezer.)

2. Add the activated yeast mixture and the kombucha to the fermentation vessel. If you're making beer, add the hops as well.

3. Put on the lid, with the airlock, and swish the contents around to mix them. Add the vodka to the airlock to prevent oxygen from getting into the brew.

4. Set the vessel in a warm, dark location; the ideal temperature range is 72–78°F (22–26°C).

## BOTTLING AND AGING

**Beer:** After 1 day, taste to determine if the hops have added enough flavor to the brew. To prevent overbittering, do not leave them in for more than 2 days. Recap and continue to ferment for another 2 to 5 days. When the beer has the preferred bitter/sweet/tart flavor, pour into bottles and cap tightly. Let sit in a cool, dark location for at least 1 week to build carbonation. The longer the bottles are left alone, the drier the flavor.

**Wine:** After 3 to 5 days, decant the wine into 750 mL bottles and cap tightly. Let sit in a cool, dark location for at least 1 week and up to a year. The longer the bottles are left alone, the drier the flavor.

**Champagne:** After 30 to 45 days, decant the champagne into 750 mL bottles and cap tightly. Let sit in a cool, dark location for at least 3 months and up to a year. The longer the fermentation time, the drier the flavor.

As with any carbonated beverage, bottle breakage can be an issue; take the necessary precautions (see Warning: Contents under Pressure!, page 135).

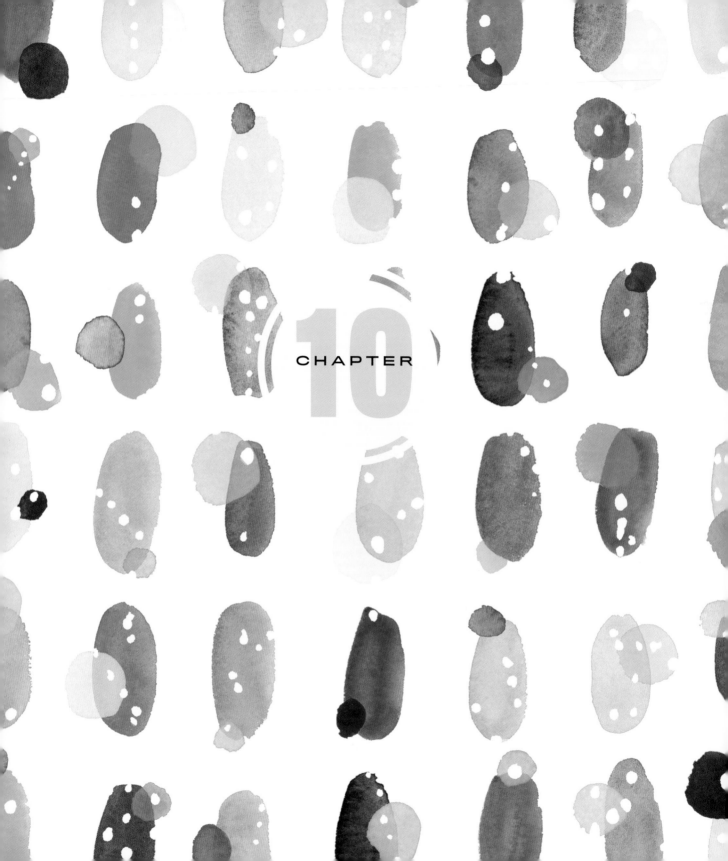

CHAPTER

10

# Troubleshooting

**B**rewing kombucha is a fun and easy hobby, but every once in a while something may go wrong. Kombucha is a forgiving culture, which makes correcting the brew quite simple. What follows are ways to self-correct as you go along making your kombucha. Find your problem here, follow these tips to fix a batch brew for the next round or figure out how to make adjustments with a CB, and you will be back on track in no time!

# Common Brewing Mistakes
## and How to Correct Them

### FORGOT TO ADD SUGAR?

*How to Fix It:* Remove the SCOBY, add the sugar, and stir to dissolve.

*What to Do Next Time:* Add the sugar as soon as you remove the loose tea or tea bags. The hot tea will help dissolve the sugar.

### FORGOT TO SAVE STARTER LIQUID FOR THE NEXT BATCH BREW?

*How to Fix It:* Add the SCOBY to 2 to 4 cups of sweet tea and allow it to ferment as usual for 7 to 10 days. Then use that SCOBY with all the liquid and new SCOBY growth to start a ½- or 1-gallon batch.

If you added flavoring to your kombucha before you realized that you forgot to save some as starter, select the flavor of kombucha with the least amount of essential oils (such as fruit or ginger) and use some of that as a starter.

*What to Do Next Time:* Save 2 cups of starter liquid from the top of the previous batch for the next batch before decanting the kombucha into bottles.

### FORGOT TO ADD WATER TO THE SWEET TEA?

*How to Fix It:* If it's within the first five days after starting the batch, go ahead and add water, up to the amount you should have used. If it's been five days or more since you started the batch, don't add the water; just taste the kombucha regularly until it's reached the desired flavor (it may ferment more quickly than usual). Then begin a new batch.

*What to Do Next Time:* Add the required amount of water to the sweet tea immediately after dissolving the sugar.

### LEFT A BREW ALONE FOR MONTHS — NOW WHAT?

*How to Fix It:* Check for mold, which grows on top of the brew and is fuzzy. If there is none, use the SCOBY and some of the liquid brew to start a new batch, and save the rest of the sour kombucha for a SCOBY Hotel (page 37), fruit fly traps (page 169), cooking with vinegar (chapter 14), or household uses (chapter 17).

*What to Do Next Time:* As long as the SCOBY stays moist, the kombucha is covered, and the liquid does not completely evaporate, there is no issue with letting a batch ferment indefinitely.

## HEATING UNIT RAISED THE BREW TEMPERATURE ABOVE THE RECOMMENDED RANGE?

**How to Fix It:** Reduce the temperature to 75 to 85°F (24 to 29°C) and monitor the brew. The organisms won't be damaged unless the brew has sustained temperatures of over 108°F (42°C).

**What to Do Next Time:** Monitor the brew more closely to maintain the proper temperature.

## SCOBY DRIED OUT IN A HOTEL — IS IT STILL VIABLE?

**How to Fix It:** Add the SCOBY to 2 to 4 cups of sweet tea and allow it to ferment as usual for 14 to 30 days. If the SCOBY was completely dried out, sprinkle a few tablespoons of distilled (pasteurized) vinegar over the liquid to help prevent mold.

As long as the rehydration process is mold-free, the SCOBY and the fermented liquid can be used to start a ½- or 1-gallon batch.

**What to Do Next Time:** Always keep the SCOBY hydrated; add sweet tea to refresh the hotel as needed.

## SCOBY AND STARTER LIQUID WERE REFRIGERATED

**How to Fix It:** If the SCOBY and starter liquid were refrigerated for less than two weeks, allow them to sit at room temperature for at least one week, then move to a fresh glass container, add 2 cups of sweet tea, cover, and leave them alone for five to seven days. This small amount of sweet tea will give the SCOBY a chance to recalibrate itself after refrigeration without exposing it to too much sweet tea, which might lead to mold. Once the beginnings of SCOBY growth and yeast formation appear at the top of the vessel, try brewing as normal. If SCOBY activity is not apparent after five to seven days, the culture and starter are no longer viable.

**What to Do Next Time:** Always store SCOBYs and SCOBY Hotels at room temperature in a dark location.

## DROPPED SCOBY ON THE FLOOR

**How to Fix It:** Best choice: rinse the SCOBY in well-fermented kombucha from a SCOBY Hotel. The second best choice is distilled white vinegar; the third is filtered water.

**What to Do Next Time:** Try not to drop SCOBYs!

# Issues with Flavor

Taste is king! Kombucha can range in flavor from sweet to sour to bitter to fruity to spicy based on the ingredients and environment. Most flavor issues require just a simple tweak to get the brew back on track. Brewing is an art, so even those with experience end up with a bad batch now and again. No worries, just make an adjustment and try again!

## Too Sweet

If the brew has a flavor that is sweeter than your palate prefers, it may be a sign of poor fermentation, weak culture, or simply impatience!

### BREWING CYCLE IS TOO SHORT

The less time fermenting, the more sugar that remains. As the brew continues to mature, it will grow sourer over time. Let it ferment a while longer. Taste it on a daily basis until it has the flavor you are looking for.

If the brew remains sweet or the flavor seems weak or watery after several weeks, the issue is likely inactive bacteria. That could mean either weak SCOBYs (see page 161) or low temperatures. Drain out some kombucha and top off with fresh sweet tea to wake up the SCOBY, and check that the temperature is in the appropriate range (see below).

### TEMPERATURE IS TOO LOW

The recommended temperature range for kombucha is 75 to 85°F (24–29°C), with the ideal being between 78 and 80°F (26 and 27°C). Maintaining the correct temperature range is most important in the first 7 to 10 days of the fermentation, but for the most even, rounded flavors, it should be maintained until the brew is ready. If the temperature range starts out too low, adding heat later in the process can sometimes help a slow-maturing batch recover.

### TOO MUCH LIQUID DRAINED FROM CB TOO SOON

New brewers are often eager to begin consuming their kombucha, yet patience during the early life of the brew is critical for long-term flavor. The CB performs best with a base of well-fermented kombucha. Overdraining during the first few batches increases the likelihood of throwing off the balance of yeast and bacteria, which may leave a sweeter flavor to the brew. Allow the brew to mature during the first four to five weeks of a new cycle by leaving the brewer about three-quarters full when harvesting kombucha.

## Too Sour

Sour is a flavor that signals nutrition, but it can be tough to swallow. For the new homebrewer, it might feel like it's too hard to get it right, but with persistence, success is often just a batch away.

### BREWING CYCLE WENT TOO LONG

Kombucha can sometimes quickly progress from too sweet to too sour, so it is important to taste it regularly when brewing (daily or even twice a day), especially once the brew is close to completion.

### TEMPERATURE IS TOO HIGH

If maintained above 85°F (29°C) for an extended time, a kombucha brew may become imbalanced, leading to sour, bitter, or otherwise off flavors. Maintain the ideal temperature range of 75 to 85°F (24–29°C) for best results.

### VESSEL WAS HEATED FROM THE BOTTOM

Especially with CB, it is important to heat kombucha from the sides of the vessel to prevent yeast overgrowth. As yeast go through their life cycle, they ultimately fall to the bottom of the vessel, where the temperature should be cooler. But if the bottom is heated, they may continue to be active, thereby throwing the fermentation process out of balance. If you are batch brewing for short cycles and scrupulously cleaning out the jar between batches, it can be okay to heat from below. But if you are brewing for eight days or longer, or doing CB, heat from the sides for best results.

### TOO MANY SCOBYS AND/OR TOO MUCH YEAST

As a CB ages, a large amount of SCOBY forms at the top while a great deal of yeast collects near the bottom. In between lives the delicious kombucha we covet. Once the culture becomes too large or the amount of yeast becomes too great, it is difficult to maintain the flavor of the kombucha. This means it's time to clean and reset the brew. (For complete instructions, see page 124.)

### TOO MUCH FUEL

Use up to one-third less sugar or one-third less tea in the primary fermentation. Reducing the fuel for the yeast and bacteria results in a less-acidic brew, but also one that contains fewer enzymes, vitamins, and healthy acids. SCOBY growth and flavor may also be thinner with this method.

### DILUTE IT

Adding water instantly raises the pH to a more drinkable range, greatly minimizing the bite of overfermented kombucha. Juice is packed with fructose, and even an ounce or two can significantly cover the flavor of sour booch. Adding sour kombucha to a smoothie camouflages the taste while allowing the benefits to live on.

### FINE IT

Adding fining agents (see page 136) can shift the pH of the brew or mellow the acidity. Try not to overdo it, though, or fining could throw the flavor too far in the wrong direction.

### MAKE VINEGAR

If the flavor is simply too sour to enjoy or if you have too much sour kombucha on hand, there are nearly unlimited uses for kombucha vinegar (see page 256).

## Too Weak

If the brew is not reaching the desired flavor intensity, the first option is always to allow more brewing time. If leaving the kombucha for a few more days does not improve the depth or acidity of the flavor, there are a few other potential causes.

### SCOBY IS DYING OR DEAD

Retire the culture to the compost and start over with a new one.

### YEAST ARE INSUFFICIENT

Use yeasty starter liquid from the bottom of a SCOBY Hotel for the next batch only.

### TEMPERATURE IS TOO LOW

Maintain the fermentation temperature at 75 to 85°F (24–29°C).

### TEA ISN'T STRONG ENOUGH

Increase the amount of tea leaves in the sweet tea, or steep the tea longer.

### NOT ENOUGH SUGAR

Use more! You can add up to 50 percent more than the standard 1 cup per gallon, if desired.

### STARTER LIQUID IS WEAK

Use starter liquid from a SCOBY Hotel that has grown very sour.

---

**A KOMBUCHA LEGEND:** Kargasok Tea

The well-documented pockets of centenarians clustered around the Caucasus Mountains are widely celebrated, but they exist also in other areas. According to one legend, in a rural Russian region called Kargasok resides a hardy population of folk who often live to be well over 100. Here, elders are revered as active and valued members of society and family. These Russian centenarians attribute their longevity not only to their work habits, but also to their consumption of kombucha, the traditional "yeast enzyme tea" that forms part of their dairy- and vegetable-rich diet.

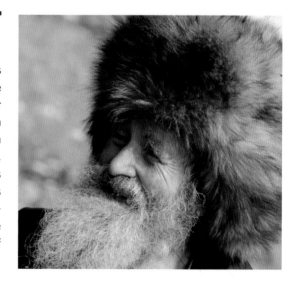

# Issues with SCOBYs

SCOBYs are the mother ship and come in different shapes, colors, and textures. Some will be familiar whereas others may inspire questions. Here are some of the common SCOBY concerns and how to deal with them.

## Poor SCOBY Growth

Each batch of kombucha should produce a new SCOBY, but if growth is weak or nonexistent after five days, it may indicate an issue with either the brew or the environment.

### TEMPERATURE IS TOO LOW

The recommended temperature range for kombucha is 75 to 85°F (24–29°C), with the ideal being between 78 and 80°F (26 and 27°C). Brewed at lower temperatures, the SCOBY may fail to thrive, and the result may be a flatter, more "dirty"-tasting kombucha that lacks the appley, sour bite of a delicious, properly brewed kombucha. Try using a heating mat around the sides of the brewing vessel to maintain the optimal temperature.

Allowing the brew to ferment longer at lower temperatures (mid to upper 60s°F [18–21°C]) will help it grow sourer and should still produce a safe, drinkable beverage. Attempting to ferment at less than 64°F (18°C) may produce a weak beverage, and the SCOBY may be susceptible to mold because the bacteria will slow down and have a difficult time protecting themselves.

### INSUFFICIENT SCOBY OR STARTER LIQUID

Without the proper ratio to begin the brew, the bacteria may struggle to reproduce quickly enough to build a proper SCOBY, especially in the first batch. As long as mold does not develop, a longer fermentation cycle should produce more growth, especially after the liquid has fully fermented and then more sweet tea is added.

### BACTERIA ARE DEAD OR DYING

If the culture is completely dead, mold will grow. But if the yeast are alive and the bacteria are dead or greatly weakened, the brew will ferment without forming a new SCOBY, producing a yeast brew that may or may not be healthy. Causes include refrigerating a SCOBY, placing a SCOBY in very hot liquid (108°F [42°C] or higher for an hour or longer), or letting a SCOBY stagnate in a hotel for more than six months. If the bacteria are completely dead, start over with a new culture.

### YEAST ARE DOMINATING

This is similar to the above scenario in that the yeast are producing the most visible aspects of fermentation. The difference is that in this case we see some signs of SCOBY reproduction and bacterial life, and so we may address the situation by reducing the yeast, which will allow the bacterial population to recover. Possible reasons for short-term yeast domination include using starter liquid from the bottom of the brew, reusing the vessel without rinsing from batch to batch, or continuously brewing for too many consecutive batches, resulting in yeast overgrowth at the bottom. (See Rebalancing the Brew, page 166.)

### VINEGAR EELS ARE PRESENT

These nematodes will nibble at the edges of the SCOBY growth, causing an initially promising culture to degrade as the brew matures, leaving a thin web of yeast connecting the culture to the edge of the vessel. (See Dealing with Vinegar Eels, page 173.)

## SCOBY Is Climbing Out of the Vessel

Sometimes a SCOBY will creep up the sides of the fermentation vessel, leaving a gap of air between itself and the liquid. Often a sort of umbilical cord of yeast and/or culture will connect the SCOBY to the brew, allowing it to maintain a source of hydration and nutrition. This strange phenomenon occurs when more carbon dioxide builds up than can remain dissolved in the liquid, combined with perfectly even SCOBY growth (no holes) that maintains the seal as the culture is pushed up by the gas.

### PUSH IT BACK DOWN

Simply press the SCOBY down until it releases. It is impossible to hurt the culture, so press down as hard as is necessary. The SCOBY may sink or float, but either way, new growth will occur on top of the brew.

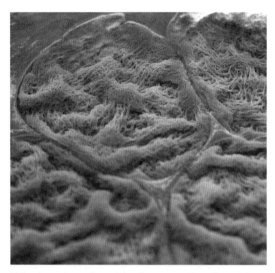

Kahm yeast is not harmful to humans and can be safely removed from most ferments while the remainder is consumed. With kombucha, however, it is an indicator that the brew is weak, and so it is best to dispose of it entirely and start a new batch with a fresh culture from your SCOBY Hotel.

# Issues with Carbonation

Try the methods outlined in Carbonation Tips and Techniques (page 148) first. If those basic techniques fail, these more advanced techniques may be required.

## Not Enough Fizz in Brew

Even if the $CO_2$ is able to escape via blowholes or from the sides of the SCOBY, some amount of bubbles ought to be apparent in the primary fermentation. Often they are visible pushing up against the bottom of the SCOBY; if they are completely absent, it may be a sign that something is off.

### USE STARTER LIQUID FROM THE BOTTOM

Starter liquid is usually pulled from the top of the vessel, where less yeast reside, in order to preserve a healthy balance of bacteria and yeast. One way to increase the fizz in your brew is to boost the yeast quotient. The best place to find them is hanging out around the bottom of the vessel.

Pull 2 cups of yeasty starter liquid from the bottom of the brewing vessel. Brew the kombucha as normal, using the yeasty bottom-based starter liquid. If 2 cups of starter liquid is more than you need, use less water in your brew to accommodate the extra liquid. If you need more than 2 cups of starter liquid, use regular starter liquid for the rest.

For best results, place the vessel near a source of warmth (heating mat, a warm spot near the stove, in a slow cooker set on low, for example) to keep the yeast active. You should notice more carbonation within one or two brewing cycles. As soon as carbonation reappears, discontinue pulling starter liquid from the bottom and return to pulling it from the top to maintain the right balance.

### INCREASE THE AMOUNT OF TEA

Extra caffeine stimulates the yeast, keeping them active rather than taking their normal rest cycle. Add another 1 to 2 teaspoons or tea bags of green or black tea to your tea blend (for a batch brew) or top-off tea (for CB) to achieve the desired result. If you've been using herbal teas, the brew may require a cycle or two to return to a state of vigor.

### INCREASE THE TEMPERATURE

Maintaining a fermentation temperature range of 75 to 85°F (24-29°C) creates the right conditions for carbonation, whether in the brew or in the bottle, with the ideal being between 78 and 80°F (26 and 27°C).

## Not Enough Fizz in Bottles

Fizz — most people just can't get enough of it! Considering that it is an ancient signal of the nutrition present (yeast!), it is understandable why we crave it in our drinks. Sometimes carbonation eludes us in the brewing process, leading to tasty but not fully realized kombucha. Here are some tips to boost the bubbles.

### STIR THE POT

With a CB, before bottling, slip a long-handled spoon underneath the SCOBY and give a good stir to rouse the yeast strands up off the bottom of the brewer. Decant immediately to capture some yeast in each bottle. Stir occasionally throughout the bottling process for even carbonation.

### INCREASE FERMENTATION TEMPERATURE

Maintaining a temperature range of 75 to 85°F (24–29°C) during fermentation creates the right conditions for carbonation, whether in the brew or in the bottle, with the ideal being between 78 and 80°F (26 and 27°C).

### INCREASE BOTTLE STORAGE TEMPERATURE

If yeast are too cold, they simply cease activity, which can lead to little or no carbonation. Even if your kombucha had bubbles prior to entering the bottle, extended time in cold storage, such as a refrigerator, can deflate the yeast.

If your bottles are in the fridge, bring them to room temperature and allow them to sit for 15 to 30 minutes, until bubbles are again visible at the top, before serving. Alternatively, store bottles in a cool but not cold spot (60–70°F [16–21°C]), and pour over ice if a cold glass is desired. Keeping the yeast at a comfortable temperature creates more fizz.

### BOTTLE SLIGHTLY TOO SWEET BREW

Bottling a little earlier in the fermentation process when the brew is somewhat sweeter than you would like should lead to more bubbles; as the yeast continue to consume the sugar, the bacteria rest in the oxygen-free second fermentation.

### CHECK BOTTLE CAPS

Carbon dioxide dissipates, so if the bottles are not as well carbonated as they should be, it could be that the lids are not secure enough. Many people find that swing-top bottles with an attached cork are best to hold in the carbonation.

### ADD SUGAR MORE SLOWLY

If the yeast are exposed to more sugar than they can consume, they may become sluggish, which slows fermentation and reduces carbonation.

If you've been using more than the standard 1 cup of sugar per gallon of kombucha, cutting back on the sugar should clear up any sluggish fermentation. However, if the yeast continue to underperform, adding the sugar gradually over the course of the first three days of the fermentation, rather than all at once at the beginning, should prevent the issue from recurring. This provides the yeast the chance to keep up with the amount of glucose present in the tea. Usually by the next batch they have recovered to the point where these steps are unnecessary.

The measurements below are based on 1 cup of sugar per 1 gallon of nutrient solution. Scale to fit the size of your batch.

- **Day 1:** Add just 25 percent of the sugar (¼ cup) with the brewed tea, SCOBY, and starter liquid
- **Day 2:** Add another 25 percent (¼ cup) of the sugar

- **Day 3:** Add the remaining 50 percent (½ cup)

There is no need to stir the brew when adding the sugar, but distributing it evenly on the bottom of the vessel allows for faster absorption. Also, be sure to move the SCOBYs out of the way so the sugar does not rest on them.

## Too Much Carbonation

While most would say there is never too much carbonation, once they've experienced a geyser that splatters fruit on the ceiling, they may sing another tune. As long as the bottles don't explode, simply allowing them to continue fermenting eventually reduces the bubbles to manageability, though sourness will become an issue. A quick stay in the fridge, from 30 minutes minimum up to 24 hours, can often dampen the deluge as well. But if you are still losing too much of your brew down the drain upon opening, try these steps to rein it in so more of the booch ends up in your belly.

### TOO MUCH FLAVORING

A little bit of flavoring in a bottle of kombucha goes a long way. As the yeast come back to life in second fermentation, they churn out lots of $CO_2$, and the more sugar they have to eat, the more bubbles they make. High-sugar flavoring agents such as fruits and rhizomes such as ginger usually provide a big burst of bubbles, so use them in small amounts. Use puréed fruit *very* sparingly.

### TOO MUCH YEAST

If the brew is yeasty, a large amount of yeast can get bottled with the brew, and this can cause eruptions or explosions. Consider filtering the brew at bottling time if this is a regular issue.

### TEMPERATURE TOO HIGH

Warmer temperatures in the second fermentation, especially above 85°F (29°C), lead to active, restless, extremely hungry yeast. Once they start eating the flavorings, the pressure builds.

### VINEGAR EELS

A side effect of these harmless-to-humans nematodes making it into the bottles is the increased potential for explosions as they eat the bacteria, allowing the yeast to thrive. If a bottle explodes for no obvious reason, check the brew for vinegar eels. (See Dealing with Vinegar Eels, page 173.)

# Rebalancing the Brew

As stewards for the kombucha brewing process, we are the keepers of the balance. While the bacteria and yeast work in symbiosis, they are also in competition. If a brew goes out of balance, usually the best option is to start fresh, whether that means you give it another go with the "problem" culture or start over with a new culture.

## Too Much Bacteria

Symptoms of too much bacteria include excessively thick SCOBYs with a brew that produces little carbonation and lacks depth of flavor or takes too long to sour. Here are a few tips to counterbalance the bacteria with a healthy yeast population.

### ADD YEASTY STARTER LIQUID

The fastest way to increase the yeast is to use starter liquid from the bottom of the brew, where yeast typically congregate.

### USE MORE TEA

Using more tea per batch and increasing the proportion of black tea if you're using a blend will also spur the yeast to reproduce more robustly.

### RAISE THE TEMPERATURE

Brew at 85°F (29°C), especially at the beginning of the fermentation process, to maximize yeast growth while minimizing — but not damaging — bacterial reproduction.

### STARVE THE YEAST

A little less sugar forces the yeast to be more efficient. This may seem counterintuitive, since we know that more sugar provides more fuel for the brew. But introducing sugar gradually, rather than all at once, allows the yeast to consume what is available without being overwhelmed, which leads to more active yeast and better balance. (See Add Sugar More Slowly, page 164.)

## Too Much Yeast

Struggling bacteria result in poor SCOBY growth and murky liquid teeming with extra yeast bodies. This can lead to a sour brew with off flavors. Here are some tips to minimize the yeast and rebuild the bacterial population.

### FILTER THE STARTER LIQUID

If the normal routine of using starter liquid from the top of the previous brew is not keeping yeast in check, filtering the starter liquid to further reduce the yeast content may help. Clean cheesecloth or a fine-mesh sieve should suffice.

### REDUCE THE TEMPERATURE

Maintaining the brew at the low end of the ideal kombucha range — around 75°F (24°C) — allows the bacteria to benefit as the yeast become less active.

### REDUCE FUEL FOR YEAST

To reduce the level of purines and caffeine, both of which stimulate the yeast, steep the tea for less time or blend in lighter teas such as white and green or even some herbals.

### INCREASE FUEL FOR BACTERIA

Substitute dextrose for 25 percent of the sugar. It is less sweet and will provide instant food for the bacteria, leading to a more balanced brew. Dextrose, available in powder form, is usually derived from corn.

## Starter Liquid Is Used Up

Sometimes you find yourself without starter liquid. Perhaps you bottled up every last drop of the brew? However it happened, there are a few ways to recover starter liquid and brew a new batch successfully.

### USE BOTTLED BREW

If you have some kombucha in bottles, "steal" some from the ones filled most recently. Unflavored is best, but if that is not available, select a fruity flavor or ginger flavor; avoid kombucha flavored with herbs that are rich with essential oils, coffee, strong spices, or other flavorings that could damage the culture.

### FILTER STARTER LIQUID FROM THE BOTTOM

If you still have the dregs from the bottom of the previous batch, they're likely filled with yeast clouds, thick, and murky, but you can try filtering this liquid and using it for your next batch. But remember to reserve starter from the top of that next batch to avoid using yeasty starter again.

### CREATE YOUR OWN

If you received a SCOBY without any liquid or somehow all the liquid has been lost, it may be possible to salvage it, provided the culture hasn't fully dehydrated. Place the SCOBY in a glass vessel with 1 to 2 cups of sweet tea and a teaspoon of distilled white vinegar. Cover with a cloth and let sit undisturbed for five to seven days. If a new SCOBY forms successfully, use both SCOBYs and all the liquid in the vessel to start a small batch, just a quart or half gallon, to slowly build up the strength of the liquid.

**Note:** We do not recommend substituting vinegar for starter liquid as some sources suggest. Using distilled vinegar will not assist the bacteria and yeast in reproducing, though it will help prevent mold in the very early stages. And using raw vinegar will contaminate the kombucha culture with the vinegar's own bacteria and yeast. If the SCOBY is weak or simply does not contain enough bacteria and yeast to reproduce, no amount of vinegar will help. If a SCOBY cannot produce 1 to 2 cups of strong starter liquid on its own, discard it in favor of a new SCOBY packed in strong starter liquid.

# Off Odors

Kombucha has a lovely aroma that is at once sweet and tart. Most people don't even notice the smell of their kombucha most of the time, but if a funky odor wafts out of the brewing vessel, it may be time to take a closer look. The cause is often with the yeast: lacking the right nutrients or conditions, they may become sick, leading to a variety of off smells and flavors. Once optimal brewing conditions are restored, these problems disappear quickly. Other times, simply leaving the brew alone will allow it to self-correct. Here are some of the ways sick yeast may show up.

## ODOR OF ACETONE

A smell similar to that of nail polish remover is usually created by ethyl acetate, an organic compound made up of acetic acid and ethanol. Typically this smell is a sign that the yeast are sick or don't have the right nutrition. Here are some of the contributing factors:

- Cohabitation by certain lager and other bottom-fermenting yeast strains
- Temperatures above the recommended range for kombucha
- Using raw honey, which has microorganisms that compete with the kombucha culture
- Lack of oxygen to kick-start the ferment

Toss the batch and start over with a SCOBY from your hotel.

## ODOR OF SULFUR

The smell of rotten eggs is generally a by-product of hydrogen sulfide production, believed to be overproduced by some yeast that have been exposed to extremely warm temperatures. The smell may or may not self-correct if given more time to ferment, but it can be worth trying if the temperature can be properly regulated.

The smell could also be due to sulfur-producing bacteria in the water (usually well water). In this case the odor does not reduce if the brew is given additional time, and it may intensify. Toss the batch, and for future batches, boil the water for 10 minutes before using it, filter it, or find another water source.

## ODOR OF VOMIT (BUTYRIC ACID)

This rare issue stems from bacterial overproduction of butyric acid (see appendix 1, page 358). (It's worth noting that bacteria that produce butyric acid are also found in the human gut — hence the acid's relationship to the smell of vomit.) This issue is not dangerous, despite its unappetizing smell. Fortunately, it is generally corrected by tossing the smelly brew and starting a new batch to let the acids balance out.

## SYRUPY OR VISCOUS BREW

This condition is rare. In the few cases we've come across, using a heater to maintain the proper temperature range normalized the brew within about a week. If the brew remains thick, there may be issues with yeast balance. If it doesn't self-correct with optimum conditions, pitch it and start over.

# Dealing with Fruit Flies

Fruit flies, also known as vinegar flies, *love* kombucha, and it's not uncommon for them to infest a SCOBY. They won't prevent fermentation, nor are they harmful to humans, but they are certainly unpleasant and icky (the larvae look like wiggly grains of rice).

### MILD INFESTATION

Gently remove the infested culture from your brew. Try not to let any of the larvae fall into the liquid. Rinse the culture in filtered water to remove the eggs and larvae. If necessary, filter the tea to remove any flies, eggs, or larvae that may have fallen in and restart the brew.

### SEVERE INFESTATION

Dispose of the infested cultures in the garbage, or compost and pour out the tea. Scrub the vessel to remove any residue. Restart the brew with a new culture. If there are several layers together, as in a CB, you may be able to dispose of the top layer with the eggs and retain the lower layers to continue the process forward.

## Make a Fruit-Fly Trap

There are plenty of more complicated methods of creating fruit fly traps that use items such as a paper cone or cut-up plastic bottle to improve the capture rate. Years of experiments have yielded the best results with this simple setup: a small dish of fermented kombucha with a drop of dish soap. The flies are lured by the tea, and dish soap breaks the surface tension of the water so that they fall in and can't escape. For best results, refresh after several flies have been captured.

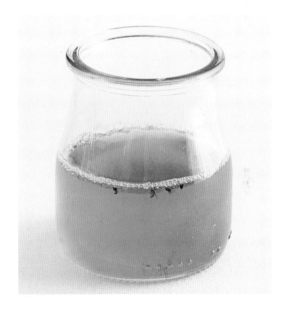

# Dealing with Mold

While intimidating and viscerally unpleasant, mold is actually a friend to the homebrewer, an easy-to-read sign that something is not right in the brewing environment or with the culture. Mold is extremely rare and easy to spot and is a blessing in disguise as it lets us know that the kombucha brew is not safe to drink and the SCOBY should be discarded. It looks exactly like the mold found on other rotting foodstuffs: it can be blue, black, or white, but most important, it is dry and fuzzy and located on top of the SCOBY, never under the surface of the liquid.

If mold occurs, the only appropriate action is to dispose of the entire batch — throw away the moldy new SCOBY growth, the mother SCOBY (even if no mold is present on the culture), and all the liquid. Start over with a fresh culture and starter liquid from your SCOBY Hotel. It is disheartening when this occurs, but before throwing the baby out with the kombucha, first confirm that what you're seeing is actually mold.

New brewers often mistake normal yet strange-looking SCOBY or yeast growth for mold. Brown yeast strands float in the liquid or embed in the SCOBY, causing dark spots that show through the translucent culture. Tea leaves sometimes remain in the liquid and get lodged in the SCOBY, causing bumps or spots. The culture grows unevenly, with lumps and wrinkles that may look unusual but are perfectly fine. (To learn more about healthy culture growth, see the Gallery of Healthy SCOBYs on page 43.)

## Causes of Mold

Mold spores are not visible to the human eye and can lie dormant or survive in extreme conditions. That is why you can't simply wash off a moldy SCOBY in water or vinegar; it won't remove the underlying culprits. Here are some conditions that may contribute to mold.

### COLD TEMPERATURES

Brewing below the optimal range of 75 to 85°F (24–29°C) causes the bacteria to become sluggish and prevents the batch from acidifying quickly enough to stop mold from developing.

### NOT ENOUGH CULTURE OR STARTER LIQUID

Skimping on SCOBY and starter liquid is one of the most common causes of mold, especially when it occurs in combination with cold temperatures. Without enough culture or starter, the brew is in a race against time to fully acidify before other organisms discover the food source.

### CONTAMINATED BREWING ENVIRONMENT

Perhaps mold is growing in the area around the brewing location. Some flowering houseplants release pollen that can carry native yeast and mold spores. Keep blooming plants

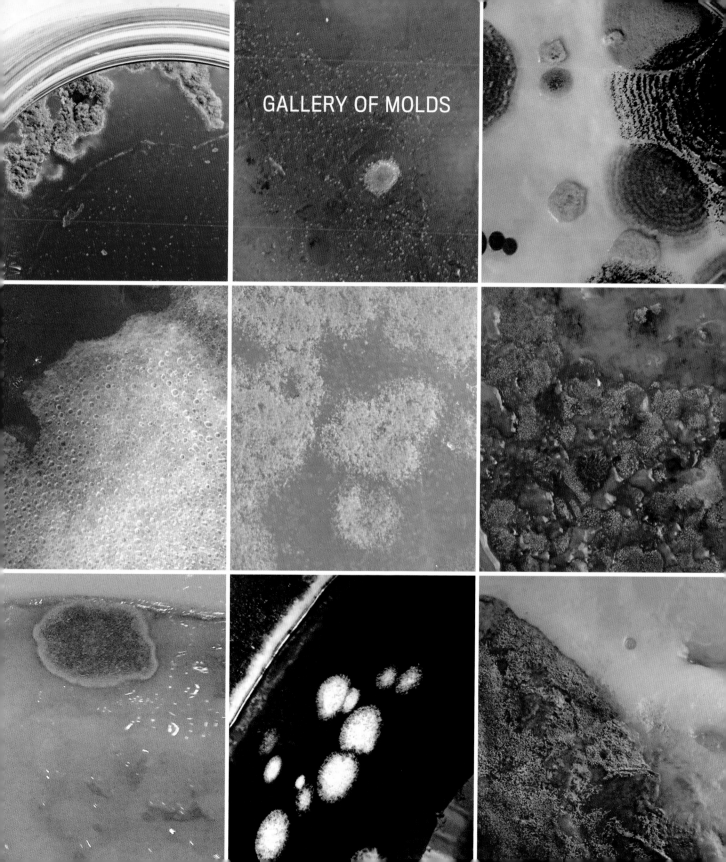

GALLERY OF MOLDS

at least 3 feet away from the brewing vessel and ideally in another room to prevent cross-contamination. (And note that even though it's not mold, cigarette smoke is another hazard that can kill cultures.)

### CONTAMINATED INGREDIENT

Tea, like any crop, may contain pesticides or other environmental residues that negatively affect the SCOBY. Water supplies can be tainted. Some sugars are simply not fermentable. If mold strikes, brew a fresh batch, adhering as closely to the original recipe and using the highest-quality ingredients as possible in order to eliminate likely culprits.

### EXCESSIVE HUMIDITY

Humidity fosters the growth of certain wild bacteria and yeast. Some of those are pathogenic to the kombucha culture and may lead to mold. If you are brewing in a tropical climate, use a fan to improve airflow around your brewing setup.

### COMPROMISED CULTURE

Refrigerated, frozen, or dehydrated SCOBYS do not brew well and can give rise to mold.

## Preventing Mold

It is rare for mold to develop in kombucha after the initial three or four days of fermentation, as the bacteria and yeast by that time have populated the brew thoroughly enough to keep invaders at bay. Therefore, it's critical to maintain optimum conditions during those first few days, when the culture is working to colonize the brew, to prevent pathogens from gaining a foothold. Starter liquid is the first line of defense: pour it on top of the SCOBY, and it acidifies the upper portion of the brew, protecting against mold and other contaminants. But there are other steps you can take:

- Use only mature starter liquid from your SCOBY Hotel or some very old kombucha. Young kombucha is not acidic enough to offer adequate protection.
- Use more starter liquid. Ten percent (total, by volume) is the minimum amount to use for protecting the brew. If the starter liquid is not as strong as desired, use more. In extreme cases, augment the starter with 1 to 2 tablespoons of distilled vinegar.
- Use a heating pad on the sides of the vessel. Many brewing problems can be solved by maintaining a temperature range of 75 to 85°F (24–29°C). Remember that 78 to 80°F (26–27°C) is the sweet spot.
- Maintain a clean environment. Keep houseplants in a separate room. Don't expose the brew to cigarette smoke.
- Improve airflow. Open the cupboard or move the brew to a countertop. Use a cloth cover made of cotton or other breathable material; avoid polyester and other synthetic fabrics.

# Dealing with Vinegar Eels

These nonparasitic nematodes (*Turbatrix aceti*) enjoy the highly acidified environment of vinegar and kombucha; many people discover vinegar eels infesting older bottles of raw apple cider vinegar. Though harmless to humans, they feed on kombucha cultures and destroy them. They are considered a blight in the vinegar industry and are eradicated by the use of sulfur dioxide or pasteurization. Imagine an unsuspecting brewer, acting on bad advice, adding raw apple cider vinegar to a kombucha brew to "help" it. Even worse, that person may then unwittingly pass infested SCOBYs and brew on to others.

Vinegar eels are the main reason that raw vinegar should never be used with kombucha. There is no way to save or disinfect a SCOBY that has vinegar eels. Everything must be thrown away, and all the equipment must be soaked in bleach before being used again.

## Signs of Vinegar Eels

- New SCOBY will not completely form.
- White, chalky residue (from nematode eggs) appears on the sides of the vessel.
- SCOBYs have a "dead" appearance and float strangely in the brew.
- Yeast proliferate excessively as the bacteria are decimated.
- The brew remains sweet even after weeks of brewing as the acetic acid is consumed by the eels.

## Checking for Vinegar Eels

Vinegar eels are extremely rare, but here's how to inspect your kombucha if you suspect their presence.

1. Remove a few ounces of kombucha from the top of the brewing vessel into a clear glass cup.

2. Hold the vessel up to a bright light.

3. Wipe the very edge of the liquid with a finger to remove any carbonation bubbles.

4. Look at the meniscus (the spot where the top surface of the liquid clings to the edge of the vessel). Yeast particles float but do not move of their own accord. Vinegar eels, however, will be moving

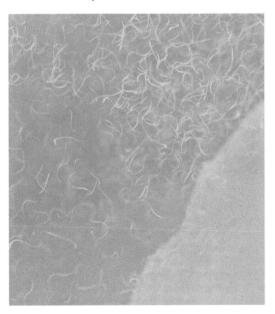

independently of the motion of the liquid. Hold the cup as still as possible to detect any movement of the pale nematodes. A bad infestation will be immediately obvious, but one that has just begun may take a little more patience to spot.

### GETTING RID OF VINEGAR EELS

1. Dump all SCOBYs, starter liquid, and kombucha from the infected batch immediately.

2. If you're using a vessel with spigot, remove the spigot, clean it thoroughly, and then soak it in a 10 percent bleach solution for 24 hours. Scrub the vessel itself with a bleach solution or another heavy-duty cleanser to remove all traces of eels, which may live in the seams of the vessel. Rinse all brewing items thoroughly and let air-dry for 24 hours.

3. Start over with confirmed clean starter liquid and SCOBY.

**A KOMBUCHA LEGEND:**
## Genghis Khan's Soldiers

Some claim that a vinegary fermented drink filled the flasks of Genghis Khan and his traveling armies. The nomadic nature of the Mongols meant that they were accustomed to extended periods of subsistence on a diet of milk, meat, and various ferments. The drink may have been koumiss (fermented mare's milk), kombucha, or some other ancient beverage.

By the way, Genghis Khan's armies are also credited with inventing barbecue, hamburgers (called steak tartare by the Russians), and hot pot, a staple of Chinese cuisine. Just as SCOBYs reproduce like mad, so too did Genghis Khan — some 16 million people are purported to be descendents of his.

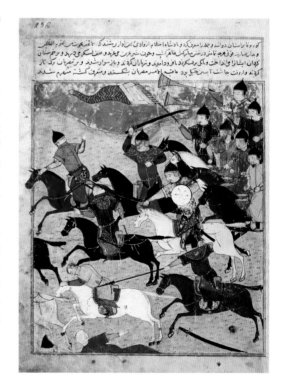

# Testing Tools and Protocols

Testing your brew for compliance with various parameters can be useful and fun, whether you are just learning the ways of fermentation or developing into a serious hobbyist. Of course many homebrewers make successful batches for years without testing, but as they learn more, many yearn to understand the brew more completely.

Those brewing larger batches or many batches at once, especially commercial brewers, may use testing to develop certain metrics and standards. Others simply want to know more about the contents of their specific brew. Here are the primary tools available for testing kombucha and what they can help you accomplish, as well as their limitations.

## Testing for Consistency

### pH STRIPS AND METER

The pH of kombucha can be checked (and should be if mold develops) to confirm that the brew is progressing safely. The simplest method is to use pH strips made of litmus paper, which changes color when it reacts with the acids in a solution (in this case, a drop of kombucha). Use strips specifically designed to measure a pH of 0 to 6; this yields a higher degree of accuracy than using broad-range pH strips. For those who want to track their pH more finely, a pH meter can give a reading to at least a tenth of a decimal.

While pH alone does not indicate that fermentation is complete, we can pair that knowledge with other factors such as the length of the fermentation cycle, time of year, taste, and Brix (estimated sugar levels) to develop metrics to consistently produce brews that have our preferred characteristics.

For example, a brew that has been fermented for 7 days and has a pH of 3.2 may taste better to you than a brew that has been fermented for 14 days and has a pH of 2.8. Tasting and testing the pH frequently and logging the readings will lead to a deeper appreciation of the pH value and what information it provides.

### REFRACTOMETER

Commonly used in the beer and wine industries, a refractometer reads changes in light waves as they pass through a solution (the refractive index). To obtain a Brix reading that enables you to estimate the sugar or alcohol content of a beverage, you can either add a few drops to a manual refractometer and hold it up to the light or test a sample in a digital refractometer with an LED. This produces a Brix reading that is used to estimate the sugar or alcohol content.

Although kombucha brewers can use this information to help determine the right time for bottling (or it could be useful for those needing to monitor sugar intake), the estimates provided by refractometers for both alcohol and sugar in kombucha must always be adjusted down. This is because kombucha contains bacteria that transform ethanol into organic acids, and because other residual solids present (such as yeast and bacterial cellulose) will skew density readings higher.

Without expensive lab testing, it is impossible to know for sure, but average alcohol estimates for kombucha are about double (so follow the formula provided by the manufacturer, and then divide the end result by two). Sugar estimates skew 25 to 50 percent high, and of course the device cannot provide any information as to the percentages of sucrose, fructose, and glucose, all of which have very different effects on the body.

Still, a refractometer is a useful tool for the brewing professional who knows specific readings to look for in conjunction with other testing tools and lab sample confirmations. It is relatively inexpensive, requires just a few drops to get a reading, and is very easy to use.

### HYDROMETER

By means of a graduated cylinder filled with the desired liquid and a weighted bulb that settles at a density reading, a hydrometer measures the specific gravity (relative density) of a solution. Readings taken before and after fermentation can be compared to estimate how much sugar has been converted into alcohol.

But as with a refractometer, because kombucha is a symbiotic ferment, this device cannot properly account for the conversion of ethanol into healthy acids by the bacteria. Moreover, when dealing with very low amounts of alcohol (anything under 3% ABV), it is extremely tricky to obtain an accurate reading as reproducing yeast, dissolved solids, and other particulates contribute to density. Another potential drawback for this method is

the amount of liquid needed to fill the cylinder for each reading.

Again, Brix readings tend to skew 25 to 50 percent higher than actual sugar content. To get a ballpark figure of the potential alcohol content, measure the specific gravity of the sweet tea solution; then measure again after the fermentation process is complete. Apply the formula provided with your particular unit and divide by two.

### TITRATABLE ACIDITY

When balanced with minerals, sugar, and trace amounts of alcohol, the acids in kombucha represent the most prevalent and unique part of the flavor profile. The ones that contribute most to the flavor include acetic, gluconic, malic, and tartaric.

Whether the goal is a sweeter brew, a balanced sweet-sour brew, or a more mature, vinegar-forward brew, titratable acidity (in conjunction with taste buds of course!) gives the professional brewer a specific metric for estimating that flavor balance. This advanced technique is rarely used by homebrewers, but home testing kits intended for wine are available.

### DNA SEQUENCING

DNA sequencing can provide an in-depth peek into the brew to help brewers understand the amazing microbial diversity of their kombucha. Older technologies were significantly more costly and involved isolating organisms on plates, then using a formula to guess at the number of organisms that would be present in the actual sample. With recent improvements in testing technology, prices for DNA sequencing have come down and offer far more precise results. This testing method identifies the actual organisms in the sample, counting them until it can determine with confidence their identity and percentage present. This complex testing must be completed at a lab.

## Testing for Alcohol

A trace amount of alcohol is a normal by-product of every fermentation process. In unflavored kombucha, that amount is typically between 0.2 and 1.0% ABV, similar to that of unpasteurized fruit juice. In the secondary fermentation stage, it is possible for the alcohol level to temporarily increase if sugar is added and the bottle is capped, but because the bacteria consume the ethanol, converting it to acids, the amount of alcohol produced by kombucha is self-limiting and is never inebriating, and over time the low levels will go down again.

As mentioned above, a hydrometer or refractometer may be used to estimate the potential alcohol content of the brew, but for more precise readings, lab testing is required.

### COMMERCIAL TESTING METHODS

Commercial brewers selling nonalcoholic kombucha must conduct testing as part of their quality control procedures as well as to ensure compliance with federal labeling laws. All types of methods may be used for estimating those tests in-house, from the most basic hydrometer to very expensive machines that can test wine and beer samples at the touch of a button. But all these methods come up against the same problem — using the density of the liquid to estimate the alcohol present. Those organic acids, and the bacteria that continue to produce them from ethanol, throw off even the pricey equipment, requiring adjustments. Moreover, the high degree of sediment in kombucha can also throw off the readings.

For accurate, repeatable ethanol testing, very sophisticated lab testing must be employed. Analytical chemists and other experts working closely with kombucha have confirmed that it is more complicated to test than ferments like beer and wine. And because the amounts of alcohol in kombucha are already so low, the testing process becomes even more difficult.

While beer and wine scientists have honed their methods for hundreds of years, kombucha scientists have only just begun. At present, the most viable method requires measuring the ethanol present in the airspace between the liquid and the cap inside the bottle, called headspace gas chromatography, which can only be done by a lab. Gas chromatography (GC) is the method used to detect blood alcohol levels for toxicology reports, and is considered to be accurate to plus or minus 0.1 percent.

While homebrewers never need to be concerned about the naturally low levels of alcohol as they are not selling their brew, for commercial brewers offering a product that can naturally range from 0.2 to 1.0% ABV (0.5% ABV and higher is considered an alcoholic beverage according to federal law), there is little room for error. Developing a proper testing standard for kombucha's particular challenges is an important and natural step in progress from folk remedy to international beverage industry.

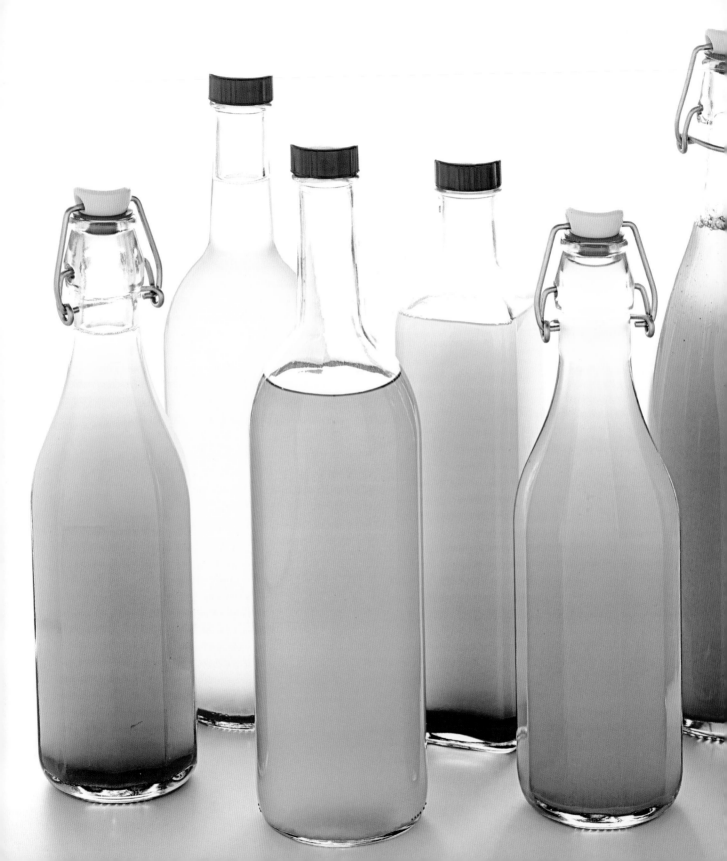

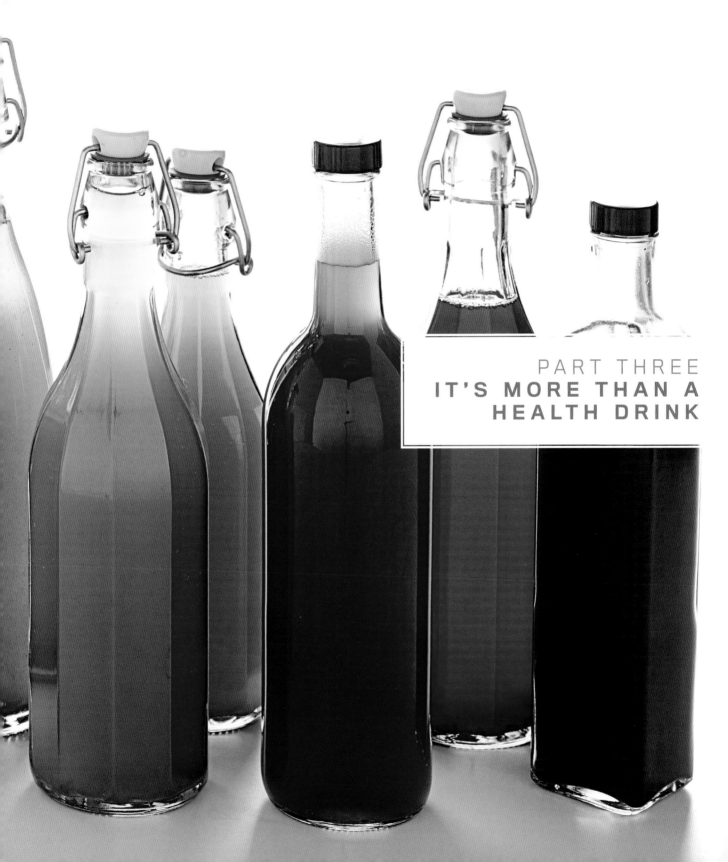

PART THREE
# IT'S MORE THAN A HEALTH DRINK

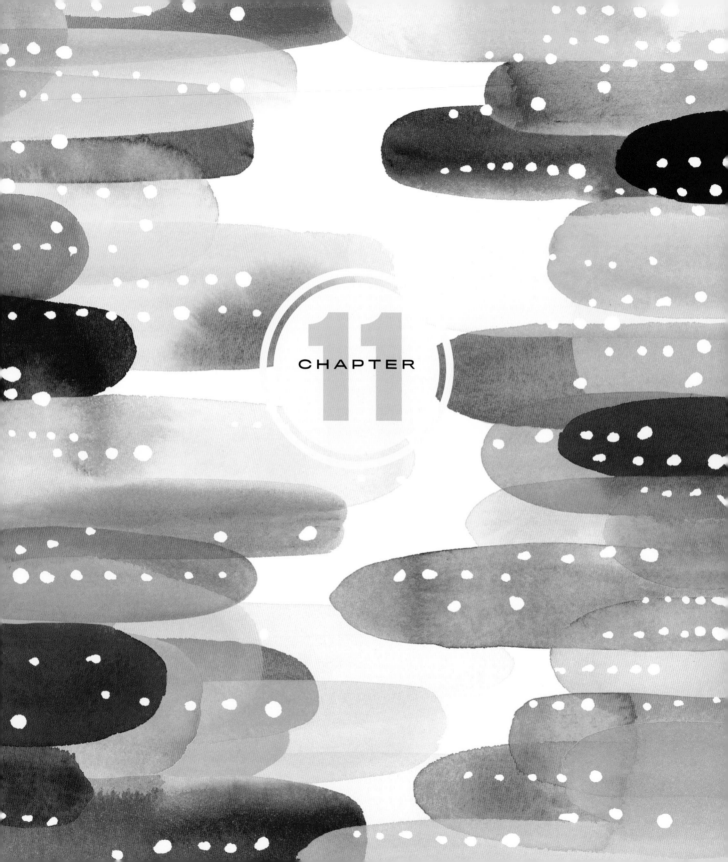

CHAPTER 11

# Flavor Inspirations

Plain kombucha has a lovely taste, but flavoring the brew is one of the most fun and creative parts of the process. Also, kombucha extracts flavonoids and vitamins from the flavoring agent and passes all that good stuff on to you. From mildly astringent to lip puckering, sweet to savory, and mild to wild, you can achieve nearly any flavor of kombucha with a little imagination. These suggestions are merely a jumping-off point, so feel free to experiment. We've tried every single one of these, and we're sure there is a flavor to please every palate!

With kombucha, a little bit of flavoring goes a long way — typically 5 percent or less of the bottle's capacity is a good amount. Surface area also plays a role in how intensely or subtly the flavor is expressed. The smaller the pieces of flavoring, the more surface area, and the easier it is for the fermentation process to break down the flavoring agents. Fruit purées and juices, along with powdered herbs and spices, are the flavoring mediums with the most surface area, so reduce the amount used or open those bottles with caution as brews can become quite carbonated.

We prefer to use fresh pieces of fruit and fresh herbs as much as possible, giving them a rough chop or tearing them to allow the plant phenols to enter the brew.

Flavors are grouped by the dominant ingredient (Fruit [page 182], Herbals [page 196], Superfoods [page 206], Savory [page 211], and Medicinal [page 216]), with measurements given for both 16 ounces and 1 gallon. Many of the suggestions mix a bit of this and a little of that, so check for various ingredients by name. These are intended to be tweaked to your personal preference — use the Brew Minder Log (page 371) to keep notes on which flavors you and your family like best!

# FRUIT

## *Apple*

The versatile apple is a fantastic flavor match for kombucha. We use fresh apples, skin on, cored, and diced, but there are many other options. If using applesauce with added sugar, add half the amount recommended for fresh fruit. Use juice sparingly to achieve a delightful apple flavor without too much sourness.

### Apple Melon

**APPLE JUICE**
2 tablespoons / ¼ cup

**WATERMELON, CHOPPED**
2 tablespoons / ¾ cup

### Apple Pie

**APPLE, DICED**
¼ cup / 1 cup

**CHAI SPICE BLEND (PAGE 197)**
½ teaspoon / 1 tablespoon

## Master Cleanse

*(inspired by the Master Cleanse Lemonade Diet popularized by Stanley Burroughs)*

**APPLE, DICED**
¼ cup / 1 cup

**MAPLE SYRUP, GRADE B**
2 teaspoons / 2 tablespoons

**LEMON ZEST**
⅛ teaspoon / 1 teaspoon

**CAYENNE**
1 pinch / ¼ teaspoon

## *Apricot*

We prefer fresh produce, but nectar and dried apricots are also terrific. More sugar in those products means using less to achieve the desired flavor.

*Amar al-dīn* is a traditional Egyptian drink served during Ramadan to mark the break from fasting.

## Apricot

*Use any one of these options:*

**FRESH APRICOT, DICED**
¼ cup / 1 cup

**APRICOT NECTAR**
1 tablespoon / ½ cup

**DRIED APRICOT, DICED**
1 tablespoon / ½ cup

### Amar Al-Dīn

**DRIED APRICOT, DICED**
1 tablespoon / ½ cup

**HONEY**
1 teaspoon / 1 tablespoon

### Apricot Rose

**FRESH APRICOT, DICED**
¼ cup / 1 cup

**ROSE PETALS, DRIED**
1 tablespoon / ¼ cup

### Take It Easy

A little bit of flavoring goes a long way. A tablespoon of fruit or a pinch of herb may be all that is needed. Keep in mind that the smaller the surface area, the more flavor — juice packs the most concentrated flavor, while a rough chop of fruit imparts a more delicate aroma. Jam, jelly, and juice all work fine, but we prefer to use fresh fruit. (See Using Frozen Fruit, page 184.)

Quantities listed are for 16 ounces / 1 gallon

# Banana

Bananas give kombucha a subtle sweetness that's both recognizable and hard to place. The riper the banana, the more sweetness and carbonation it will add. Dried bananas are bland — stick with fresh for the best flavor. Use them alone, mix it up, or rock out with the Elvis Special ("Uh-huh, thank you, thank you very much!").

## Strawberry Banana

**BANANA, MASHED**
2 tablespoons / ½ cup

**STRAWBERRY JAM**
1 tablespoon / ¼ cup

## Choco-Banana

**BANANA, MASHED**
2 tablespoons / ½ cup

**RAW CACAO POWDER**
1 teaspoon / 1 tablespoon

## Elvis Special

**BANANA, MASHED**
2 tablespoons / ½ cup

**PEANUT BUTTER**
1 teaspoon / 2 tablespoons

# Blackberry

High in vitamins C and K, blackberries impart a gorgeous color along with a nutritional punch. Try mellowing the tart bite of the berry with some fresh sage.

## Wise Berry

**BLACKBERRIES, QUARTERED**
2 tablespoons / ¾ cup

**FRESH SAGE, ROUGHLY CHOPPED**
1 leaf / 4 leaves

## Berry Medley

**BLACKBERRIES, QUARTERED**
1 tablespoon / ½ cup

**RASPBERRIES, LIGHTLY MASHED**
2 teaspoons / ¼ cup

**STRAWBERRIES, CHOPPED**
2 teaspoons / ¼ cup

## Midnight Fire

**BLACKBERRIES, QUARTERED**
2 tablespoons / ¾ cup

**FRESH GINGER, DICED**
1 teaspoon / 1 tablespoon

# Blood Orange

Blood oranges are a wonderful complement to kombucha. Naturally sweet, their beautiful purple flesh is an unmistakable mutation that has afforded them a special place in the hearts of citrus lovers everywhere. First discovered in Italy, these delicious fruits add a twist of the exotic.

## Blood Orange Italian Soda

**BLOOD ORANGE JUICE**
1 tablespoon / ¼ cup

**FRESH SAGE, ROUGHLY CHOPPED**
2 leaves / 4 leaves

**FRESH THYME**
1 sprig / 2 sprigs

## Rock the Casbah

**BLOOD ORANGE JUICE**
1 tablespoon / ¼ cup

**FRESH GINGER, DICED**
½ teaspoon / 1 teaspoon

**CLOVES, WHOLE**
¼ teaspoon / ½ teaspoon

## Citrus Mist

**BLOOD ORANGE ZEST**
¼ teaspoon / 1 teaspoon

**LEMON ZEST**
¼ teaspoon / 1 teaspoon

**GRAPEFRUIT ZEST**
¼ teaspoon / 1 teaspoon

## Juice vs. Zest

Some citrus fruits are easier to enjoy than others depending on how sour or bitter they are. Many of the suggestions here call for the juice of a particular fruit, which adds more sugar and therefore tends to produce a stronger flavor. If the flavor created by using juice is too overpowering, try using just the zest in your next batch. The zest, or grated peel, is where the essential oils reside, imparting a lovely floral/citrus flavor. Use just the colored part of the peel, not the white pith, which is quite bitter.

Quantities listed are for 16 ounces / 1 gallon

# Blueberry

Small but mighty, this tiny fruit deserves its reputation as a superfood. It gives kombucha a nice tart punch-up and a deep purple hue. Love Potion 99 is Hannah's favorite flavor: the rose and lavender lend lovely floral notes that perfectly balance the berries.

## Love Potion 99

**BLUEBERRIES, HALVED**
¼ cup / 1 cup
**ROSE PETALS, FRESH OR DRIED**
½ teaspoon / ¼ cup
**LAVENDER, FRESH OR DRIED**
⅛ teaspoon / ⅛ cup

## Holy Boly

**BLUEBERRIES, HALVED**
2 tablespoons / ¾ cup
**HOLY BASIL (TULSI)**
⅛ teaspoon / ½ teaspoon

## Blue Apple

**BLUEBERRIES, HALVED**
1 tablespoon / ¼ cup
**APPLE, DICED**
⅛ cup / ¾ cup

# Cherry

High levels of antioxidants and anti-inflammatory agents make this delicious little fruit an excellent flavoring option. Bings and maraschinos will provide a sweeter flavor, but tart cherries like morellos can also be used. Add a pinch of sugar to balance the tartness and boost carbonation.

## Cherry Up

**CHERRIES, HALVED**
1 tablespoon / ½ cup

## Cherry Cream Soda

**CHERRIES, HALVED**
1 tablespoon / ½ cup
**WHOLE VANILLA BEAN, SLICED**
¼ bean / ¾ bean
**HONEY**
½ teaspoon / 1 tablespoon

## Super C

**CHERRIES, HALVED**
1 teaspoon / ½ cup
**DRIED, SWEETENED CRANBERRIES, CHOPPED**
1 teaspoon / ¼ cup
**ROSE HIPS, DRIED**
1 teaspoon / 1 tablespoon

# Cranberry

This naturally antibacterial fruit is packed with fiber, full of vitamins C and E, and bursting with antioxidants. The Pilgrims, who learned about it from Native Americans, called it *craneberry* because the small, pink blossoms resemble the head and bill of a Sandhill crane.

Dried, sweetened cranberries are the best choice for kombucha as the sweetness balances the tartness. Use fresh cranberries in Cranberry Citrus Spice for a truly lip-puckering flavor sensation.

## Cran-bucha

**DRIED, SWEETENED CRANBERRIES, CHOPPED**
2 teaspoons / 2 tablespoons

## Cranberry Citrus Spice

**DRIED, SWEETENED CRANBERRIES, CHOPPED**
2 teaspoons / 2 tablespoons
**FRESH ORANGE JUICE**
1 tablespoon / ¼ cup
**CLOVES, GROUND**
⅛ teaspoon / ½ teaspoon

## Cran-banapple

**DRIED, SWEETENED CRANBERRIES, CHOPPED**
2 teaspoons / 2 tablespoons
**BANANA, MASHED**
1 teaspoon / 1 tablespoon
**APPLE, DICED**
1 tablespoon / ¼ cup

## Using Frozen Fruit

Fruit tastes best when it is in season, but the growing season is short, and our desire for blueberry kombucha might be a year-round phenomenon. Don't fret — frozen fruit to the rescue! Simply add it directly to the kombucha; if you let it thaw first, it will be easy to mash or cut up.

Quantities listed are for 16 ounces / 1 gallon

# Date

The date palm, its fruit rich in a variety of vitamins, is as ancient as humankind. According to an Arabic legend, God molded man from the earth, and then created the date palm from the remaining material and placed it in the garden of paradise. Naturally sweet, dates add terrific carbonation and a lovely tang. Allow a bottle to ferment longer for a unique vinegar.

## Inun-date

**DATES, CHOPPED**
1 tablespoon / ¼ cup

## Hot Date

**DATES, CHOPPED**
1 tablespoon / ¼ cup

**CAYENNE**
⅛ teaspoon / 1 teaspoon

## Turkish Coffee

**DATES, CHOPPED**
1 tablespoon / ¼ cup

**BREWED COFFEE**
1 tablespoon / ½ cup

**CARDAMOM, GROUND**
⅛ teaspoon / 2 teaspoons

**CLOVES, GROUND**
⅛ teaspoon / 2 teaspoons

# Elderberry

For centuries the elderberry was known as "the medicine chest of the country people" because it was used to cure just about everything! We use dried elderberries, but elderberry syrup can also be used. If using syrup, divide the amount in half, and eliminate any additional sugar as the syrup has enough to make a fizzy brew.

## Black Beauty

**DRIED ELDERBERRIES**
½ teaspoon / 1 tablespoon

**SUGAR**
¼ teaspoon / 1 teaspoon

## Cold Fighter

**DRIED ELDERBERRIES**
½ teaspoon / 1 tablespoon

**FRESH GINGER, DICED**
½ teaspoon / 1 tablespoon

**LEMON ZEST**
¼ teaspoon / 1 teaspoon

## Berry Mint

**DRIED ELDERBERRIES**
½ teaspoon / 1 tablespoon

**FRESH MINT, ROUGHLY CHOPPED**
½ teaspoon / 2 teaspoons

**FRESH SAGE, ROUGHLY CHOPPED**
½ teaspoon / 2 teaspoons

# Fig

A good source of fiber, iron, and calcium, figs were one of the first foods ever cultivated by humans. These recipes call for dried figs, which are usually easier to come by. If using fresh, double the amount to yield a similar flavor.

## Spiced Fig

**DRIED FIGS, CHOPPED**
2 tablespoons / ¼ cup

**BLACK PEPPER**
⅛ teaspoon / ¾ teaspoon

**WHOLE VANILLA BEAN, SLICED**
¼ bean / ¾ bean

## Fig Leaf

**DRIED FIGS, CHOPPED**
2 tablespoons / ¼ cup

**FRESH BASIL, ROUGHLY CHOPPED**
½ teaspoon / 1 tablespoon

## Fig 'n' Pig

**DRIED FIGS, CHOPPED**
2 tablespoons / ¼ cup

**BACON, COOKED AND CRUMBLED**
1 tablespoon / 4 tablespoons

Quantities listed are for 16 ounces / 1 gallon

# Grape

Grapes, which were considered a medicine rather than a food in ancient times, boost the nutritional value of kombucha, as well as adding major fizz and packing a tangy, grape-soda punch.

## Full Concord

**CONCORD GRAPE JUICE**
2 tablespoons / ½ cup

## Mediterranean Delight

**RED GRAPES, SLICED**
2 tablespoons / ½ cup
**FIGS, CHOPPED**
1 tablespoon / ¼ cup
**BALSAMIC VINEGAR**
½ teaspoon / 1 tablespoon

## Thinker's Punch

**RED GRAPES, SLICED**
2 tablespoons / ½ cup
**BRAIN BREW BLEND (PAGE 196)**
¼ teaspoon / 1 teaspoon

# Grapefruit

What happens when you add notoriously sour grapefruit to already tart kombucha? Perhaps surprisingly, the flavors complement each other to create citrusy, floral notes. We prefer Ruby Reds as they have a naturally sweeter taste that pairs nicely with herbs and other botanicals for a refreshing second ferment. Juice may be used if fresh fruit is not available; strain out the pulp to prevent bitterness.

## Ruby Sage

**RUBY RED GRAPEFRUIT JUICE**
2 tablespoons / ½ cup
**FRESH SAGE, ROUGHLY CHOPPED**
½ teaspoon / 2 teaspoons

## Grapefruit Elderflower

**RUBY RED GRAPEFRUIT JUICE**
2 tablespoons / ⅓ cup
**DRIED ELDERFLOWER BLOSSOMS**
½ teaspoon / 2 teaspoons

## Ruby Root Punch

**RUBY RED GRAPEFRUIT JUICE**
2 tablespoons / ½ cup
**FRESH GINGER, DICED**
⅛ teaspoon / 1 teaspoon
**HIBISCUS PETALS, DRIED**
⅛ teaspoon / 1 teaspoon

# Guava

Guava fruits contain more vitamin C than oranges and are a good source of copper as well as vitamins $B_3$ (niacin) and $B_6$. Guava nectar is thick and sweet. If using fresh guava fruit, double the amount called for and add a pinch of sugar.

## Pure Guava

**GUAVA NECTAR**
1 tablespoon / ¼ cup

## Tropical Delight

**GUAVA NECTAR**
2 teaspoons / ¼ cup
**PINEAPPLE JUICE**
1 teaspoon / ⅛ cup
**PAPAYA NECTAR**
1 teaspoon / ⅛ cup

## Guava-nut

**GUAVA NECTAR**
2 teaspoons / ¼ cup
**COCONUT WATER**
1 tablespoon / ½ cup

## Keep It Whole

Others may prefer to use juice, purées, essential oils, or other flavoring agents, but we feel that whole fruit and herbs allow the kombucha to extract maximum nutrition, though the flavor may be more subtle. Play with different forms to find what works best for your palate.

Quantities listed are for 16 ounces / 1 gallon

LOVE potion 99

pink LEMONADE

ROCK the CASBAH

KUMQUAT

BUDDHA'S Delight

Super C

APPLE pie

Elderberry

# Honeydew

The sweet flavor of the honeydew makes for a light note in the kombucha, while the fruit itself is rich in folate, potassium, and vitamins C and B$_6$.

## All in Dew Thyme

**HONEYDEW, DICED**
2 tablespoons / ¾ cup

**FRESH THYME**
1 sprig / 2 sprigs

## Honey Tang

**HONEYDEW, DICED**
2 tablespoons / ¾ cup

**FRESH TANGERINE JUICE**
2 tablespoons / ¼ cup

## Melon-riffic

**HONEYDEW, DICED**
1 tablespoon / ¼ cup

**WATERMELON, CHOPPED**
1 tablespoon / ¼ cup

**CANTALOUPE, DICED**
1 tablespoon / ¼ cup

# Kiwi

Full of vitamin C and potassium, kiwi kombucha is powerful in both flavor and nutrition. Remove the fuzzy skin but don't strain the seeds; they are full of vitamin A. Use dried kiwi in half the amounts called for.

## Kiwi Berry

**KIWI, PEELED AND CHOPPED**
2 tablespoons / ¾ cup

**BLACKBERRIES, QUARTERED**
2 tablespoons / ¾ cup

## Peach Fuzz

**KIWI, PEELED AND CHOPPED**
2 tablespoons / ¾ cup

**PEACH, PEELED AND DICED**
2 tablespoons / ½ cup

## Green Goddess

**KIWI, PEELED AND CHOPPED**
2 tablespoons / ¾ cup

**FRESH MINT, ROUGHLY CHOPPED**
1 teaspoon / 1 tablespoon

**CARDAMOM, GROUND**
⅛ teaspoon / 1 teaspoon

# Kumquat

Originally considered part of the citrus family, kumquats were reclassified to their own genus, *Fortunella*, in 1915. They are high in vitamin C, fiber, calcium, potassium, and iron. Like nature's "Sour Patch Kid," kumquats are an inside-out citrus with sour flesh and a sweet rind.

## Golden Good Fortune

**KUMQUAT RIND OR ZEST**
1 rind / 3 rinds

**DRIED THYME**
½ teaspoon / 2 teaspoons

## Kumquat Persimmon

**KUMQUAT RIND OR ZEST**
1 rind / 3 rinds

**PERSIMMON, DICED**
2 teaspoons / ¼ cup

## Plumquat

**KUMQUAT RIND OR ZEST**
1 rind / 3 rinds

**PLUM, DICED**
2 teaspoons / ¼ cup

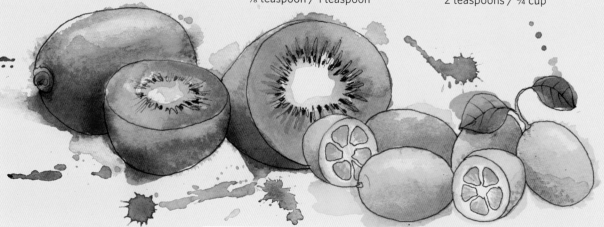

Quantities listed are for 16 ounces / 1 gallon

# Lemon

The lemon, in all its various forms, may be the most commonly consumed fruit flavor in the world. We like to use the juice and zest for kombucha; the pith is extremely bitter. For more lemon flavor, use the juice; for a lighter citrus hint, the zest is best. We like to combine lemon with other herbs for unique, subtle bursts of flavor that tantalize the tongue. Meyer lemons offer the sweetest flavor and are our go-to version in the following recipes.

## Lemon Basil

**FRESH LEMON JUICE**
2 tablespoons / ¾ cup

**FRESH BASIL, ROUGHLY CHOPPED**
2 teaspoons / ¼ cup

## Lemon Zing

**FRESH LEMON JUICE**
1 tablespoon / ¼ cup

**FRESH GINGER, DICED**
½ teaspoon / 2 teaspoons

**LEMON ZEST**
¼ teaspoon / 1 teaspoon

## Lavender Lemonade

**LEMON ZEST**
½ teaspoon / 2 teaspoons

**DRIED LAVENDER FLOWERS**
¼ teaspoon / 1 teaspoon

# Lime

Lime is the lemon's sweeter, greener cousin. Packed with the awesome superpowers of all citrus fruits, lime can be found in everything from food and drink to beauty and health-care products. The zest and juice provide a burst of citrus with a hint of floral that is the perfect backdrop to ingredients both exotic and mundane for a refreshing kombucha brew.

## Lime in the Coconut

**FRESH LIME JUICE**
1 teaspoon / 1 tablespoon

**COCONUT WATER**
4 tablespoons / ¼ cup

## Berry Cherry Lime

**FRESH LIME JUICE**
1 teaspoon / 1 tablespoon

**BLUEBERRIES, HALVED**
2 teaspoons / ¼ cup

**CHERRIES, HALVED**
2 teaspoons / ¼ cup

## Limeade

**LIME ZEST**
½ teaspoon / 2 teaspoons

**HONEY**
1 teaspoon / 1 tablespoon

# Lychee

A tropical fruit tree native to southern China, the lychee contains an abundance of oligonol, which is thought to have antioxidant and anti-influenza actions. The firm flesh has a grapelike texture and even sweeter taste that imbues a lightly floral fragrance into the kombucha. Fresh ones are typically available in the United States only at Asian markets and some farmers' markets. We use the canned variety, which is often packed in a sweet syrup that may be used to sweeten a glass of kombucha or for making a shrub (see page 236).

## Lychee Love

**LYCHEE FRUIT, DICED**
1 tablespoon / ¼ cup

**LYCHEE JUICE**
1 teaspoon / 1 tablespoon

## China Punch

**LYCHEE FRUIT, DICED**
1 tablespoon / ¼ cup

**BANANA, MASHED**
1 teaspoon / 1 tablespoon

**PINEAPPLE, DICED**
1 teaspoon / 1 tablespoon

## Lychee Rose

**LYCHEE FRUIT, DICED**
1 tablespoon / ¼ cup

**ROSEWATER**
1 teaspoon / ⅛ cup

Quantities listed are for 16 ounces / 1 gallon

# Mango

Best used fresh or frozen, mango adds color and luscious flavor. Dried mango or juice is okay, but use about half the amount called for to balance the extra sugar.

## Buddha's Delight

**MANGO, DICED**
¼ cup / ¾ cup

## Heart Fire

**MANGO, DICED**
¼ cup / ¾ cup

**CAYENNE**
2 pinches / ½ teaspoon

## Mango Spice

**MANGO, DICED**
¼ cup / ¾ cup

**WHOLE VANILLA BEAN, SLICED**
¼ bean / 1 whole bean

**CINNAMON BARK CHIPS**
1 teaspoon / 1 tablespoon

# Orange

Freshly squeezed orange juice marries beautifully with kombucha, and a touch of rind imparts a floral essence. Store-bought is acceptable (use pulp-free). To use fresh fruit, chop segments into pieces and double the amount called for.

## Oranjulius

**FRESH ORANGE JUICE**
1 tablespoon / ¼ cup

**WHOLE VANILLA BEAN, SLICED**
¼ bean / 1 whole bean

## Dreamy Orange

**FRESH ORANGE JUICE**
1 tablespoon / ¼ cup

**WHOLE VANILLA BEAN, SLICED**
¼ bean / 1 whole bean

**HONEY**
1 teaspoon / 1 tablespoon

## Mint Squeeze

**FRESH ORANGE JUICE**
1 tablespoon / ¼ cup

**FRESH MINT, ROUGHLY CHOPPED**
1 teaspoon / 1 tablespoon

# Papaya

This luscious, musky native of the New World contains tons of vitamin C along with plenty of carotenoids, folate, and dietary fiber. Use ripe fruit that is buttery in texture rather than mealy. Green papaya, used in Asian cooking, doesn't offer enough flavor and is not recommended. If fresh papaya is unavailable, use frozen or dried fruit.

## Banana Papaya

**PAPAYA, FRESH OR FROZEN, DICED**
1 tablespoon / ½ cup

**BANANA, MASHED**
2 teaspoons / ¼ cup

**CINNAMON BARK CHIPS**
¼ teaspoon / 1 tablespoon

## P3

**PAPAYA, FRESH OR FROZEN, DICED**
1 tablespoon / ½ cup

**PINEAPPLE JUICE**
2 teaspoons / ⅛ cup

**CAYENNE**
⅛ teaspoon / ½ teaspoon

## Pop-aya

**PAPAYA, FRESH OR FROZEN, DICED**
1 tablespoon / ½ cup

**SPINACH, CHOPPED**
1 teaspoon / ⅛ cup

**FRESH GINGER, DICED**
¼ teaspoon / 1 tablespoon

Quantities listed are for 16 ounces / 1 gallon

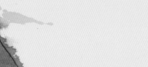

# Passion Fruit

This sweet-sour fruit kicks up levels of vitamin A, vitamin C, and iron. Pierce the fresh pulp with a fork to release the nectar. The seeds are edible. Store-bought juice tends to be cloying, so use less.

## Tropical Passion

**PASSION FRUIT, CHOPPED**
1 tablespoon / ½ cup
**MANGO JUICE**
1 teaspoon / ⅛ cup
**FRESH GINGER, DICED**
¼ teaspoon / 1 tablespoon

## Passionberry

**PASSION FRUIT JUICE**
2 teaspoons / ¼ cup
**RASPBERRIES, LIGHTLY MASHED**
1 teaspoon / ⅛ cup
**ORANGE ZEST**
¼ teaspoon / 1 tablespoon

## V.P.

**PASSION FRUIT JUICE**
2 teaspoons / ¼ cup
**WHOLE VANILLA BEAN, SLICED**
¼ bean / ¾ bean

# Peach

Peaches calm sour stomachs and promote good digestion. We prefer fresh, peeled peaches when they are in season and frozen slices when they are not. Use half the amount of canned peaches or nectar.

## Peachy Keen

**PEACH, PEELED AND DICED**
2 tablespoons / ½ cup
**CHAI SPICE BLEND (PAGE 197)**
¼ teaspoon / 1 teaspoon

## Pêche Rouge

**PEACH, PEELED AND DICED**
2 tablespoons / ½ cup
**RASPBERRIES, LIGHTLY MASHED**
1 tablespoon / ¼ cup

## Peach Cobbler

**PEACH, PEELED AND DICED**
2 tablespoons / ½ cup
**WHOLE VANILLA BEAN, SLICED**
½ bean / 1 bean
**CINNAMON**
1 pinch / 1 teaspoon

# Pear

A longtime remedy for nausea, pears promote digestive health. Fresh, ripe pears are best, but canned or dried fruit or pear nectar works fine if you use half the amount specified.

## Pear

**PEAR, CHOPPED**
¼ cup / ¾ cup

## Purple Pear

**PEAR, CHOPPED**
¼ cup / ¾ cup
**RED OR PURPLE GRAPES, SLICED**
2 tablespoons / ½ cup

## Perry Cherry

**PEAR, CHOPPED**
¼ cup / ¾ cup
**CHERRIES, HALVED**
1 tablespoon / ¼ cup

# Persimmon

Naturally high in catechins and vitamin C, the ripe flesh has a divine sweetness. Although persimmons are most frequently consumed fresh, dried ones can be found online or in Asian markets. Scoop the fruit from the skin, and add it to the second ferment for a delectable infusion reminiscent of flowers and plum.

## Persinammon

**PERSIMMON, DICED**
1 tablespoon / ½ cup
**APPLE, DICED**
1 teaspoon / ⅛ cup
**CINNAMON**
⅛ teaspoon / ½ teaspoon

## Persimmon au Chocolat

**PERSIMMON, DICED**
1 tablespoon / ½ cup
**RAW CACAO POWDER**
1 teaspoon / ⅛ cup

## Persimmon Cookie

**PERSIMMON, DICED**
1 tablespoon / ½ cup
**RAISINS, CHOPPED**
1 teaspoon / ⅛ cup
**VANILLA EXTRACT**
¼ teaspoon / 1 teaspoon

Quantities listed are for 16 ounces / 1 gallon

# Pineapple

Bromelain, an enzyme found only in pineapple, has anti-inflammatory, anticlotting, and anticancer properties. The heavenly sweet-tart, tropical flavor of pineapple sparkles on the tongue, brightening up a sweeter batch and adding balance to a tarter brew.

Fresh, canned, or frozen pineapple works well; the juice is good, but use less to avoid excess carbonation and strain it if pulpy. Combine with other tropical fruits, and take your tongue to the beach!

## Pineapple

**FRESH PINEAPPLE, CHOPPED**
¼ cup / ¾ cup

## Piña Picante

**FRESH PINEAPPLE, CHOPPED**
¼ cup / ¾ cup
**CAYENNE**
½ pinch / ⅛ teaspoon

## Pina-mint

**FRESH PINEAPPLE, CHOPPED**
¼ cup / ¾ cup
**FRESH MINT, ROUGHLY CHOPPED**
½ teaspoon / 2 teaspoons

# Plum

Plums are helpful for digestion and constipation, as well as a good source of dietary fiber; vitamins A, C, and K; and minerals such as potassium, fluoride, and iron. They deepen the flavor and natural tartness of kombucha. (See separate entry for using prunes, page 193.)

## Plum Spice

**PLUM, DICED**
2 tablespoons / ¼ cup
**CINNAMON**
½ teaspoon / 2 teaspoons
**CLOVES, WHOLE**
2 cloves / ½ teaspoon

## Plum Chutney

**PLUM, DICED**
2 tablespoons / ¼ cup
**CHERRIES, HALVED**
1 teaspoon / ⅛ cup
**FRESH GINGER, DICED**
½ teaspoon / 2 teaspoons

## Sugar Plum Flower

**PLUM, DICED**
2 tablespoons / ¼ cup
**LAVENDER, DRIED**
½ teaspoon / 2 teaspoons
**HONEY**
½ teaspoon / 1 tablespoon

# Pomegranate

This ancient fruit, long revered as a symbol of health, fertility, and eternal life, contains unique compounds that benefit the heart and has three times more antioxidants than green tea.

Pomegranate juice is preferred over the arils, which do not provide enough flavor on their own. Naturally astringent, pomegranate's bitter properties are mellowed by kombucha's acids, creating a brew with a deep purple hue.

## Pomcoco

**POMEGRANATE JUICE**
1 tablespoon / 1 cup
**COCONUT WATER**
1 tablespoon / ¾ cup

## Pom-cuke Cooler

**POMEGRANATE JUICE**
1 tablespoon / ¾ cup
**CUCUMBER, DICED**
2 teaspoons / ⅔ cup
**FRESH MINT, ROUGHLY CHOPPED**
½ teaspoon / 1 tablespoon

## Lemon PomBucha

**POMEGRANATE JUICE**
1 tablespoon / ¾ cup
**HONEY**
1 teaspoon / 1 tablespoon
**LEMON ZEST**
¼ teaspoon / 1 teaspoon

Quantities listed are for 16 ounces / 1 gallon

# Prune

Prunes are simply dried plums. Prunes are more concentrated in flavor and sugar content, so fewer are needed to achieve a deep flavor and add a pale purplish hue. Packed with antioxidants, prunes also deliver a nutritional boost. The reconstituted prune pieces are a great addition to Fermented-Fruit Kombucha Sourdough Bread (page 264).

## Desert Delight

**PRUNES, CHOPPED**
2 tablespoons / ½ cup

**DRIED APRICOT, DICED**
2 teaspoons / ¼ cup

**DATES, DICED**
1 teaspoon / ⅛ cup

## Pork au Prune

**PRUNES, CHOPPED**
2 tablespoons / ½ cup

**BACON, COOKED AND CRUMBLED**
1 tablespoon / ⅛ cup

**ORANGE ZEST**
¼ teaspoon / 1 teaspoon

## Prunella Thyme

**PRUNES, CHOPPED**
1 tablespoon / ¼ cup

**WHOLE VANILLA BEAN, SLICED**
¼ bean / ¾ bean

**DRIED THYME**
½ teaspoon / 2 teaspoons

# Pumpkin

One of the most popular crops in the United States, pumpkin makes a special holiday brew, but the flavor is great any time of year. We like to use canned pumpkin pie filling, but plain canned pumpkin is fine too. When pumpkin is added to kombucha, the result may be reminiscent of a sour pumpkin beer. Punch up the spiciness for a warmer brew or mix it with coffee and vanilla ice cream for a pumpkin Kombuffee frappé!

## Pumpkin Pie

**PUMPKIN PIE FILLING, CANNED**
2 tablespoons / ½ cup

**CINNAMON**
¼ teaspoon / 1 teaspoon

**NUTMEG, GRATED**
⅛ teaspoon / ½ teaspoon /

## Pig in a Pumpkin Patch

**PUMPKIN, CANNED**
2 tablespoons / ½ cup

**BACON, COOKED AND CRUMBLED**
1 tablespoon / ⅛ cup

**MAPLE SYRUP**
¼ teaspoon / 1 teaspoon

## Pumpkin Sage

**PUMPKIN, CANNED**
2 tablespoons / ½ cup

**APPLES, DICED**
1 tablespoon / ⅛ cup

**SAGE, DRIED**
¼ teaspoon / 1 teaspoon

# Raisin

Raisins are a classic addition during second ferment to help create carbonation via concentrated grape sugar. They not only offer a touch of sweetness but also balance more intense flavors like jalapeño or savory flavors like carrot.

## Raisin Cookie

**RAISINS, CHOPPED**
1 tablespoon / ¼ cup

**CINNAMON BARK CHIPS**
¼ teaspoon / 1 teaspoon

**VANILLA EXTRACT**
¼ teaspoon / 1 teaspoon

## Raisin' Hell-a-peño

**RAISINS, CHOPPED**
1 tablespoon / ¼ cup

**JALAPEÑO, CHOPPED**
¼ teaspoon / 1 teaspoon

**ORANGE ZEST**
¼ teaspoon / 1 teaspoon

## Raisin Slaw

**RAISINS, CHOPPED**
1 tablespoon / ¼ cup

**CARROT JUICE**
1 teaspoon / 1 tablespoon

**LEMON ZEST**
¼ teaspoon / 1 teaspoon

Quantities listed are for 16 ounces / 1 gallon

# Raspberry

Raspberries pack a pleasingly puckering punch, along with a gorgeous glow, when added to booch, but they can be on the tart side, so use them sparingly or combine with herbs that will mellow the sharp bite. We use fresh or frozen, gently mashed with a fork or tossed in whole. The unmistakable pink jewel tone signals antioxidant power for a pleasing nutritional boost.

### Raspberry

**RASPBERRIES, LIGHTLY MASHED**
1 tablespoon / ¾ cup

### Raspberry Ginger

**RASPBERRIES, LIGHTLY MASHED**
1 tablespoon / ¾ cup
**FRESH GINGER, DICED**
1 teaspoon / 2 teaspoons
**FRESH LEMON JUICE**
1 teaspoon / 1 tablespoon

### Razzlemint

**RASPBERRIES, LIGHTLY MASHED**
1 tablespoon / ¾ cup
**DRIED HIBISCUS**
½ teaspoon / 1 teaspoon
**FRESH MINT, ROUGHLY CHOPPED**
½ teaspoon / 2 teaspoons

### Razzy Bazzy

**RASPBERRIES, LIGHTLY MASHED**
1 tablespoon / ¾ cup
**HOLY BASIL (TULSI)**
⅛ teaspoon / 1 teaspoon

# Rhubarb

Rhubarb, also known as pie-plant, is extremely high in vitamin K. It was cultivated primarily for medicinal purposes until sugar became affordable in the seventeenth century, making it more popular for cooking.

### Rhubarb

**RHUBARB SAUCE**
1 tablespoon / ¼ cup

### Rhuberry

**RHUBARB SAUCE**
1 tablespoon / ¼ cup
**STRAWBERRIES, CHOPPED**
2 tablespoons / ½ cup

# Strawberry

Eaten in 94 percent of North American households, strawberries make a luscious contribution to many different recipes. Used fresh or frozen, strawberries mellow kombucha's tartness while turning it a lovely shade of pink. Pink Lemonade is what turned Alex into a convert — give it a try!

### Strawberry

**STRAWBERRIES, CHOPPED**
2 tablespoons / ½ cup

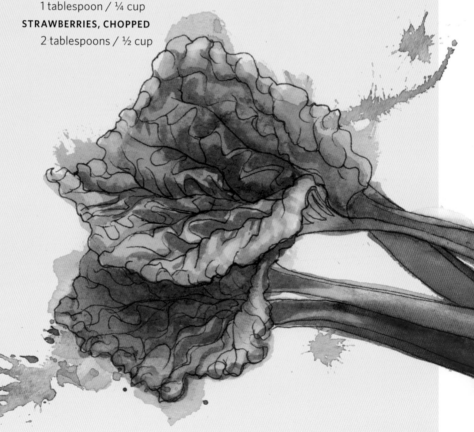

Quantities listed are for 16 ounces / 1 gallon

## Pink Lemonade
**STRAWBERRIES, CHOPPED**
  2 tablespoons / ½ cup
**FRESH THYME**
  1 sprig / 2 sprigs
**FRESH LEMON JUICE**
  1 teaspoon / 1 ounce

## Green Strawberry
**STRAWBERRIES, CHOPPED**
  2 tablespoons / ¾ cup
**CHLOROPHYLL POWDER**
  ½ teaspoon / 2 teaspoons

## Straw Apple
**STRAWBERRIES, CHOPPED**
  2 tablespoons / ¾ cup
**APPLE, DICED**
  2 tablespoons / ½ cup

# Tamarind

Used in paste form that is available online or from Asian or Latino specialty shops, this sweet-tart, antioxidant-rich pulp lends a tropical twist that tickles the taste buds.

## Tambucha
**TAMARIND PASTE**
  2 teaspoons / 3 tablespoons

## Tamarind Fire
**TAMARIND PASTE**
  2 teaspoons / 3 tablespoons
**CAYENNE**
  1 pinch / ½ teaspoon

## Cinna-tam
**TAMARIND PASTE**
  2 teaspoons / 3 tablespoons
**CINNAMON BARK CHIPS**
  ½ teaspoon / 2 teaspoons
**CAYENNE**
  1 pinch / ½ teaspoon

# Tangerine

A little tangy juice adds a lot of flavor, so go easy at first; too much will turn the booch puckeringly sour. Maybe you like that, you kombucha freak? (Us, too!) This citrus plays well with spicy and sweet combos.

## Tangabuch
**FRESH TANGERINE JUICE**
  2 tablespoons / ¼ cup

## Spicy Tangerine
**FRESH TANGERINE JUICE**
  2 tablespoons / ¼ cup
**CAYENNE**
  ½ pinch / ¼ teaspoon

## Tangerine Dream
**FRESH TANGERINE JUICE**
  2 tablespoons / ¼ cup
**COCONUT WATER**
  2 tablespoons / ¼ cup

# Watermelon

You can blend the fruit to concentrate the flavor and sugar; reduce the amount called for by half. It gives kombucha a greenish hue more reminiscent of the rind. Add some hibiscus to play up the candy flavor and color for a "jolly" kombucha brew.

## Watermelon
**WATERMELON, CHOPPED**
  2 tablespoons / ¾ cup
**DRIED HIBISCUS**
  ½ teaspoon / 1 teaspoon

## Cinna-melon
**WATERMELON, CHOPPED**
  2 tablespoons / ¾ cup
**CINNAMON**
  1 teaspoon / 1 tablespoon

## Melonilla
**WATERMELON, CHOPPED**
  2 tablespoons / ¾ cup
**WHOLE VANILLA BEAN, SLICED**
  ¼ bean / ¾ bean

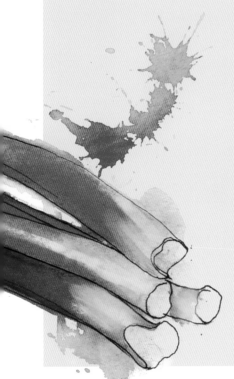

Quantities listed are for 16 ounces / 1 gallon

# HERBALS

## Brain Brew

Gingko biloba and gotu kola promote improved blood flow — this combination will go straight to your head! Use it to imbue kombucha with an uplifting herbal flavor, or drink on its own as an herbal tisane. Don't want to strain out the herbs? Steep them in hot water for 15 minutes; then use the tisane to flavor your brew. Or brew up a batch of Brain Brew booch, using an extra SCOBY from your hotel, of course. We recommend dried or fresh ginger root, not powdered or candied.

### BRAIN BREW BLEND

8 tablespoons gingko biloba leaf
8 tablespoons gotu kola leaf
2 tablespoons chopped
  ginger root
1 tablespoon dried hibiscus

Shake all ingredients together and store in an airtight container.

### Plain Brain Brew

**BRAIN BREW BLEND**
½ teaspoon / 1 tablespoon

### Rose Brain Brew

**BRAIN BREW BLEND**
½ teaspoon / 1 tablespoon
**ROSE PETALS, DRIED**
1 teaspoon / 1 tablespoon

### Elderberry Brain Brew

**BRAIN BREW BLEND**
½ teaspoon / 1 tablespoon
**DRIED ELDERBERRIES**
½ teaspoon / 2 teaspoons

## Burdock

This earthy-tasting root, an ingredient in many traditional Chinese medicine recipes, has a blend of sweet and bitter similar to its cousin the artichoke. As a good source of inulin, it is a prebiotic that provides nutrition for bacteria in your gut, and it pairs well with other herbs such as ginger and turmeric. Add some fruit to balance the earthiness.

### Burdock

**DRIED BURDOCK ROOT**
2 teaspoons / 1½ tablespoons

### Burdock Ginger

**DRIED BURDOCK ROOT**
2 teaspoons / 1½ tablespoons
**FRESH GINGER, DICED**
¼ teaspoon / 2 teaspoons

### Blue Burd

**DRIED BURDOCK ROOT**
2 teaspoons / 1½ tablespoons
**BLUEBERRIES, HALVED**
2 tablespoons / ¼ cup

Quantities listed are for 16 ounces / 1 gallon

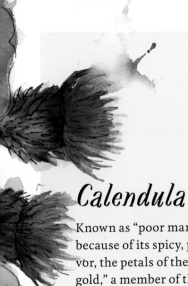

## Calendula

Known as "poor man's saffron" because of its spicy, peppery flavor, the petals of the "pot marigold," a member of the daisy family, add pizzazz and a golden hue to kombucha. Once a staple addition to broths, calendula tisane helps heal gut ulcers and soothe inflammation. Combine it with yellow or orange fruits (or turmeric, even) for a sunny kombucha ablaze with flavor.

### Golden Glow
**DRIED CALENDULA**
1 teaspoon / 1 tablespoon
**TURMERIC, GROUND**
½ teaspoon / 2 teaspoons

### Calendula Cucumber
**DRIED CALENDULA**
1 teaspoon / 1 tablespoon
**CUCUMBER, DICED**
2 tablespoons / ¼ cup

### Morning Refresher
**DRIED CALENDULA**
1 teaspoon / 1 tablespoon
**ORANGE ZEST**
¼ teaspoon / 1 teaspoon
**HONEY**
¼ teaspoon / 1 teaspoon

## Chai Spice

The origin of this popular beverage base is generally attributed to the Himalayan region, where *chai* means "tea." Recipes for chai spice have been handed down as an herbal tonic in India for over five thousand years. All the spices traditionally used to make the blend have immune-boosting and cold-fighting properties.

### CHAI SPICE BLEND

Chai mix typically includes ginger, cinnamon, cardamom, and cloves, but feel free to create your own special blend. The combination given here is just a starting place. Whether you purchase powdered spices or grind your own, choose the freshest available. When flavoring kombucha, use less of the preground spices, as they will impart more intense flavor than the coarser powder produced by hand-grinding. A good rule of thumb is 1 teaspoon of preground blend = 1 tablespoon of hand-ground.

*Yield: 2 tablespoons preground,*
*⅓ cup hand-ground*

**ALLSPICE**
2 teaspoons / 7 berries
**CARDAMOM**
2 teaspoons / 1 tablespoon pods
**CINNAMON**
2 teaspoons / 1 cinnamon stick, broken

**CLOVES**
1 teaspoon / 4 whole
**CORIANDER**
1 teaspoon / 1 tablespoon seeds
**GINGER**
2 teaspoons / ¼-inch piece, diced
**PEPPERCORN**
½ teaspoon / 1 teaspoon whole corns
**STAR ANISE**
1 teaspoon / 3 whole pods

If using powdered spices, combine them in an airtight container, cap tightly, and shake well. If using whole spices, place them all in a spice grinder and pulse until finely ground, and then transfer to an airtight container. Store at room temperature for up to a year.

### Vanilla Chai
**CHAI SPICE BLEND, HAND-GROUND**
1 teaspoon / 1 tablespoon
**WHOLE VANILLA BEAN, SLICED**
¼ bean / ¾ bean

### Honey Spice
**CHAI SPICE BLEND, HAND-GROUND**
½ teaspoon / 1 tablespoon
**HONEY**
1 teaspoon / ⅛ cup

### Moroccan Coffee
**CHAI SPICE BLEND, HAND-GROUND**
½ teaspoon / 2 teaspoons
**GROUND COFFEE**
1 teaspoon / 1 tablespoon

Quantities listed are for 16 ounces / 1 gallon

# Chamomile

One of the most popular herbs in the world, its light, earthy flavor has a hint of apple. It is often used as a sleep aid or to calm the nerves and stomach, plus it has anti-inflammatory and antifungal characteristics.

## Summer Breeze

**CHAMOMILE FLOWER, DRIED**
 1 teaspoon / 1 tablespoon
**LAVENDER, DRIED**
 ¼ teaspoon / 1 teaspoon

## Chamo-melon

**CHAMOMILE FLOWER, DRIED**
 ½ teaspoon / 2 teaspoons
**WATERMELON, CHOPPED**
 2 tablespoons / ½ cup

## Chamomile Grapefruit

**CHAMOMILE FLOWER, DRIED**
 ½ teaspoon / 2 teaspoons
**RUBY RED GRAPEFRUIT JUICE**
 1 tablespoon / ¾ cup

# Cinnamon

Chips of cinnamon bark can be added in the primary ferment to reduce acetic acid and smooth the brew, but the best use is in second ferment, where this spice blends well with mature kombucha and an almost unlimited variety of ingredients. Adding vanilla gives a result reminiscent of the creamy, cinnamon flavor of *horchata*, a traditional Mexican rice water.

## Cinnamon

**CINNAMON BARK CHIPS**
 ½ teaspoon / 1 tablespoon

## Horchata Brew

**CINNAMON BARK CHIPS**
 ½ teaspoon / 1 tablespoon
**WHOLE VANILLA BEAN, SLICED**
 ¼ bean / ¾ bean

## Cinn-tillating Mango

**CINNAMON BARK CHIPS**
 ½ teaspoon / 1 tablespoon
**MANGO, DICED**
 2 tablespoons / ¾ cup

# Clove

Actually the unopened flower buds of an evergreen tree, cloves have a distinctive taste and warm, piney smell that infuse kombucha with a sweet and aromatic flavor. Due to the pungent natural oils, only a few cloves are needed to capture the signature flavor. As a natural antiseptic and stress reliever, they are also beneficial for teeth and help boost the immune system. Ground cloves are very potent — use a small amount to gauge their spicy strength.

## Fresh Breath

**CLOVES, WHOLE**
 3 cloves / 8 cloves
**FRESH MINT, ROUGHLY CHOPPED**
 1 teaspoon / 1 tablespoon
**FENNEL SEED**
 ⅛ teaspoon / ½ teaspoon

## Clove-amon

**CLOVES, WHOLE**
 2 cloves / 4 cloves
**CINNAMON BARK CHIPS**
 ¼ teaspoon / 1 teaspoon

## Crimson and Clove

**CLOVES, WHOLE**
 2 cloves / 4 cloves
**RASPBERRY, CHOPPED**
 1 tablespoon / ¼ cup
**CANDIED GINGER, CHOPPED**
 ½ teaspoon / 2 teaspoons

# Elderflower

Flower essences are traditional additives that delight the palate and calm the mind. The flowers of elder tree signal the arrival of summer. Its creamy white blossoms, with naturally present yeast that aids carbonation, have fueled many healthful and delicious beverages throughout history.

## Sunny Delight

**DRIED ELDERFLOWER BLOSSOM**
 ½ teaspoon / 2 teaspoons
**FRESH LEMON JUICE**
 1 tablespoon / 3 tablespoons
**SUGAR, HONEY, OR OTHER SWEETENER**
 ½ teaspoon / 1 tablespoon

Quantities listed are for 16 ounces / 1 gallon

CALM balm

SUMMER breeze

maté MINT

lavender

herbes DE PROVENCE

ROOTBUCHA

## Wise Elders

**DRIED ELDERFLOWER BLOSSOM**
½ teaspoon / 2 tablespoons

**DRIED ELDERBERRIES**
½ teaspoon / 1 tablespoon

**FRESH SAGE, ROUGHLY CHOPPED**
½ teaspoon / 2 teaspoons

## Wildflower

**DRIED ELDERFLOWER BLOSSOM**
½ teaspoon / 2 tablespoons

**ROSE PETALS, DRIED**
1 tablespoon / ¼ cup

**CHAMOMILE FLOWER, DRIED**
1 teaspoon / 1 tablespoon

**LAVENDER, DRIED**
¼ teaspoon / 1 teaspoon

# Four Thieves

Legend has it that "four thieves vinegar" was used by pickpockets of dead plague victims, who doused themselves to prevent catching the dreaded disease. Chopped fresh herbs are higher in volatile oils, the compounds that give them their unique healing properties, but dried herbs can be used.

## Four Thieves #1

**LAVENDER**
1 pinch / ¼ teaspoon

**ROSEMARY**
2 pinches / ½ teaspoon

**MINT**
1 pinch / ¼ teaspoon

**SAGE**
1 leaf / ½ teaspoon

**OREGANO**
1 pinch / ¼ teaspoon

**FRESH GARLIC, DICED**
⅛ teaspoon / ½ teaspoon

## Four Thieves #2

**CLOVES, GROUND**
⅛ teaspoon / ½ teaspoon

**CINNAMON BARK CHIPS**
⅛ teaspoon / ½ teaspoon

**GARLIC, DICED**
⅛ teaspoon / ½ teaspoon

**NUTMEG, GRATED**
⅛ teaspoon / ½ teaspoon

**MINT, DRIED**
pinch / ¼ teaspoon

**LAVENDER, DRIED**
pinch / ¼ teaspoon

**ROSEMARY, DRIED**
¼ teaspoon / 1 teaspoon

**SAGE, DRIED**
⅛ teaspoon / ½ teaspoon

# Herbes de Provence

This popular spice rub combines herbs from southern France; lavender is often added to American versions. It adds a lovely aroma and complexity to kombucha, creating layers of flavor that encourage continued sipping. Dried herbs are called for here, because they are often easier to source. When using fresh herbs, which also impart essential oils to the brew, double the amount called for.

## Herbes de Provence

**ROSEMARY**
¼ teaspoon / 1½ teaspoons

**THYME**
⅛ teaspoon / 1 teaspoon

**OREGANO**
⅛ teaspoon / 1 teaspoon

**BASIL**
⅛ teaspoon / 1 teaspoon

**FENNEL SEED**
1/16 teaspoon / ¼ teaspoon

**TARRAGON**
⅛ teaspoon / 1 teaspoon

*Optional:*

**LAVENDER**
⅛ teaspoon / 1 teaspoon

**CHERVIL**
⅛ teaspoon / 1 teaspoon

**BAY LEAF, CRUMBLED**
¼ leaf / 1 leaf

# Hibiscus

The hibiscus flower, with its deep pink color and tangy flavor, is consumed as a tisane around the world. It can be included in primary fermentation (see page 60), but use it sparingly until you are familiar with its strength.

## Jamaica Me Crazy

**DRIED HIBISCUS**
1 teaspoon / 1 tablespoon

Quantities listed are for 16 ounces / 1 gallon

### Ginger Punch

**DRIED HIBISCUS**
1 teaspoon / 1 tablespoon
**FRESH GINGER, DICED**
½ teaspoon / 2 tablespoons

### Hibiscus Lemonade

**DRIED HIBISCUS**
½ teaspoon / 1 tablespoon
**FRESH GINGER, DICED**
½ teaspoon / 1 tablespoon
**FRESH LEMON JUICE**
⅛ teaspoon / ½ teaspoon

# Juniper Berry

The primary flavoring in gin, juniper berries are best described as tart, resinous, and piney. Dried berries are easier to source and best used sparingly. Use juniper kombucha as a mixer to create gin-free mocktails.

### Just Juniper

**DRIED JUNIPER BERRIES**
2 teaspoons / 1½ tablespoons

### Juniper Rose

**DRIED JUNIPER BERRIES**
2 teaspoons / 1½ tablespoons
**ROSE PETALS, DRIED**
2 teaspoons / 1 tablespoon

### Spicy Juniper

**DRIED JUNIPER BERRIES**
2 teaspoons / 1½ tablespoons
**CAYENNE**
½ pinch / 1 pinch

# Lavender

With their beautiful scent and floral, slightly minty taste, lavender blossoms lend a heady flavor to the acidic nature of the booch, creating an excellent contrast. Fresh flowers and leaves offer the strongest scent, while dried petals impart a delicate note.

### Lavender

**LAVENDER FLOWER**
½ teaspoon / 1 tablespoon

### Love Melon

**LAVENDER FLOWER**
½ teaspoon / 1 tablespoon
**WATERMELON, CHOPPED**
2 tablespoons / ¾ cup

### Lavender Brain Brew

**LAVENDER FLOWER**
½ teaspoon / 1 tablespoon
**BRAIN BREW BLEND (PAGE 196)**
½ teaspoon / 1 tablespoon

# Lemon Balm

This mild-flavored plant tastes equally of lemon and mint. Known as a calming herb, it has been used for thousands of years to reduce anxiety and increase focus. Punch up the citrusy notes with lemon zest or orange juice or accentuate the herbal notes with lavender or peppermint.

### Calm Balm

**LEMON BALM, DRIED**
½ teaspoon / 2 tablespoons
**CHAMOMILE FLOWER, DRIED**
½ teaspoon / 2 tablespoons
**LAVENDER, DRIED**
¼ teaspoon / 1 tablespoon

### Peach-Mint Lemonade

**PEACH, PEELED AND DICED**
1 tablespoon / ¼ cup
**LEMON BALM, DRIED**
½ teaspoon / 2 tablespoons
**MINT, DRIED**
¼ teaspoon / 1 tablespoon

Quantities listed are for 16 ounces / 1 gallon

## Ginger Dew

**HONEYDEW, DICED**
1 tablespoon / ¼ cup

**LEMON BALM, DRIED**
½ teaspoon / 2 tablespoons

**GINGER, GROUND**
¼ teaspoon / 1 tablespoon

# Mint

Rich in antioxidants, mint contains a natural decongestant (menthol), is good for sore throats, upset stomach, and irritable bowel syndrome and has been used to whiten teeth since the 1500s. There are hundreds of varieties to choose from, but we often use the most common — peppermint and spearmint — to add cool refreshment to kombucha. Combine with other herbs for a complex brew (see Doshas, page 217), or use alone for a new twist on mint tea.

## Maté Mint

**YERBA MATÉ**
½ teaspoon / 1 tablespoon

**FRESH MINT, ROUGHLY CHOPPED**
½ teaspoon / 2 teaspoons

## Melon Cooler

**WATERMELON, CHOPPED**
2 tablespoons / ¾ cup

**FRESH MINT, ROUGHLY CHOPPED**
1 teaspoon / 2 teaspoons

## Apple Mint

**APPLE, DICED**
2 tablespoons / ¾ cup

**FRESH MINT, ROUGHLY CHOPPED**
1 teaspoon / 2 teaspoons

# Root Beer

Naturally fermented beverages such as root beer and ginger ale held an important place in our food culture before being co-opted by the sugar soda industry. Serving a natural root beer made from flavored kombucha to soda lovers restores it to its original place as a health tonic. The possible combinations are endless — experiment to find your ideal flavor!

### ROOT BEER SPICE BLEND

Root beer is uniquely American in flavor and history. Supposedly invented at the request of Samuel Adams as a beverage his children could drink, the original concoction was a small beer — a low-alcohol ferment (see Negus, page 250). The consumption of sassafras and sarsaparilla bark was also a common herbal remedy used by Native American tribes. Try making a syrup (see page 145), or simply infuse the herbs directly in the kombucha for a mellower flavor.

Whether you purchase ground spices or grind your own, choose the freshest available. When flavoring kombucha, use less of the pre-ground spices, as they will impart more intense flavor than the coarser powder produced by hand-grinding. A good rule of thumb is 1 teaspoon of preground blend = 1 tablespoon of hand-ground.

*Yield: 2 tablespoons preground*
*⅓ cup hand-ground*

**SASSAFRAS BARK, CHOPPED**
2 teaspoons / 2 tablespoons

**SARSAPARILLA BARK, CHOPPED**
1 teaspoon / 1 tablespoon

**WINTERGREEN, DRIED**
2 teaspoons / 2 tablespoons

**VANILLA BEAN POWDER, CHOPPED**
1 teaspoon / 1 pod

*Other options (mix and match):*
**ALLSPICE**
1 teaspoon / 3 berries

**BIRCH BARK, CHOPPED**
2 teaspoons / 2 tablespoons

**BURDOCK ROOT, SLICED**
2 teaspoons / 2 tablespoons

**CINNAMON STICK, BROKEN**
2 teaspoons / 1 stick

**CLOVES**
1 teaspoon / 4 whole

**DANDELION ROOT, DRIED AND CHOPPED**
1 teaspoon / 1 tablespoon

**GINGER, CHOPPED**
2 teaspoons / ¼-inch piece

**HOPS, DRIED**
½ teaspoon / 2 flowers, broken

**LICORICE ROOT, CHOPPED**
1 teaspoon / 2 teaspoons

**MINT, DRIED AND CRUMBLED**
1 teaspoon / 1 tablespoon

Quantities listed are for 16 ounces / 1 gallon

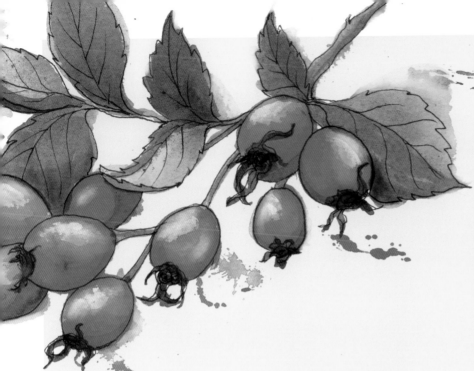

## Rose Hip

High in vitamins C and A, rose-hip jam and syrups were once given regularly to children to prevent colds. Most commonly sold dried, these potent little antioxidant powerhouses can turn booch sour fast. Use sparingly and pair them with other antioxidant rich berries or mellow with a touch of honey to create your own modern elixirs.

**STAR ANISE**
1 teaspoon / 3 whole pods
**WILD CHERRY BARK, CHOPPED**
1 teaspoon / 1 tablespoon

If using powdered spices, combine them in an airtight container, cap tightly, and shake well. If using whole spices, place them all in a spice grinder and pulse until finely ground, then transfer to an airtight container. Store at room temperature for up to a year.

### Rootbucha
**ROOT BEER SPICE BLEND, HAND-GROUND**
½ teaspoon / 1 tablespoon
*Alternative:*
**ROOT BEER SPICE BLEND, PREGROUND**
1 teaspoon / ¼ cup

### Gingerootbucha
**ROOT BEER SPICE BLEND, HAND-GROUND**
½ teaspoon / 2 teaspoons
**CANDIED GINGER, CHOPPED**
1 teaspoon / 1 tablespoon
**MOLASSES**
¼ teaspoon / 1 teaspoon

### Cherry Vanilla Root Beer
**ROOT BEER SPICE BLEND, HAND-GROUND**
1 teaspoon / ⅛ cup
**CHERRIES, HALVED**
2 teaspoons / ¼ cup
**WHOLE VANILLA BEAN, SLICED**
¼ bean / ¾ bean

### Rosehipnotic
**ROSE HIPS, DRIED**
1 teaspoon / 1 tablespoon

### Hip Goji
**ROSE HIPS, DRIED**
¾ teaspoon / 1 tablespoon
**GOJI BERRIES**
¾ teaspoon / 1 tablespoon

### Soothing C
**ROSE HIPS, DRIED**
¾ teaspoon / 1 tablespoon
**LEMON ZEST**
¼ teaspoon / 1 teaspoon
**HONEY**
¼ teaspoon / 1 teaspoon

Quantities listed are for 16 ounces / 1 gallon

# Rose Petals

Rose petals offer an intriguing flavor that varies widely from sweet to tangy to spicy, depending on the variety. They are a mild sedative, an antidepressant, and a mood-enhancing agent that is naturally high in vitamin C. Romantic and exotic, they add a hint of color and a delicate aroma to the brew. We like to use dried petals from our garden; they are also readily available at Middle Eastern and health food stores and online.

## Rose Petal
**ROSE PETALS, DRIED**
    1 tablespoon / 2 tablespoons

## Power Petal
**ROSE PETALS, DRIED**
    1 tablespoon / 2 tablespoons
**CHLOROPHYLL POWDER**
    ½ teaspoon / 2 teaspoons

## Roseberry
**ROSE PETALS, DRIED**
    1 tablespoon / 2 tablespoons
**ROSE HIPS, DRIED**
    ¼ teaspoon / 1 teaspoon
**DRIED ELDERBERRIES**
    ¼ teaspoon / 1 teaspoon

# Sassafras

Sassafras is a laurel tree whose roots and bark have been used in herbal medicine since ancient times to improve blood flow and dispel stagnation. Native to North America, it typically comes in powdered or bark form. In kombucha, it adds the signature root beer flavor characterized by safrole, the active compound in sassafras. We enjoy the distinctive flavor that sassafras brings to kombucha and include it in our Rootbucha decoction recipe (see page 145).

## Sassachino
**BREWED COFFEE**
    2 tablespoons / ¼ cup
**SASSAFRAS POWDER**
    1 teaspoon / 1 tablespoon

## Crancherry Sass
**CRANBERRY JUICE, SWEETENED**
    1 tablespoon / ⅛ cup
**CHERRY JUICE**
    1 teaspoon / 1 tablespoon
**SASSAFRAS POWDER**
    1 teaspoon / 1 tablespoon

## Molassafras
**SASSAFRAS BARK, CHOPPED**
    1 teaspoon / 1 tablespoon
**MOLASSES**
    ¼ teaspoon / 1 teaspoon
**VANILLA BEAN POWDER**
    ⅛ teaspoon / ½ teaspoon

# St. John's Wort

This plant is named after the martyr because the petals exude a reddish tinge when rubbed. Acclaimed since ancient times as a treatment for everything from wounds, headaches, and gout to anxiety and depression, this dried herb has a natural earthiness that works best in kombucha when blended with other herbs or fruit to mask the flavor.

## Holy Ghost
**ST. JOHN'S WORT**
    ¼ teaspoon / 1 teaspoon
**HOLY BASIL (TULSI)**
    ¼ teaspoon / 1 teaspoon

## Devotional Brew
**ST. JOHN'S WORT**
    ¼ teaspoon / 1 teaspoon
**DRIED CALENDULA**
    ¼ teaspoon / 1 teaspoon
**ROSE HIPS, DRIED**
    ⅛ teaspoon / ½ teaspoon

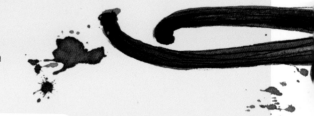

Quantities listed are for 16 ounces / 1 gallon

# Thyme

When first inventing fun flavors, I turned to my garden: the result was dubbed Garden Dew. Thyme has historically been included in cheese and alcohol, and its pungent undertone works well with other herbs or as an accent to fruits. While we prefer to use fresh thyme and other herbs, dried can be used as well; simply reduce the amount by about half.

## Garden Dew

**THYME**
¼ teaspoon / 1 teaspoon

**OREGANO**
¼ teaspoon / 1 teaspoon

**ROSEMARY**
¼ teaspoon / 1 teaspoon

**LAVENDER**
⅛ teaspoon / ½ teaspoon

## Herbal-ade

**THYME**
½ teaspoon / 1 tablespoon

**FRESH LEMON JUICE**
½ teaspoon / 1 tablespoon

**LEMON ZEST**
¼ teaspoon / 1 teaspoon

## BBT

**THYME**
½ teaspoon / 1 tablespoon

**FRESH BASIL, ROUGHLY CHOPPED**
¼ teaspoon / 1 teaspoon

**BANANA, MASHED**
1 teaspoon / ⅛ cup

# Vanilla Bean

Vanilla beans contain anti-inflammatories, reduce nausea, and are considered an aphrodisiac. Terrific in blends, the fragrant oils of the bean take the tart edge off kombucha while adding a hint of sweetness to the brew (along with a ton of black flecks, just like in real vanilla ice cream!). We prefer to use the whole bean, cut into pieces. Powdered vanilla bean can be used instead and may offer more sweetness with less mellowing oils for a tarter second ferment.

## Ruby Bean

**WHOLE VANILLA BEAN, SLICED**
¼ bean / 1 bean

**ROOIBOS TISANE**
½ teaspoon / 2 teaspoons

## 'Nilla Wafer

**WHOLE VANILLA BEAN, SLICED**
¼ bean / 1 bean

**AGAVE SYRUP**
1 teaspoon / 2 tablespoons

## Cream Soda

**WHOLE VANILLA BEAN, SLICED**
¼ bean / 1 bean

**HONEY**
1 tablespoon / ¼ cup

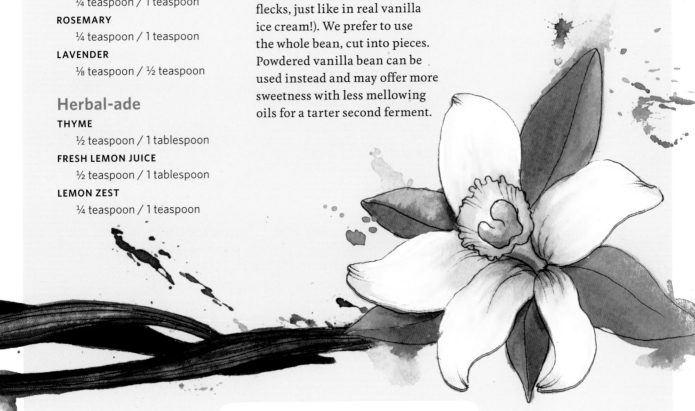

Quantities listed are for 16 ounces / 1 gallon

# SUPER-FOODS

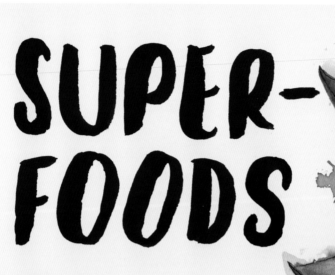

## *Aloe Vera*

This succulent has a long history of topical use to treat burns and wounds and can be taken internally for improved digestion and decreased inflammation. The juice is available at many health food stores, but the bitter taste (the name *aloe* comes from an Arabic word that means "shining bitter substance") usually requires combining with other fruits to help the medicine go down.

### Aloe Guv'nor

**ALOE JUICE**
1 tablespoon / ¼ cup

### Green Soother

**ALOE JUICE**
1 tablespoon / ¼ cup
**GREEN POWER BLEND (PAGE 210)**
½ teaspoon / 2 teaspoons
**HONEY**
1 teaspoon / 1 tablespoon

### Aloe Pomegranate

**ALOE JUICE**
1 tablespoon / ¼ cup
**POMEGRANATE JUICE**
1 teaspoon / 1 tablespoon

## *Avocado*

It's hard to find anyone who doesn't love the rich creamy flesh of the avocado, which is actually a berry. It pairs beautifully with so many flavors: tart, sweet, savory, spicy. In kombucha, it mellows the tartness and grounds the overall taste.

### Avocado

**AVOCADO, MASHED**
2 tablespoons / ½ cup

### Peppercado

**AVOCADO, MASHED**
2 tablespoons / ½ cup
**BLACK PEPPER**
1 pinch / 1 teaspoon

### Guakombucha

**AVOCADO, MASHED**
2 tablespoons / ½ cup
**TOMATO, DICED**
1 teaspoon / 1 tablespoon
**FRESH LEMON JUICE**
½ teaspoon / 2 teaspoons
**CILANTRO, ROUGHLY CHOPPED**
¼ teaspoon / 1 teaspoon

Quantities listed are for 16 ounces / 1 gallon

# Bee Pollen

Bees not only make delicious, nutritious honey but also produce pollen grains that can be incorporated into your booch to give it a healthy buzz! Bee pollen grains are nutritional power balls made of amino acids, protein, and B vitamins, intended to feed larval bees. These dense pollen and bee excretions make superfizzy kombucha with a piquant flavor reminiscent of honey, yet lacking the same sweetness. Those with bee or pollen allergies are wise to use caution when consuming bee pollen.

## Superbuzz

**BEE POLLEN, LIGHTLY CRUSHED**
1 teaspoon / 1 tablespoon
**RAW CACAO POWDER**
2 teaspoons / 1½ tablespoons
**MACA POWDER**
1 teaspoon / 1 tablespoon

## Mellowbuzz

**BEE POLLEN, LIGHTLY CRUSHED**
1 teaspoon / 1 tablespoon
**CHAMOMILE FLOWER, DRIED**
½ teaspoon / 2 teaspoons
**LAVENDER, DRIED**
¼ teaspoon / 1 teaspoon

## C-Buzz

**BEE POLLEN, LIGHTLY CRUSHED**
1 teaspoon / 1 tablespoon
**FRESH ORANGE JUICE**
2 teaspoons / ¼ cup
**LEMON ZEST**
¼ teaspoon / 1 teaspoon

# Cacao

Cacao is the pulverized form of roasted fermented cacao beans. It is high in theobromine (an alkaloid similar to caffeine), antioxidants, and amino acids such as tryptophan and serotonin. It contains no added sugar and has a slightly bitter flavor. It imparts a chocolatey tone that pairs well with sweeter fruits to create fun, new "soda" flavors. We love the malty flavor of Cuzco Chocolate, which uses lucuma, a popular fruit in South America that is readily available in powder form.

## Cuzco Chocolate

**RAW CACAO POWDER**
¼ teaspoon / 1 teaspoon
**LUCUMA POWDER**
¼ teaspoon / 1 teaspoon

## Cacao Pow

**RAW CACAO POWDER**
¼ teaspoon / 1 teaspoon
**MACA POWDER**
¼ teaspoon / 1 teaspoon

## Choco-Cherry

**RAW CACAO POWDER**
¼ teaspoon / 1 teaspoon
**CHERRY PRESERVES**
1 teaspoon / 1 tablespoon

# Chia Seeds

Native to Mexico, these seeds of a desert plant that has traditionally been used for energy are rich in omega-3s. To make the gel used in these recipes, combine 1 tablespoon of chia seeds with ¼ cup of warm water in a dish and stir well. Let sit, undisturbed, for 20 to 30 minutes or until a thick gel forms. Use the gel immediately or store in the fridge up to 1 week. The seeds will not remain suspended in the brew as in commercial versions and are best consumed within 3 days.

## Green Chia

**CHIA GEL**
2 teaspoons / ¼ cup
**GREEN POWER BLEND (PAGE 210)**
1 teaspoon / 1 tablespoon

## Cherry Garchia

**CHIA GEL**
2 teaspoons / ¼ cup
**CHERRIES, HALVED, OR PRESERVES**
1 tablespoon / ¼ cup

## Grape Chia

**CHIA GEL**
2 teaspoons / ¼ cup
**GRAPE JUICE**
1 tablespoon / ¼ cup

Quantities listed are for 16 ounces / 1 gallon

# Coconut Water

Popular in the tropics, coconut water is hydrating and refreshing. It is high in potassium and magnesium, making it a natural choice for postworkout refreshment for replenishing lost minerals. Look for brands without pulp, or filter before using.

## Coco-buch

**COCONUT WATER**
¼ cup / 1 cup

## Coco-Chai

**COCONUT WATER**
¼ cup / 1 cup
**CHAI SPICE BLEND**
¼ teaspoon / 1 teaspoon

## Cinna-coco

**COCONUT WATER**
¼ cup / 1 cup
**CINNAMON BARK CHIPS**
¼ teaspoon / 1 teaspoon

# Coffee

Adding coffee to a tea-based beverage might not seem like a great idea, but, it creates a complex flavor that will please coffee lovers. The bitter flavors balance the tanginess of the kombucha. A sweeter element such as vanilla or cacao provides a deep yet subtle aroma that will please and stimulate. For a really different twist, use coffee to brew kombucha in primary fermentation (see Kombuffee, page 230).

## Starbucha

**WHOLE VANILLA BEAN, SLICED**
¼ bean / 1 bean
**BREWED COFFEE**
⅛ cup / ⅓ cup

## Moka

**BREWED COFFEE**
⅛ cup / ⅓ cup
**RAW CACAO POWDER**
¼ teaspoon / 1½ teaspoons

## Turkish Delight

**BREWED COFFEE**
⅛ cup / ⅓ cup
**CARDAMOM, GROUND**
⅛ teaspoon / ½ teaspoon
**CINNAMON**
⅛ teaspoon / ½ teaspoon
**CLOVES, GROUND**
⅛ teaspoon / ½ teaspoon

# Goji Berry

Also known as wolfberries, these Chinese natives are most commonly found in dehydrated form. The flavor is subtle, but add these nutrient-rich berries, long associated with immortality, to your "tea," and who knows how many lifetimes of goji berry kombucha you will enjoy!

## Go, Goji

**GOJI BERRIES**
½ teaspoon / 2 teaspoons

## Tibetan Delight

**GOJI BERRIES**
½ teaspoon / 2 teaspoons
**FRESH GINGER, DICED**
⅛ teaspoon / 1 teaspoon

## Big Red

**GOJI BERRIES**
½ teaspoon / 2 teaspoons
**STRAWBERRIES, CHOPPED**
1 teaspoon / ¼ cup

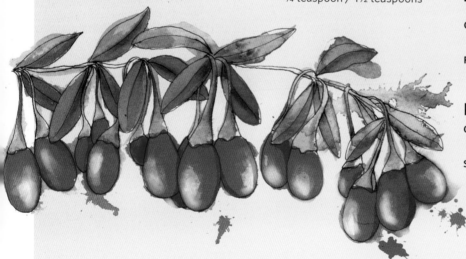

Quantities listed are for 16 ounces / 1 gallon

GO, GOJI

Coco-buch

Maui Maca

ALOE guv'nor

C-Buzz

CACAO POW

# Green Power Blend

All green foods pack a nutritional punch, and most pair well with kombucha to create a satisfying alkaline beverage. Use any of your favorite "greens" either powdered or juiced. We like wheatgrass, barley grass, spirulina, and chlorella.

## I Dream of Greenie
POWDERED GREENS
1 teaspoon / 1 tablespoon

## Green Melon
GREEN JUICE
2 teaspoons / 2 tablespoons
WATERMELON, CHOPPED
2 tablespoons / ¾ cup

## Empowermint
POWDERED GREENS
1 teaspoon / 1 tablespoon
FRESH MINT, ROUGHLY CHOPPED
½ teaspoon / 2 teaspoons

# Maca

One of several South American superfoods, this root has been consumed for centuries by Peruvians who prize it for its aphrodisiac and energy-boosting properties. It has a malted flavor reminiscent of earthy butterscotch.

## Power-Up Kombucha
MACA POWDER
1 teaspoon / 1 tablespoon
BEE POLLEN, LIGHTLY CRUSHED
1 teaspoon / 1 tablespoon
RAW CACAO POWDER
2 teaspoons / 1½ tablespoons

## Banana Maca
MACA POWDER
1 teaspoon / 1 tablespoon
BANANA, MASHED
2 tablespoons / ½ cup

## Goji Maca
MACA POWDER
1 teaspoon / 1 tablespoon
GOJI BERRIES
½ teaspoon / 2 teaspoons

# Maqui Berry

The fruit of an evergreen, maqui berries are similar in flavor to blackberries. Research indicates that they may be a potent anti-inflammatory that could reduce the risk of a variety of inflammation-triggered diseases.

## Maqui
MAQUI BERRY, POWDERED OR DRIED
1 teaspoon / 4 berries
4 teaspoons / 16 berries

## Maqui Mint
MAQUI BERRY, POWDERED OR DRIED
1 teaspoon / 4 berries
4 teaspoons / 16 berries
FRESH MINT, ROUGHLY CHOPPED
1 teaspoon / 2 teaspoons

## Maqui Maca
MAQUI BERRY, POWDERED OR DRIED
1 teaspoon / 4 berries
4 teaspoons / 16 berries
MACA POWDER
1 teaspoon / 1 tablespoon

Quantities listed are for 16 ounces / 1 gallon

# SAVORY

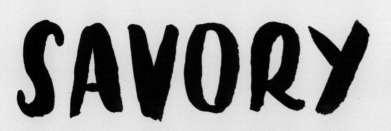

## Bacon

Bacon is awesome, it's delicious, it's fun, and yep, you can add it to your kombucha. This works with salty vegan bacon too.

### Maple Pork Soda
**BACON, COOKED AND CRUMBLED**
½ teaspoon / 1 tablespoon
**MAPLE SYRUP**
¼ teaspoon / 1 teaspoon

### Apple Bacon
**BACON, COOKED AND CRUMBLED**
½ teaspoon / 1 tablespoon
**THYME, DRIED**
¼ teaspoon / 1 teaspoon
**APPLE, DICED**
½ teaspoon / 1 tablespoon

### Cherry Pig Pop
**BACON, COOKED AND CRUMBLED**
½ teaspoon / 1 tablespoon
**CHERRIES, HALVED**
1 teaspoon / ⅛ cup
**ORANGE ZEST**
⅛ teaspoon / ½ teaspoon

## Beet

This root is high in folate and manganese and also contains a lot of sugar. Its sweet, earthy flavor can quickly overwhelm the kombucha taste with intense sweetness if too much is added. Use raw beet, peeled and chopped. It also adds great color.

### Can't Be Beet!
**FRESH BEET, CHOPPED**
1 tablespoon / ¼ cup

### Pep-a-Beet
**FRESH BEET, CHOPPED**
1 tablespoon / ¼ cup
**BLACK PEPPER**
1 pinch / ⅛ teaspoon

### Root Tonic
**FRESH BEET, CHOPPED**
1 tablespoon / ¼ cup
**CELERY, CHOPPED**
1 tablespoon / ¼ cup

Quantities listed are for 16 ounces / 1 gallon

## Carrot

While perhaps not an obvious flavoring choice, carrots are bursting with nutrition and versatile enough to pair with both savory and sweet. Shredded carrot offers more earthiness but less sweetness than juice, which can quickly take the bite out of most any sour kombucha brew, making it an excellent flavoring choice for newbie drinkers.

### Fire Carrot

**CARROT JUICE**
 1 tablespoon / ¼ cup
**CAYENNE**
 ⅛ teaspoon / ½ teaspoon

### Vital C

**CARROT JUICE**
 1 tablespoon / ¼ cup
**ORANGE ZEST**
 ⅛ teaspoon / ½ teaspoon
**THYME, DRIED**
 ¼ teaspoon / 1 teaspoon

### Carrot Pie

**CARROT JUICE**
 1 tablespoon / ¼ cup
**CINNAMON**
 ¼ teaspoon / 1 teaspoon
**VANILLA BEAN POWDER**
 ⅛ teaspoon / ½ teaspoon

## Cayenne

Most commonly used in powdered form, cayenne increases blood flow and speeds metabolism while offering an obviously hot kick to any recipe. Just a little bit can nicely spice up the tang of kombucha — and it makes a great addition to kombucha vinegar.

### Fire Melonade

**CAYENNE**
 ½ pinch / ¼ teaspoon
**WATERMELON, CHOPPED**
 ¼ cup / ¾ cup

### SizzLemon

**CAYENNE**
 ½ pinch / ¼ teaspoon
**LEMON JUICE**
 ½ teaspoon / 2 teaspoons
**LEMON ZEST**
 ⅛ teaspoon / ½ teaspoon
**CUCUMBER, DICED**
 2 teaspoons / ¼ cup

### Summer Heat

**CAYENNE**
 ½ pinch / ¼ teaspoon
**TOMATO, DICED**
 2 teaspoons / ¼ cup
**FRESH BASIL, ROUGHLY CHOPPED**
 ¼ teaspoon / 2 teaspoons

## Cucumber

This member of the melon family adds a surprising amount of vitamin K and sneaks in quite a lot of flavor when paired with the right partners. We toss unpeeled cuke with herbs to capture the essence of the summer garden.

### English Garden

**CUCUMBER, DICED**
 2 tablespoons / ¼ cup
**DRIED ELDERFLOWER BLOSSOM**
 1 teaspoon / 1 tablespoon
**FRESH MINT, ROUGHLY CHOPPED**
 ½ teaspoon / 2 teaspoons

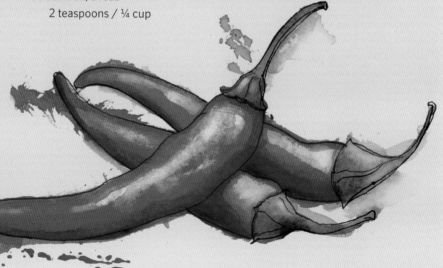

Quantities listed are for 16 ounces / 1 gallon

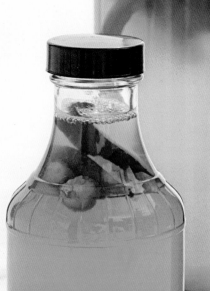
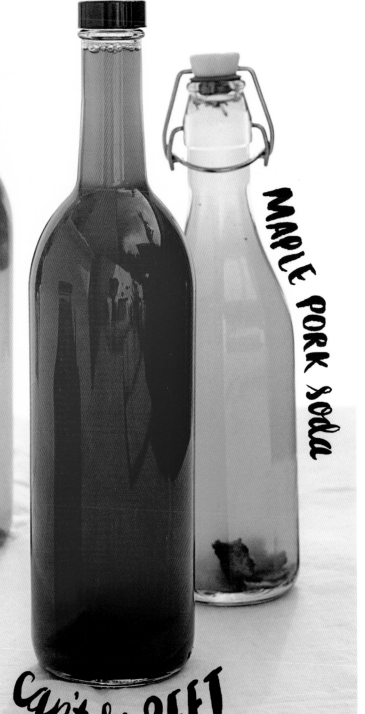

SPICY 'MATO

SHIITAKE sour

Can't be BEET

MAPLE PORK soda

### Cuke Marie

**CUCUMBER, DICED**
2 tablespoons / ¼ cup

**ROSEMARY, DRIED**
⅛ teaspoon / ¼ teaspoon

**LEMON ZEST**
⅛ teaspoon / ¼ teaspoon

### Cool Melon

**CUCUMBER, DICED**
1 tablespoon / ¼ cup

**HONEYDEW, DICED**
1 tablespoon / ¼ cup

**PEPPERMINT, DRIED, CRUMBLED**
¼ teaspoon / 1 teaspoon

# Garlic

This may seem like a surprising addition to kombucha, but the correct usage yields a nicely balanced spicy and savory note that plays off other elements. Use fresh for the best flavor. The longer it ages, the more intense the garlic aroma.

### Garlicious

**GARLIC, DICED**
½ teaspoon / 2 teaspoons

**LEMON ZEST**
⅛ teaspoon / ½ teaspoon

### Pizza Booch

**GARLIC, DICED**
½ teaspoon / 2 teaspoons

**FRESH TOMATO, CHOPPED**
2 tablespoons / ¼ cup

**OREGANO, DRIED**
⅛ teaspoon / ¼ teaspoon

### Purple Gold Tonic

**GARLIC, DICED**
½ teaspoon / 2 teaspoons

**FRESH BEET, DICED**
1 tablespoon / ¼ cup

**FRESH LIME JUICE**
½ teaspoon / 1 tablespoon

# Jalapeño

A spicy booch clears the sinuses and is also great for making mixed drinks or combining with savory juices. These recipes call for just the flesh of the pepper but you can add a few seeds to your brew if you want to kick it up a notch.

### Peño Cucumber

**JALAPEÑO, CHOPPED**
½ teaspoon / 1 tablespoon

**CUCUMBER, DICED**
2 tablespoons / ¼ cup

### Spicy Tomato

**JALAPEÑO, CHOPPED**
½ teaspoon / 1 tablespoon

**FRESH TOMATO, CHOPPED**
2 tablespoons / ¼ cup

**CILANTRO, ROUGHLY CHOPPED**
¼ teaspoon / 1 teaspoon

### Mango Salsa

**JALAPEÑO, CHOPPED**
½ teaspoon / 1 tablespoon

**MANGO, DICED**
2 tablespoons / ¼ cup

**FRESH LIME JUICE**
¼ teaspoon / 1 teaspoon

**LEMON ZEST**
⅛ teaspoon / ½ teaspoon

# Mushrooms

A rich, hearty, brothy booch may not be ideal all the time, but we really enjoy these flavors of kombucha with a heavy meal or as an afternoon snack all on their own. Dried or fresh mushrooms can be used in the same proportions.

### Funga-mintal

**OYSTER MUSHROOMS, DICED**
1 teaspoon / 2 teaspoons

**SHIITAKE MUSHROOMS, DICED**
1 teaspoon / 2 teaspoons

**MINT, DRIED**
¼ teaspoon / 1 teaspoon

### Herbed Mushroom

**MUSHROOMS, ANY TYPE, DICED**
1 tablespoon / ¼ cup

**ROSEMARY, DRIED**
⅛ teaspoon / ½ teaspoon

**THYME, DRIED**
⅛ teaspoon / ½ teaspoon

### Shiitake Sour

**SHIITAKE MUSHROOMS, DICED**
1 tablespoon / ¼ cup

**LEMON JUICE**
½ teaspoon / 2 teaspoons

Quantities listed are for 16 ounces / 1 gallon

# *Tomato*

Adding an acidic fruit like tomatoes to sour kombucha might seem redundant, but with the right spices, the combination can be delightful, as it highlights the natural sweetness of the tomato. Savory kombuchas have a variety of uses that extend beyond a mere beverage; they complement vinaigrettes, add body to soups, and give a splash of vibrancy to other savory dishes.

## Pico de Boocha

**FRESH TOMATO, CHOPPED**
2 tablespoons / ¼ cup

**ONION, CHOPPED**
⅛ teaspoon / ½ teaspoon

**JALAPEÑO, CHOPPED**
⅛ teaspoon / ½ teaspoon

**CILANTRO, ROUGHLY CHOPPED**
1 teaspoon / 1 tablespoon

**GARLIC, DICED**
1 pinch / ⅛ teaspoon

**BLACK PEPPER**
1 pinch / ⅛ teaspoon

## ZorBucha the Greek

**CUCUMBER, DICED**
2 tablespoons / ¼ cup

**FRESH TOMATO, CHOPPED**
2 tablespoons / ¼ cup

**OREGANO, DRIED**
1 teaspoon / 1 tablespoon

## Maters 'n' Peppers

**FRESH TOMATO, DICED**
2 tablespoons / ¼ cup

**BLACK PEPPER**
⅛ teaspoon / ½ teaspoon

**JALAPEÑO**
½ tablespoon / 1½ tablespoon

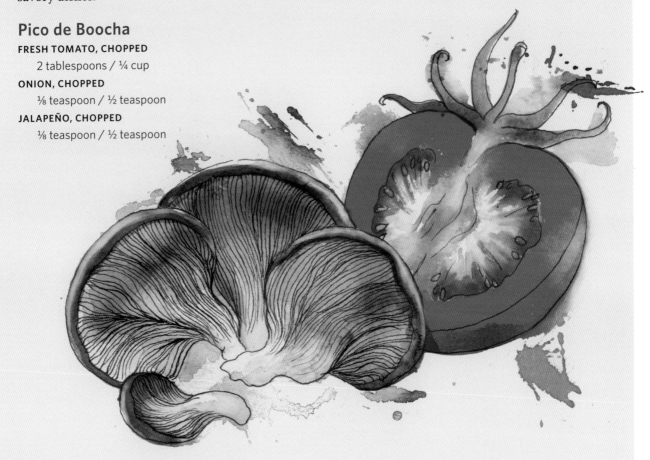

Quantities listed are for 16 ounces / 1 gallon

# MEDICINAL

*Traditional Chinese Medicine (TCM) and Ayurveda*

## Angelica

Also known as *dang-gui*, or "women's ginseng," angelica root has warming properties and is used to relax muscle tissue, balance hormones, and improve digestion. The root can be powdered or sliced, but the powdered version in capsules is easiest to source. Increase sliced root amount by 25 percent.

### Wonder Brew

**ANGELICA, DRIED**
1 teaspoon / 1 tablespoon
**DRIED APRICOT, DICED**
1 tablespoon / ¼ cup
**LAVENDER, DRIED**
¼ teaspoon / 1 teaspoon

### Angel and the Devil

**ANGELICA, DRIED**
1 teaspoon / 1 tablespoon
**FRESH GINGER, DICED**
1 tablespoon / ¼ cup

### Plumgelica

**ANGELICA, DRIED**
1 teaspoon / 1 tablespoon
**PLUM, DICED**
2 tablespoons / ½ cup

## Astragalus

Astragalus, or *huang qi*, is a warming agent that supports the immune system and combats fatigue. Its slightly sweet taste pairs well with bitter herbs. Astragalus comes in a variety of forms. We find capsules provide the easiest means of using and storing it. To use dried astragalus root, substitute 1 teaspoon for every capsule.

### Astragalus

**ASTRAGALUS ROOT**
1 capsule / 4 capsules

### Blue Astragalus

**ASTRAGALUS ROOT**
1 capsule / 4 capsules
**BLUEBERRIES, HALVED**
2 tablespoons / ¾ cup

## Rhizzzome Power

**ASTRAGALUS ROOT**
1 capsule / 4 capsules
**CANDIED GINGER, CHOPPED**
1 teaspoon / 1 tablespoon
**BEE POLLEN, LIGHTLY CRUSHED**
¼ teaspoon / 1 teaspoon

## Ayurvedic Blends

Ayurveda is the ancient Indian herbal medicine practice that arose simultaneously with TCM. The two systems share many commonalities, being based on the elements of nature while treating the patient as a whole system rather than focusing on the disease.

## Use Herbs with Caution

Herbs were used in medical practice for thousands of years and are the root of many modern pharmaceutical formulations; as such they should be used with caution. Consult a qualified professional for long-term use as a kombucha flavoring agent. Experimental brews should always be consumed with caution, and special attention to biofeedback is encouraged. You may discover a new favorite flavor, but conscientiousness is required to utilize herbs successfully.

Quantities listed are for 16 ounces / 1 gallon

## Doshas

The doshas of Ayurveda represent the energy of the human body and mind. According to Ayurveda, a person achieves maximum health when all of the doshas are in balance. The three doshas are *vata, pitta,* and *kapha.* Most people tend to reflect the energy of one dosha more than the others, though all of the elements of each are present. There are specific foods, herbs, and activities that strengthen and balance each of the doshas.

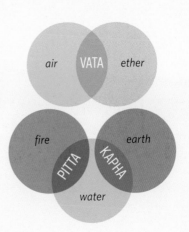

### PITTA

These herbs help balance *pitta,* the dosha that controls metabolism through digestion, nutrition, and body temperature. Fire is the dominant element of *pitta* and when in balance leads to contentment and intelligence.

**CARDAMOM, GROUND**
⅛ teaspoon / ½ teaspoon
**HIBISCUS, DRIED**
⅛ teaspoon / ½ teaspoon
**FRESH PEPPERMINT, ROUGHLY CHOPPED**
2 leaves / 6 leaves
**SARSAPARILLA, DRIED**
⅛ teaspoon / ½ teaspoon
**HOLY BASIL (TULSI)**
¼ teaspoon / ¾ teaspoon
**LEMON ZEST**
1 teaspoon / 2 teaspoons
**PEACH, PEELED AND DICED**
½ tablespoon / 2 tablespoons

### KAPHA

These herbs support *kapha,* the dosha that controls growth, supports immunity, and moisturizes the skin. Water is the dominant element of *kapha* and when in balance is expressed as love and forgiveness.

**CLOVES, WHOLE**
⅛ teaspoon / ½ teaspoon
**FRESH GINGER, DICED**
⅛ teaspoon / ½ teaspoon
**CINNAMON**
⅛ teaspoon / ½ teaspoon
**PEPPERMINT, DRIED**
⅛ teaspoon / ½ teaspoon
**CARDAMOM, GROUND**
⅛ teaspoon / ½ teaspoon
**ALLSPICE, GROUND**
$1/16$ teaspoon / ¼ teaspoon
**ORANGE ZEST**
$1/16$ teaspoon / ¼ teaspoon
**BLACK PEPPER**
$1/16$ teaspoon / ¼ teaspoon

### VATA

This combination supports *vata,* the dosha that controls motion, blood circulation, and breathing. Air is the dominant element of *vata* and when in balance is expressed as creativity and vitality.

**CHAMOMILE FLOWER, DRIED**
¼ teaspoon / 1 teaspoon
**DRIED LICORICE ROOT, CHOPPED**
⅛ teaspoon / ¾ teaspoon
**FRESH GINGER, DICED**
⅛ teaspoon / ¾ teaspoon
**FENNEL SEED**
⅛ teaspoon / ¾ teaspoon
**MINT, DRIED**
½ teaspoon / 1 teaspoon
**ROSE PETALS, DRIED**
¼ teaspoon / 1 teaspoon
**ROSE HIPS, DRIED**
⅛ teaspoon / ¾ teaspoon
**HOLY BASIL (TULSI)**
⅛ teaspoon / ¾ teaspoon
**ORANGE ZEST**
⅛ teaspoon / 1 teaspoon

Quantities listed are for 16 ounces / 1 gallon

# Black Pepper

With its warming properties, black pepper is used to treat cough, cold, indigestion, gum problems, hoarseness, dysentery, and indigestion. Piperine, an alkaloid in pepper, has been shown to have antifever, anti-inflammatory, and pain-relieving benefits.

## Cherry Spice

**CHERRIES, HALVED**
1 tablespoon / ½ cup

**BLACK PEPPER**
½ teaspoon / 2 teaspoons

**CINNAMON BARK CHIPS**
¼ teaspoon / 1 teaspoon

## Heaven Scent

**CARDAMOM, GROUND**
⅛ teaspoon / ½ teaspoon

**CLOVES, WHOLE**
3 cloves / 10 cloves

**FRESH GINGER, DICED**
¼ teaspoon / 1 teaspoon

**BLACK PEPPER**
½ teaspoon / 2 teaspoons

## Pepper Berry

**STRAWBERRIES, CHOPPED**
1 tablespoon / ½ cup

**RASPBERRIES, LIGHTLY MASHED**
1 tablespoon / ½ cup

**BLACK PEPPER**
½ teaspoon / 2 teaspoons

# Ginger

Highly revered in both TCM and Ayurveda, ginger has a long history of use in treating digestive issues, increasing circulation, and creating warmth. Its spicy sweetness pairs particularly well with kombucha and can be combined with myriad other flavoring agents to create any number of flavors. Readily available fresh, dried, ground, or candied, ginger can be used in any form as a flavor agent. Some recipes specify a particular type, but fresh ginger, finely chopped, gives the most flavor. No need to peel it, either!

## Apple Ginger

**APPLE, DICED**
¼ cup / 1 cup

**FRESH GINGER, DICED**
¼ teaspoon / 1 teaspoon

## Ginger Buzz

**FRESH GINGER, DICED**
¼ teaspoon / 2 teaspoons

**HONEY**
1 teaspoon / 1 tablespoon

**BEE POLLEN, LIGHTLY CRUSHED**
⅛ teaspoon / 1 teaspoon

## Jade Dragon

**GREEN JUICE**
2 teaspoons / 2 tablespoons

**FRESH GINGER, DICED**
¼ teaspoon / 2 teaspoons

**CAYENNE**
⅛ teaspoon / ½ teaspoon

# Ginseng

The Chinese word for ginseng, *rénshēn*, means "person root," a description of the way the fleshy, forked root often resembles a person with two legs. Sweet and slightly warming, with a hint of bitterness, it acts as an aphrodisiac, invigorates spleen and lung *qi*, promotes the production of body fluids, and calms the nervous system.

Ginseng comes in a variety of forms. We find capsules are the easiest and most affordable source. If using dried ginseng root, substitute 1 teaspoon for every capsule.

## Just Ginseng

**GINSENG CAPSULE**
1 capsule / 4 capsules

## Panax Pie

**GINSENG CAPSULE**
1 capsule / 4 capsules

**APPLE, DICED**
1 tablespoon / ½ cup

**CINNAMON BARK CHIPS**
¼ teaspoon / 1 teaspoon

## Mint-seng

**GINSENG CAPSULE**
1 capsule / 4 capsules

**FRESH PEPPERMINT, ROUGHLY CHOPPED**
1 teaspoon / 1 tablespoon

Quantities listed are for 16 ounces / 1 gallon

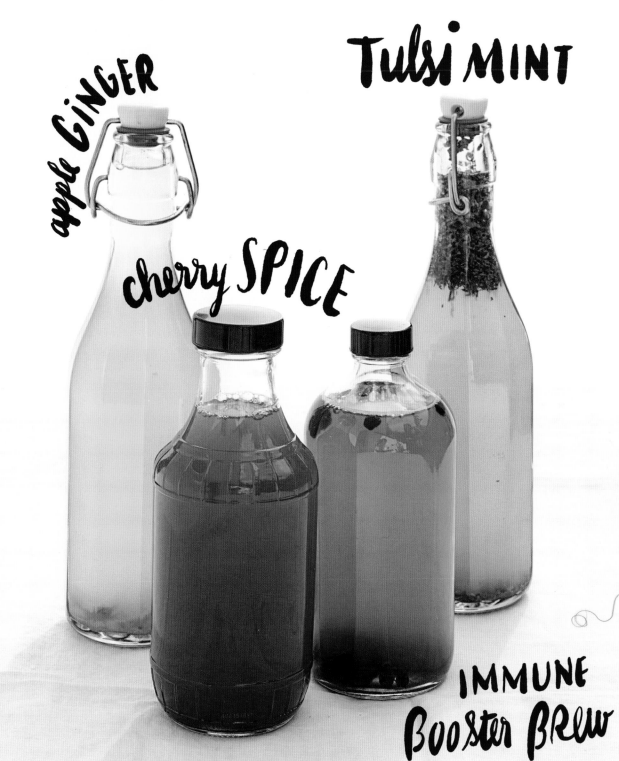

apple GINGER

Tulsi MINT

cherry SPICE

IMMUNE
Booster BRew

# Holy Basil (Tulsi)

Holy basil is highly revered in the Indian tradition, where it is considered the incarnation of the goddess Tulsi and therefore offers divine protection to those who cultivate it. The stalks are often dried and used as rosary beads in meditation malas (prayer beads). A warming herb, it promotes purity and lightness in the body, alleviates gas and indigestion, and cleanses the respiratory tract. It is most commonly available dried in tea bags.

## Holy Melon

**HOLY BASIL (TULSI)**
2 teaspoons / 1 tablespoon
**WATERMELON, CHOPPED**
¼ cup / ¾ cup

## Flower Goddess

**HOLY BASIL (TULSI)**
2 teaspoons / 1 tablespoon
**ROSE PETALS, DRIED**
1 tablespoon / ¾ cup
**CHAMOMILE FLOWER, DRIED**
1 tablespoon / ½ cup

## Tulsi Mint

**HOLY BASIL (TULSI)**
2 teaspoons / 1 tablespoon
**ROOIBOS TISANE**
¼ teaspoon / 1 teaspoon
**FRESH MINT, ROUGHLY CHOPPED**
1 teaspoon / 1 tablespoon

# Licorice

Licorice's naturally sweet flavor comes from the glycyrrhizin in the hard, fibrous root. Other herbs like anise and fennel have a similar flavor and are easier to use. Called *gāncǎo* in TCM, this sweet, neutral herb clears heat from a sore throat, alleviates pain, and prevents spasms in the legs or abdomen, as well as being an antidote for toxins. Be aware that licorice uses up potassium in the body, so supplement potassium intake when consuming licorice regularly.

## Sweet Spice

**DRIED LICORICE ROOT, CHOPPED**
1 teaspoon / 1 tablespoon
**CINNAMON BARK CHIPS**
¼ teaspoon / 1 teaspoon

## Berry Licorice

**DRIED LICORICE ROOT, CHOPPED**
1 teaspoon / 1 tablespoon
**RASPBERRY, DICED**
1 tablespoon / ¼ cup
**BLUEBERRIES, HALVED**
1 tablespoon / ¼ cup

## Tang-orice

**DRIED LICORICE ROOT, CHOPPED**
1 teaspoon / 1 tablespoon
**FRESH TANGERINE JUICE**
1 tablespoon / ¼ cup

# Schizandra Berry

Schizandra berry, or *wǔ wèi zǐ* (five-flavor seed), has the unique distinction of containing all the classic flavors (see chart, facing page). Its properties are sour and warm, and its uses include treating diarrhea, cleansing lung and kidney *qi*, balancing the nervous system, and supporting the production of sexual fluids. The flavor and fizz it lends to kombucha is a testament to its power. A little tart and bitter, it is best paired with fruits or other, sweeter herbs (vanilla, licorice, rooibos) for balance.

## Schizandra

**SCHIZANDRA BERRIES, DRIED**
⅛ teaspoon / 1 teaspoon

## Elder Zandra

**SCHIZANDRA BERRIES, DRIED**
⅛ teaspoon / 1 teaspoon
**DRIED ELDERBERRIES**
1 teaspoon / 1 tablespoon

## Immune Booster Brew

**SCHIZANDRA BERRIES, DRIED**
⅛ teaspoon / 1 teaspoon
**DRIED ELDERBERRIES**
1 teaspoon / 1 tablespoon
**FRESH GINGER, DICED**
¼ teaspoon / 1 teaspoon
**CINNAMON BARK CHIPS**
¼ teaspoon / 1 teaspoon

Quantities listed are for 16 ounces / 1 gallon

# *Turmeric*

Turmeric, sometimes called *kanchani* ("golden goddess") in India, can be applied topically or taken internally and is valued in Ayurvedic medicine for its balancing and healing properties, in particular for respiratory complaints, wounds, and skin ailments. A natural preservative, it can be used in cosmetics and makes an effective insect repellent.

Most noted for the presence of curcumin, this orange rhizome adds oomph to the brew. It is widely available in powder form, but we use fresh root from our health food store. Use 25 percent more of the fresh root (diced) than the powder. Turmeric kombucha has the tang of fresh OJ with the zing of a rhizome for a palate-pleasing punch.

## Orange Blastoff

**TURMERIC, POWDERED**
½ teaspoon / 1½ teaspoons
**FRESH ORANGE JUICE**
1 tablespoon / ¼ cup
**CINNAMON BARK CHIPS**
½ teaspoon / 2 teaspoons

## Soothing Sunrise

**TURMERIC, POWDERED**
½ teaspoon / 1½ teaspoons
**CHAMOMILE FLOWER, DRIED**
1 teaspoon / 1 tablespoon

**FRESH LIME JUICE**
1 teaspoon / 1 tablespoon
**FRESH GINGER, DICED**
½ teaspoon / 1 tablespoon

## Righteous Rhizome

**TURMERIC, POWDERED**
¼ teaspoon / 1 teaspoon
**FRESH GINGER, DICED**
½ teaspoon / 2 teaspoons

## Five Flavors, Five Organs, Five Elements

| Flavor | Organ | Element |
| --- | --- | --- |
| Sweet | Stomach & digestive system | Earth |
| Bitter | Heart & cardiovascular system | Fire |
| Sour | Liver & nervous system | Wood |
| Salty | Kidney & endocrine system | Water |
| Pungent | Lungs, lymph & immune system | Metal |

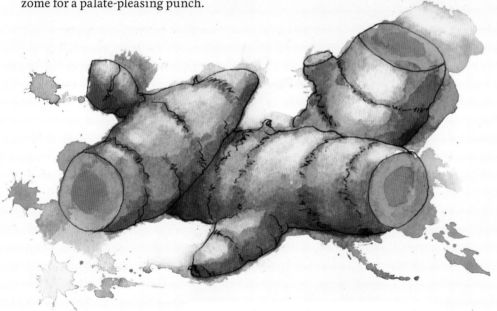

Quantities listed are for 16 ounces / 1 gallon

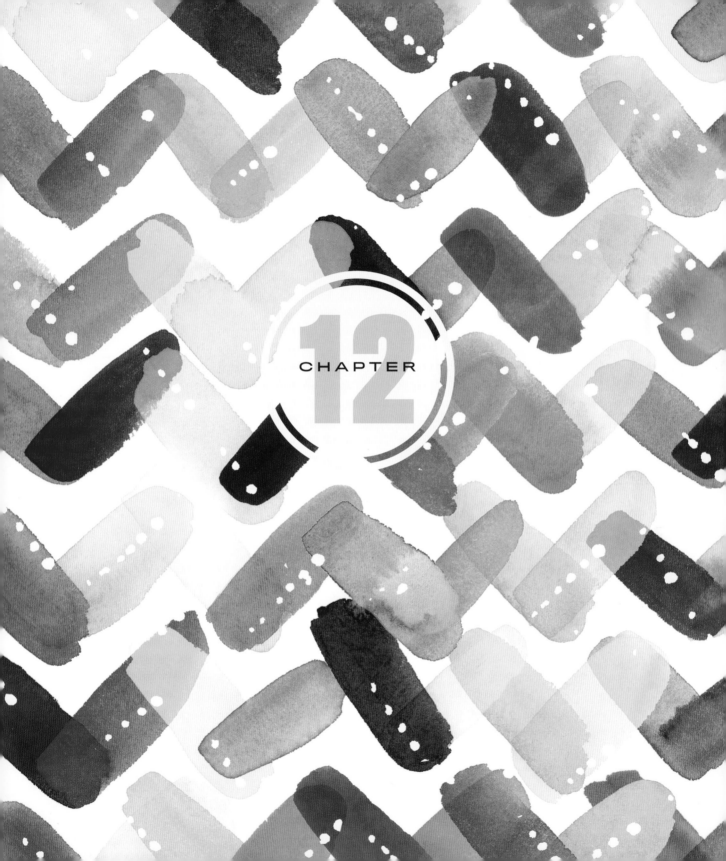

CHAPTER

12

# Smoothies, Sodas, and Spritzers

As consumers gain more awareness of the artificial flavorings, sweeteners, and colorings that make up the average soft drink, the era of soda pop continues to wane. But we still like a sparkly, scintillating alternative to plain water, so now what do we drink? The answer is clear: people are rediscovering fermented beverages. After all, root beer and ginger ale used to be fermented from actual roots, herbs, and spices that delivered authentic flavor with a nutritional boost. The neat thing about rediscovering fermentation technology is that it also inspires us to invent new drinks, using our own unique recipes.

This collection of beverages provides a fun foundation to be creative and tickle your palate. Plus the real foods used to make them add a nutritional boost that simply cannot be found on most grocery shelves these days.

While you're at it, you can power up your morning joe with a little kombucha twist as well. Some coffee drinks and smoothies really fall more in the dessert category of shakes, but hey, we all scream for ice cream once in a while! And you don't need to feel too guilty when you're adding the extra digestive oomph of kombucha to your frozen dessert.

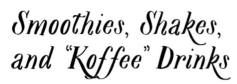

# Smoothies, Shakes, and "Koffee" Drinks

## Basic Fruit 'n' Kombucha Smoothie

Smoothies are a staple for many on-the-go families. Quick, easy, and packed with nutrition, smoothies are practically a meal in a cup, and now you can make them with a natural boost of kombucha power. Mix and match at least one selection from each category below, give the blender a whirl, and voilà!

*Yield: 2 servings*

### FRUIT

bananas, cherries, strawberries, mango, pineapple, peaches, raspberries

### KOMBUCHA

unflavored, ginger-flavored, Power-Up Kombucha (page 210), or experiment

### BOOSTERS

maca powder, protein powder, raw cacao, green powder (chlorophyll, blue-green algae, wheatgrass), bee pollen, nut butter, fruit juice

Ice cubes

Combine 2 cups of fruit, 8 ounces of kombucha, and 1 to 2 tablespoons of boosters in a blender. Add 1 to 2 cups of ice cubes and blend well, adding more kombucha if necessary for a smooth texture. Extra smoothie can be stored in the fridge for up to 24 hours.

## Kombucha Kefir Smoothie

Power up with the probiotic duo of kombucha and kefir. This drink is smooth, creamy, and loaded with nutrition, plus you can mix and match fruits and flavors to create a zillion combos.

*Yield: 2 servings*

    1½ cups mixed berries, frozen or fresh
    ⅔ cup Super C Kombucha (page 184), plus
        more as needed
    ⅓ cup pomegranate juice
    3 tablespoons kefir cheese (see page 271)
        or Greek yogurt
    Ice cubes

Combine the berries, kombucha, juice, and kefir cheese in a blender. If you're using fresh berries, add 1 to 2 cups of ice cubes; skip the ice cubes if you're using frozen berries. Blend well, adding more kombucha if necessary for a smooth texture. Extra smoothie may be stored in the fridge for up to 24 hours.

**KOMBUCHA MAMMA SEZ**

### Freeze!

"Sneaking probiotics into drinks is easy with kombucha ice cubes. Simply pour your favorite kombucha into an ice tray and freeze. Then whenever you need a flavor or health boost, toss a couple of cubes into your drink or smoothie."

# KOMBUCHA KEFIR smoothie

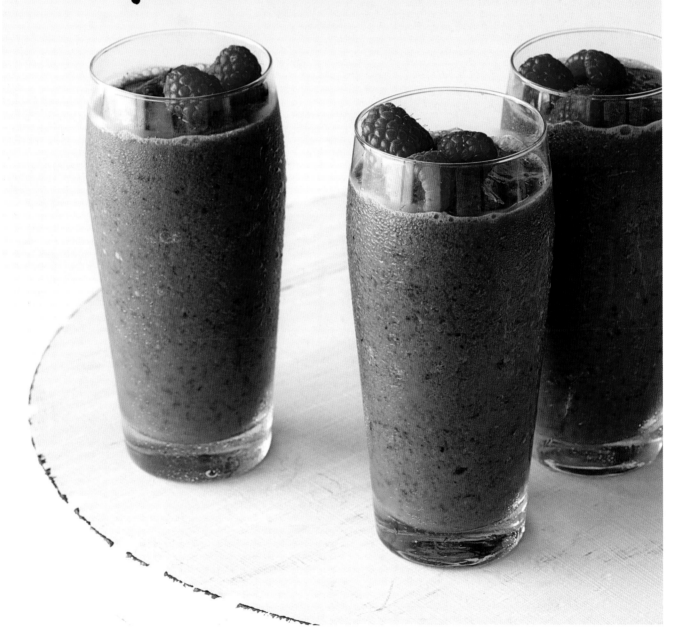

## Kombucha 'n' Kale Smoothie

This nutrient-dense combo is even better than Popeye's spinach trick! The acidity of the kombucha and orange juice gently softens the intensity of the kale, while the banana gives good texture and the berries add a hint of sweetness.

*Yield: 2 servings*

    1 medium banana
    1 whole orange, peeled and seeded
    1 cup fruit (pineapple, strawberries, cherries,
        blueberries, peaches, mangoes)
    1 cup spinach or baby chard
    3 large kale leaves, stems removed
    1 cup I Dream of Greenie kombucha
        (page 210), plus more as needed
    Ice cubes

Combine the banana, orange, fruit, spinach, kale, and kombucha in a blender. Top off with 1 to 2 cups of ice cubes, and blend well, adding more kombucha if necessary for a smooth texture. Extra smoothie can be stored in the fridge for up to 24 hours.

## Kombucha Nut Smoothie

The high fat content of the nuts lends a creaminess to this cool nondairy treat. Fruity kombucha pairs well with creamy cashews, but try it also with Brazil nuts, almonds, or hazelnuts. Soaking the nuts softens them and breaks down phytic acid, an anti-nutrient that impedes digestion and absorption of protein.

*Yield: 2 servings*

    ½ cup raw nuts
    1 cup Raspberry kombucha (page 194), plus
        more as needed
    2 teaspoons maple syrup (grade B, if available)
    2 cups ice cubes

Soak the nuts in water for about 2 hours. Drain and rinse well.

Combine the soaked nuts in a blender with the kombucha, maple syrup, and ice cubes. Blend slowly, adding more kombucha as needed for a smooth texture.

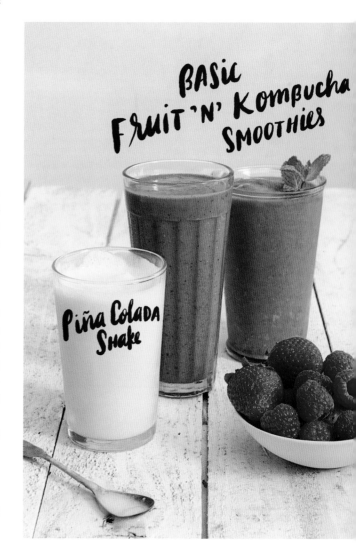

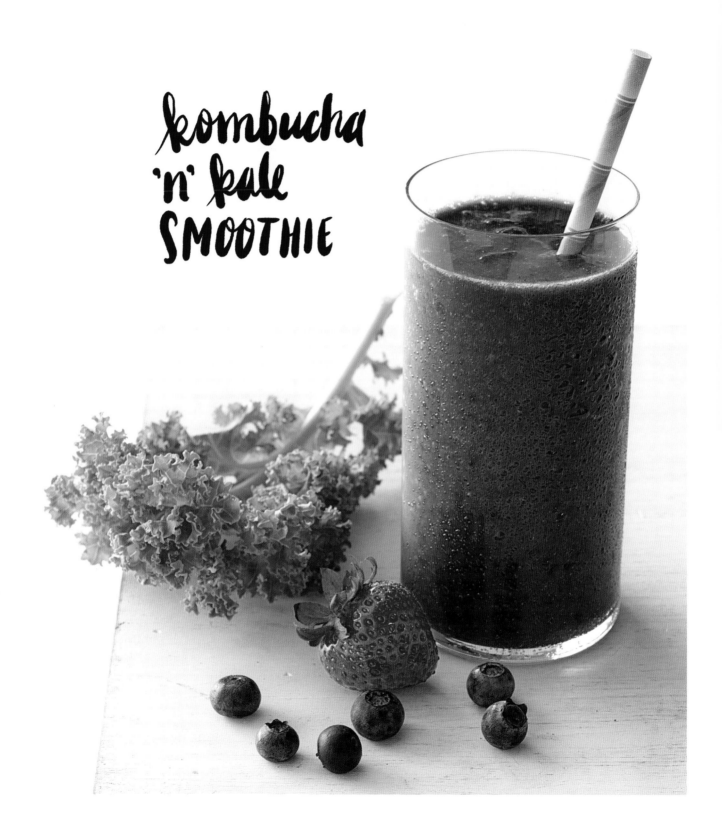

kombucha 'n' kale SMOOTHIE

## Piña Colada Shake

Let your taste buds relax as they float down a river of vanilla and coconut, while the sweet tang of pineapple and kombucha in this frothy treat quenches your thirst for the exotic.

*Yield: 1 serving*

1 cup vanilla ice cream
¼ cup Lime in the Coconut kombucha (page 189)
2 tablespoons pineapple juice
½ cup ice cubes
1 tablespoon flaked coconut
Fresh pineapple slice, for garnish

Scoop ice cream into a blender and pour in the kombucha and pineapple juice. Top off with the ice cubes and coconut flakes. Blend until smooth and serve garnished with a pineapple slice.

## Rootbucha Float

Update this classic summer cooler with a healthy twist. The ice cream balances the medicinal and tangy notes of the Rootbucha. It's easy to invent other fun floats by mixing and matching flavors of ice cream and kombucha.

*Yield: 1 serving*

2 scoops ice cream, sherbet, or frozen yogurt
1½–2 cups Rootbucha (page 145 or 203)

Scoop the ice cream into a tall glass. Slowly pour enough Rootbucha over the ice cream to fill the glass. It may foam up, but you can top off with more kombucha as you slurp it down. Two straws = more fun!

## Chocolate Cherry Kombucha Float

Bitter, tart, and sweet flavors combine to perfection in this decadently dreamy quaff. Omit the coffee to mellow the intensity.

*Yield: 1 serving*

2 scoops of ice cream, sherbet, or frozen yogurt
¼ cup espresso or dark roast coffee
¼ cup Choco-Cherry kombucha (page 207)
Whipped cream, chocolate sprinkles, and cherry, for garnish

Scoop the ice cream into a tall glass. Pour the coffee and kombucha over the ice cream. Spoon a dollop of whipped cream on top, followed by chocolate sprinkles and a cherry.

## Chai Latte Float

Spicy and sweet meet in a creamy treat that can't be beat! Dial up the spice by adding more chai, as desired.

*Yield: 1 serving*

2 scoops of ice cream, sherbet, or frozen yogurt
¼ cup brewed chai tea, cold
¼ cup Chai Spice kombucha (page 197)

Scoop the ice cream into a tall glass; then pour in the chai tea and kombucha.

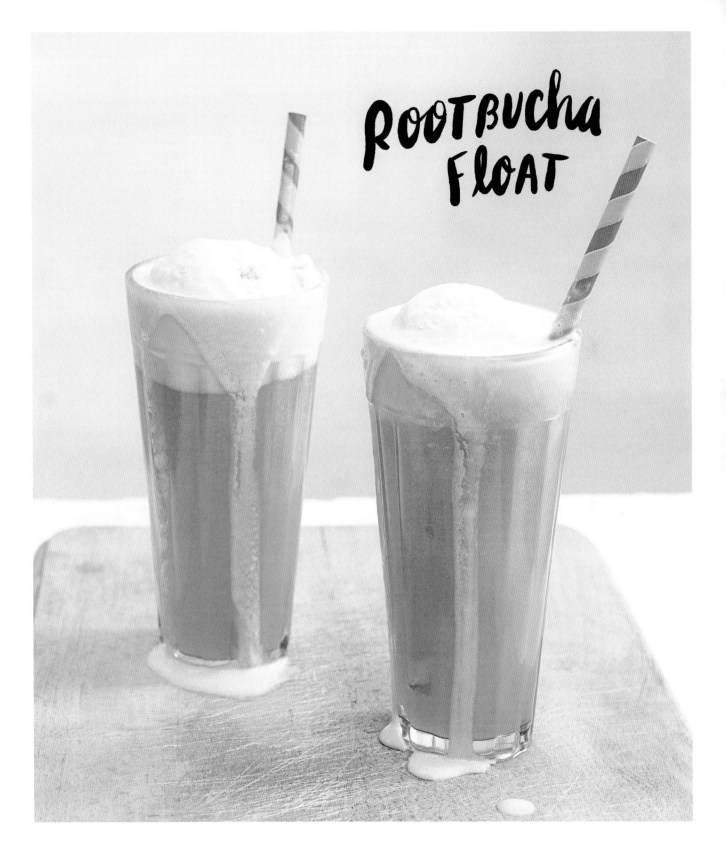

ROOTBUCHA FLOAT

## Kombuffee

The coffee bean's harsh, acidic tones smooth to produce chocolate undertones and a surprisingly sweet aroma. For deeper flavor, increase the ground coffee to ½ cup. We enjoy Kombuffee on its own and use it to make a healthier version of lattes and mochas.

*Yield: 1 gallon*

4 quarts water
⅓ cup ground coffee
1 cup sugar
1 SCOBY
1 cup starter liquid

**1.** Bring 1 quart of water almost to boiling; then remove from the heat. Pour the hot water over the coffee in a large heat-proof bowl and let steep for 5 to 7 minutes. Strain out the grounds and stir the sugar into the hot brew until dissolved.

**2.** Pour the remaining 3 quarts water into a brewing vessel. Add the sweetened coffee and test the temperature with your hand. When it reaches body temperature, add the SCOBY and starter liquid, and then cover and set aside as usual.

**3.** Start tasting the brew after 5 days. Coffee tends to mellow the acetic acid, so it may not taste as tart as regular booch.

**4.** When the brew is ready, remove the SCOBY. If you intend to brew another batch of Kombuffee, you may reuse the SCOBY, but we recommend real kombucha tea as starter liquid rather than brewed kombuffee. If not, compost the culture or store it in a separate SCOBY Hotel.

**5.** Decant the Kombuffee into bottles. We recommend flavoring with complementary tastes like cacao, vanilla bean, and cherry. Let sit at room temperature for 1 to 4 days until it has the flavor and carbonation level desired.

## Iced Kombuffee Latte

Give your morning cuppa a probiotic face-lift. Plus, you save money making this "coffee treat" at home.

*Yield: 1 serving*

1 cup Kombuffee
¼ cup kefir or yogurt
1 teaspoon honey, or to taste
½ cup ice cubes

Combine the Kombuffee, kefir, honey, and ice in a blender. Blend until the mixture has the texture of a Frappa-you-know-what.

**KOMBUCHA MAMMA SEZ**

### Make Mine a Mocha

"Add 2 teaspoons of chocolate syrup to your Iced Kombuffee Latte for an even richer treat. Sprinkle with cinnamon for a gourmet touch."

# Healthy Sparkling Drinks

## Kombuchade

The main problem with commercial energy and sports drinks is that they are loaded with chemicals and sugar. Make your own sports drink that actually replenishes the body and reduces lactic acid buildup.

*Yield: 1 quart*

3½ cups Berry Medley kombucha (page 183)
½ cup apple juice (preferably organic)
¼ teaspoon salt (preferably Himalayan pink salt or Celtic sea salt)

Combine the kombucha, juice, and salt in a quart jar and shake gently. Store in the refrigerator for up to 1 month.

## Kombucha Palmer

Golf great Arnold Palmer used to enjoy a combo of lemonade and iced tea at home. When he ordered one at the bar at the U.S. Open in 1960, a woman nearby requested "that Palmer drink," thus naming it. Use a fruity iced tea with the Lemon Zing booch to hit a thirst-quenching hole in one.

*Yield: 2 quarts*

6 cups iced tea
2 cups Lemon Zing kombucha (page 189)
⅓ cup sugar (optional)
Ice cubes
Sprigs of mint, for garnish

Combine the tea and kombucha in a pitcher. Stir in the sugar until it is completely dissolved. Fill serving glasses with ice. Pour the iced tea mixture over the ice and serve garnished with a sprig of mint.

## Warm Kombucha Cider

When you feel a chill in the air, gently heat a warm mug of kombucha cider. The mulling spices have warming properties that linger within even after the mug is empty. Tie them into a square of muslin or a reusable tea bag.

*Yield: 2 quarts*

### MULLING SPICES

3 cinnamon sticks, broken into pieces
1 tablespoon whole allspice
1 tablespoon whole cloves
2 slices fresh ginger, ½ inch thick
Zest of 1 orange or dehydrated orange peel, chopped as needed

### MAKE THE CIDER

1 quart apple cider
1 cup diced dried apple
½ cup dried cranberries
1 packet mulling spices
1 quart Cinnamon kombucha (page 198)
Cinnamon sticks, for garnish

Combine the apple cider, apple, cranberries, and mulling spices in a pot. Bring to a boil; then reduce the heat and simmer, uncovered, for 20 minutes. Remove from the heat and let cool for 5 minutes. Remove the spice packet.

Stir the kombucha into the warm cider. Ladle into mugs, and garnish with a cinnamon stick.

# warm KOMBUCHA Cider

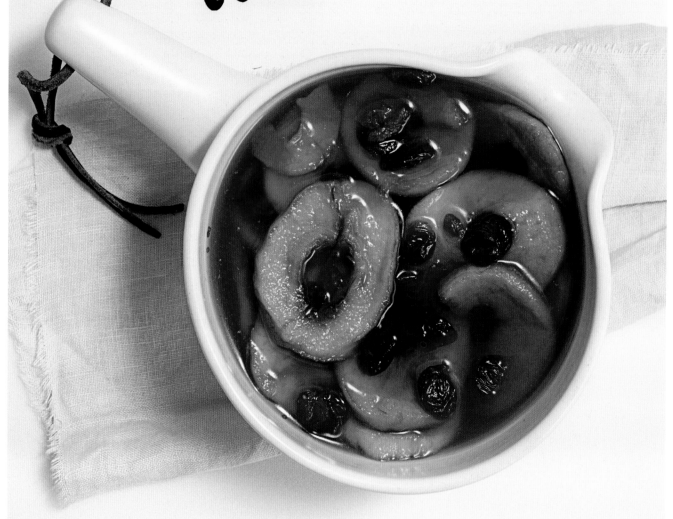

## KombuChia Boba Tea

Boba tea, or pearl tea, is an Asian treat that adds texture by including chewy balls of tapioca or taro root. Chia seeds lend a similar texture when added to kombucha. Native to Mexico, chia seeds come from a desert mint plant and have been cultivated since Mayan and Aztec times. The name *chia* comes from a Nahuatl word that means "oily," and indeed, the seeds are rich in omega-3 fatty acids, along with calcium and antioxidants. They are valued for their energy-giving properties. Chia is popular with runners, as purportedly it was traditionally consumed by warriors and messengers to give them stamina on long journeys.

*Yield: ¼ cup of gel, enough for several servings*

1 tablespoon chia seeds
¼ cup warm water
1 cup flavored kombucha

Combine the chia seeds and warm water in a dish and stir well. Let sit, undisturbed, for 20 to 30 minutes, or until a thick gel forms. Use the gel immediately or store in the fridge for up to 1 week.

For a single serving, mix the kombucha with 1 teaspoon of chia gel in a glass and enjoy! Consume KombuChia within a couple of days for the best flavor. If using chia gel for secondary ferment, the chia seeds, unlike store-bought versions, may not remain suspended in the liquid. Stir to distribute the seeds evenly prior to consuming.

If KombuChia is stored for a period of time, the chia seeds will absorb the sweetness of the kombucha, yielding a flatter, blander flavor in the drink. In this case, add a tablespoon or two of juice or ¼ teaspoon sugar to boost the flavor.

## Kurley Temple

Envious of the fruit in the strictly adult old-fashioned, America's favorite curly-haired starlet requested a fun drink of her own. A Hollywood bartender whipped up a tasty concoction featuring ginger ale and maraschino cherries, and the iconic child's mocktail was born. The kombucha adds a touch of sparkle.

*Yield: 1 serving*

Ice cubes
1 cup ginger-flavored kombucha or Lemon Zing kombucha (page 189)
¼ cup sparkling water or mineral water
2 tablespoons Grenadine Kombucha Shrub (page 246)
Maraschino cherry and orange wheel, for garnish

Fill a highball glass with ice. Add the kombucha, sparkling water, and shrub, and stir. Drop in a cherry and garnish the rim with a slice of orange.

## Mellow Kombujito

Quench your thirst with this refreshingly mellow kombucha mojito mocktail. It's perfect for a midday energy boost that tastes like a cocktail but won't get you in trouble with the boss.

*Yield: 1 serving*

Ice cubes
2 fresh mint leaves
2 tablespoons simple syrup (page 246)
⅛ teaspoon lime zest
¾ cup Lime in the Coconut kombucha (page 189)

Fill a rocks glass with ice. In a separate glass, muddle together the mint, simple syrup, and lime zest. Strain into the rocks glass and top with the kombucha.

## Green Apple Spritz

Power up with a megadose of green goodness in this refreshing palate cleanser.

*Yield: 1 serving*

  Ice cubes
 2 fresh basil leaves
 2 fresh mint leaves
 ¼ cup apple juice
 ¾ cup Apple Mint kombucha (page 202)
    Granny Smith apple slice and a sprig of fresh
    mint, for garnish

Fill a rocks glass with ice. In a separate glass, muddle together the basil and mint with the apple juice. Strain into the rocks glass and add the kombucha. Garnish with an apple slice and a sprig of mint.

## Tropical Slow Burn

Tamarind and pineapple offer sweet and sour notes, while the cayenne slowly ignites a fire from within. Burn, baby, burn!

*Yield: 1 serving*

  Ice cubes
 ½ cup Tamarind Fire kombucha (page 195)
 ½ cup pineapple juice
    Maraschino cherries and pineapple wheel,
    for garnish

Fill a rocks glass with ice. Add the kombucha and juice. Garnish with maraschino cherries and a pineapple wheel.

## Strawb'rita

Nothing will come between you and this lovely 'rita, chock-full of flavor for smooth sipping any time of day, any day of the week.

*Yield: 2 servings*

    Sea salt and sugar, to rim the glass
 1 cup Pink Lemonade kombucha (page 195)
 ½ cup Lemon-Lime shrub (page 239)
 1 cup frozen strawberries
 1 cup ice cubes
 2 lime wheels

Rim 2 rocks glasses with a 50:50 mix of salt and sugar.

Combine the kombucha, shrub, strawberries, and ice in a blender. Pulse until slushy, adding more kombucha as needed to achieve the desired texture.

Pour the drink into the rimmed glasses, and garnish each with a lime wheel.

## Tuesday Night Sangria

If sangria on a weeknight is too much to handle, try this "sin vino" version to avoid whining on a Wednesday. Make it in the morning and sip it with dinner.

*Yield: 1 quart*

 2 cups Plum Spice kombucha (page 192)
 ¾ cup orange juice
 1 cup halved red grapes
 1 sweet red plum, sliced thin
 1 cup sparkling water
    Orange wheels, for garnish

Combine the kombucha, orange juice, grapes, and plum slices in a quart jar. Cap it and let it sit on a counter overnight (8–12 hours). It may be fizzy the next day, and you can let it sit for even longer if you want more carbonation. When the fizz and flavor are to your liking, add the sparkling water, stir very gently, and pour into rocks glasses, garnished with orange wheels.

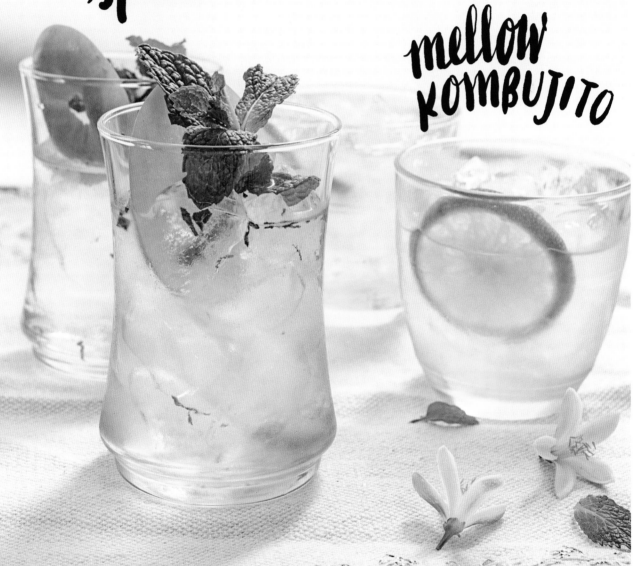

GREEN APPLE
spritz

mellow
KOMBUJITO

# Making and Using Shrubs

Shrubs, which are simply sweetened fruit syrup preserved in vinegar, have refreshed and delighted humankind since ancient times. One way of preserving the fruits of the season, shrubs are high in vitamin C content, making them useful for preventing scurvy aboard seafaring vessels. Shrubs gained popularity during the Temperance movement in the United States, as evidenced by the many recipes found in nineteenth- and twentieth-century housekeeping manuals.

The rise in popularity of "farm-to-bar" cocktails has inspired a reemergence of these tasty, healthful nonalcoholic syrups. Whenever the whistle desires whetting, shrubs provide a tangy, refreshing quaff, whether added to a cocktail or just a plain old glass of water. Using kombucha instead of vinegar adds another layer of flavor and benefit. These easy-to-make syrups are sure to become family favorites, whether they're destined for homemade sodas or for cocktails.

## BASIC SHRUB RECIPE

Shrubs follow a fairly standard ratio of 1 part fruit, 1 part sugar, and 1 part vinegar. However, since kombucha vinegar is less acidic than traditional vinegars, the ratio for a kombucha shrub is 1 part fruit, 1 part sugar, and 2 parts kombucha vinegar. Any type of fresh fruit works — try berries, peaches, plums, rhubarb, apricots, apples, melons, cherries, you name it!

Kombucha vinegar (page 256) — the tarter the better — yields the best flavor, but unflavored kombucha can be used in a pinch as it will continue

*WORD NERD:* **Shrub**

*The word* shrub *comes from Arabic* sharāb, *meaning "wine" (or any beverage), and* shariba, *meaning "to drink." Other words with the same root include* sherbet *(not the frozen dessert but a powder used to make effervescent drinks) and* syrup. *In the oldest definition,* shrub *referred specifically to drinks made of citrus juice, sugar, and rum, or other liquor. In the mid-1800s, the meaning extended to the vinegar/sugar/fruit cordial that is returning to popularity today.*

to ferment, even in the fridge. Try using a spiced kombucha such as Chai Spice (page 197), Herbes de Provence (page 200), or one of the Ayurvedic blends (page 216). Using aromatics and spices adds depth and intensity.

The cold and hot methods described on the following page have plusses and minuses. We prefer the cold shrub method to maintain the maximum health benefit of the fruit and flavorings. If the party is tonight, however, you can use the hot process to whip up a quick batch.

With either method, the sugar will recrystallize on the bottom of the bottle when left undisturbed for an extended period of time. If that happens, shake well to dissolve the sugar in the liquid. Over time the acids in the vinegar and fruit will dissolve all of the sugar crystals.

Taste shrubs frequently. They do mellow, so frequent tasting will allow you to observe how the flavor changes over time. Shrubs keep for up to 2 months in the fridge.

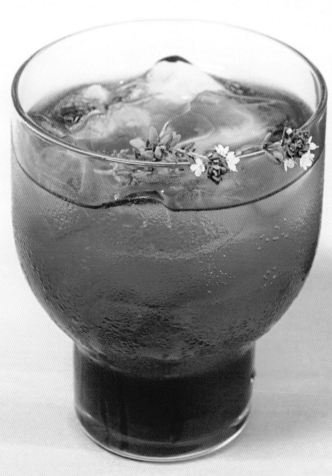
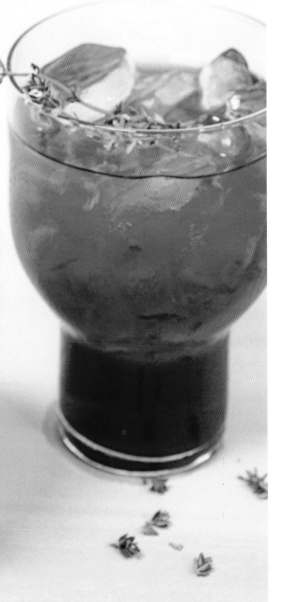

beet AND lemon Shrub

## COLD SHRUBBING

1 cup chopped fruit, pitted if necessary

1 cup sugar

2 cups kombucha vinegar

Combine the fruit and sugar in a bowl and toss gently. Cover and let sit at room temperature for at least a few hours, and up to 24 hours. Stir occasionally to redistribute the sugar over the fruit.

The sugar will pull liquid from the fruit, creating a sweet syrup. Strain the syrup into a 1-quart glass container through a sieve or cheesecloth, pressing to release as much juice as possible from the solids. Scrape any bits of sugar left in the bowl into the syrup. Add the kombucha vinegar and stir to dissolve any residual sugar.

Store in the fridge, where the shrub will keep for up to 2 months or longer. Shake prior to using.

## HOT SHRUBBING

1 cup water

1 cup sugar

1 cup chopped fruit, pitted if necessary

2 cups kombucha vinegar

Combine the water and sugar in a saucepan over medium heat; stir until the sugar dissolves.

Add the chopped fruit to the pan and bring to a boil; then reduce the heat and let simmer for 8 to 15 minutes, until the fruit gives up its juice into the syrup. When the fruit takes on a mushy appearance, it is exhausted of its juice; remove the pan from the heat and let cool completely.

Strain the syrup through a sieve or cheesecloth, pressing to release as much juice as possible from the spent fruit. Pour the syrup into a 1-quart glass bottle and top with the kombucha vinegar. Store in the fridge, where the shrub will keep for up to 2 months or longer.

# How to Enjoy Shrubs

You can create many healthy homemade sodas by simply adding 2 to 4 ounces of shrub syrup to 6 to 8 ounces of sparkling mineral water. Some may prefer more intense flavors, whereas others desire a mellower mix, so customizing for personal tastes is easy. The number of flavor combinations is limited only by your imagination!

Shrubs also add depth and complexity to a cocktail, but use them sparingly at first until you get a feel for the flavor. This is especially true when you're using other sour additives like citrus juice. See more on making cocktails in the following chapter.

**KOMBUCHA MAMMA SEZ**

## Careful with That Fruit

**“**Using fruit left over from a secondary fermentation is *not* recommended for shrubs, because you want the full flavor of the fruit, and fruit from a second ferment will already have had much of its flavor extracted. However, using older or blemished fruit not only saves money but also salvages fruit otherwise headed for the compost pile. Often blemished fruit may be purchased for a discount at farmers’ markets — just ask!”

# shrub flavor SUGGESTIONS

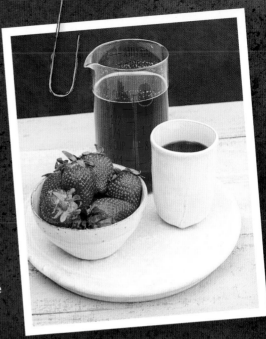

Shrubs can show off a single fruit, multiple fruits, or fruit and herb or spice combinations. The fruit can be fresh or frozen. Below are some suggested combinations to inspire your imagination.

### Apple Cinnamon
1 cup diced apple
1 teaspoon ground cinnamon

### Beet and Lemon
1 cup chopped beets
2 teaspoons lemon zest

### Black 'n' Rasp
½ cup blackberries
½ cup raspberries

### Cucumber Watermelon
½ cup chopped cucumbers
½ cup mashed watermelon
      pieces

### Elderberry Ginger
1 cup dried or fresh elderberries
1 tablespoon diced fresh ginger

### Ginger
1 cup sliced or chopped fresh
      ginger

### Lavender Lemon
1 tablespoon dried lavender
1 teaspoon lemon zest
1 cup lemon juice

### Lemon-Lime
1 cup lemon and lime slices

### Mixed Berry and Lavender
1 cup diced berries
1 tablespoon fresh lavender

### Peach Spice
1 cup sliced peaches
1 teaspoon chai spice, hand
      ground (page 197)

### Plum Spice
1 cup sliced plums
½ teaspoon ground cinnamon
¼ teaspoon ground cloves
⅛ teaspoon ground allspice

### Strawberry and Rhubarb
fresh berries and diced rhubarb

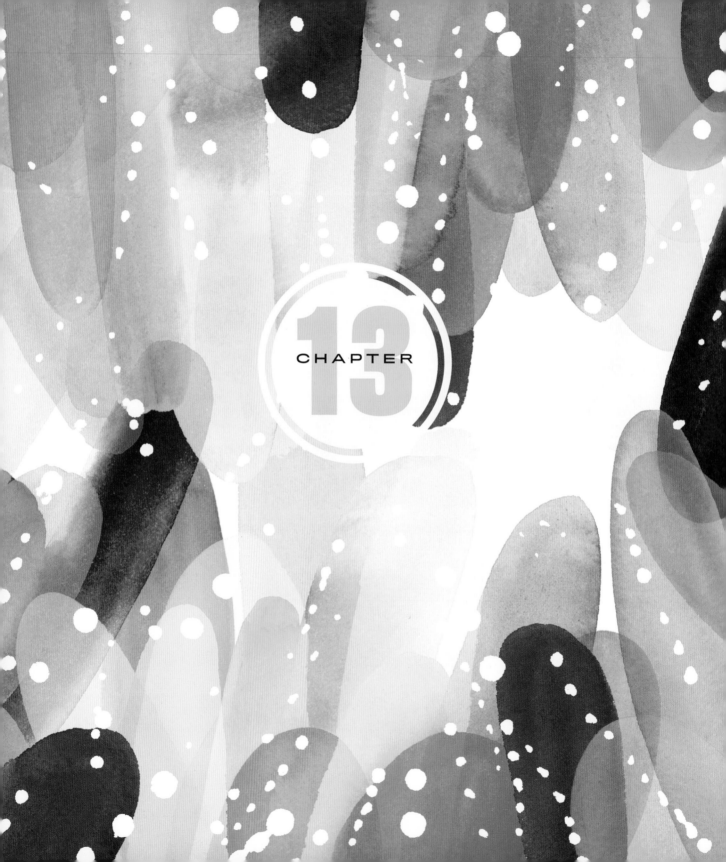

CHAPTER

13

# Kick Back with a "Kocktail"

Though often maligned in modern society, alcohol holds significant cultural, social, historical, nutritional, medical, and even evolutionary importance. It is normal for humans to crave alcohol because it has deep roots in our physical well-being, and this chapter celebrates that craving.

Kombucha takes on the flavor and benefits of whatever is infused into it, making it the perfect mixer. Straight up, in a shrub, or as a cocktail, kombucha imbues complex flavor for deeply satisfying drinks. Kombucha is so low in alcohol that it's pretty much impossible to get a buzz. But Kombucha Kocktails are a great way to marry the goodness of the booch to a little extra alcohol for additional relaxation. Many find that drinking kombucha quells their desire for harder beverages, thanks in part to its living profile.

Another reason kombucha is the perfect cocktail mixer is that it provides a built-in hangover cure — a little "antidote with the poison," as we always say. This is due to the B vitamins, which prevent nausea and enhance mood. Glucuronic acid also assists the liver, where alcohol is metabolized, in expelling toxic molecules.

This recipe collection features many American classics with a kombucha twist. So raise a glass and toast to the healing benefits of nature's gifts and enjoy the relaxation and peace of mind that comes from conscious and balanced consumption. As they say in Russia, "Za zdarov'e!" (to your health).

# Beer Drinks

## Kombucha Shandy

> 4 ounces ginger-flavored kombucha
>
> 4 ounces beer (preferably a lighter beer such as wheat beer or lager)

Combine the kombucha and beer in a cold glass.

## Spicy en Chelada

> Salt, for rimming a glass
>
> 6 ounces Master Cleanse kombucha (page 182)
>
> 4 ounces beer
>
> 2 ounces Clamato (tomato juice with clam broth; optional)
>
> Lime wedge, for garnish

Rim a cold glass with salt. Add the kombucha, beer, and Clamato (if using) and garnish with a lime wedge.

## Red Beerd

> 6 ounces Pico de Boocha (page 215) or other tomato-based kombucha
>
> 4 ounces beer (preferably a lighter beer such as wheat beer or lager)
>
> 2 ounces tomato or veggie juice
>
> Salt
>
> Lime wedge, for garnish

Pour the kombucha, beer, and tomato juice into a cold glass and add salt to taste. Stir and garnish with a lime wedge.

*WORD NERD:* **Shandy**

*Shandies were created by German bartenders who on hot summer days mixed lemonade and beer to serve more people with a limited beer supply. Enjoy a Kombucha Shandy any time of year!*

# Bourbon and Whiskey Drinks

## Bourbon 'n' Booch

> 2 ounces bourbon
>
> 4 ounces ginger-flavored kombucha or Lemon Zing kombucha (page 189)
>
> 1 slice fresh ginger
>
> Lemon wedge, for garnish

Pour the bourbon and kombucha into an ice-filled glass and stir gently. Squeeze the ginger into the glass through a garlic press and garnish with a lemon wedge.

## New-Fashioned

> 2 orange slices
>
> 3 maraschino cherries
>
> 2 dashes bitters
>
> Ice cubes
>
> 2 ounces bourbon
>
> 4 ounces Cherry Up kombucha (page 184) or Orange Blast-Off kombucha (page 221)

Muddle one orange slice, two cherries, and the bitters in a rocks glass. Remove the orange slice, leaving the cherries, and fill the glass with ice cubes. Add the bourbon, top with kombucha, and stir. Garnish with the remaining slice of orange and cherry.

## Jack 'n' Booch

> Ice cubes
>
> 3 ounces Jack Daniel's whiskey
>
> 3 ounces Cream Soda kombucha (page 205)

Fill a rocks glass with ice. Pour in the Jack Daniel's and kombucha and stir.

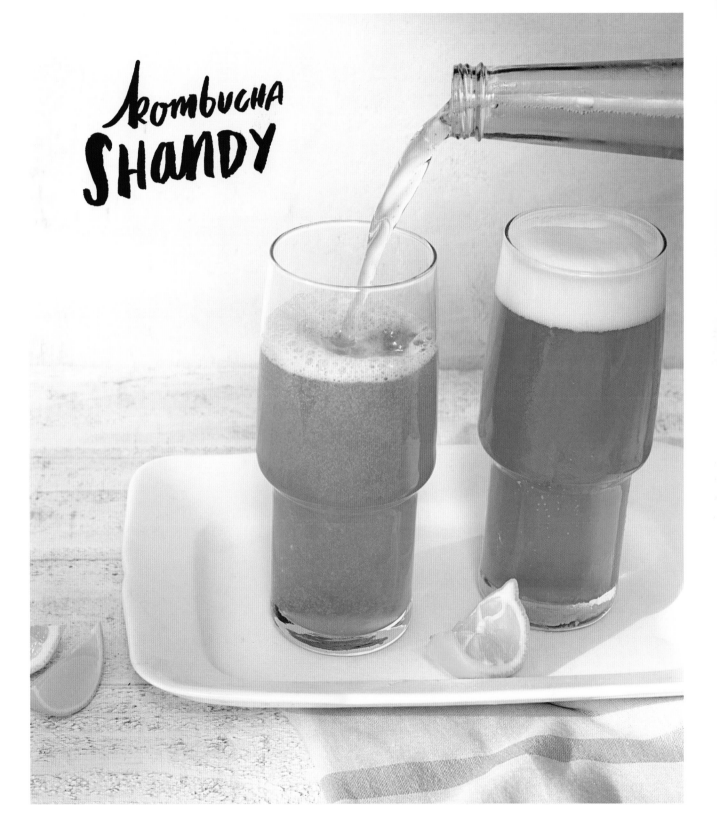

Kombucha
SHANDY

### Rock the Bourb

Ice cubes

2 ounces bourbon

6 ounces Rock the Casbah kombucha
(page 183)

Blood orange slice, for garnish

Fill a glass with ice, add the bourbon, and top with the kombucha. Garnish with a slice of blood orange.

### Peach Spice Bourbon Shrub

Ice cubes

2 ounces bourbon

1 ounce cherry liqueur

1 ounce Peach Spice kombucha shrub
(page 239)

6 ounces sparkling water

Fill a highball glass with ice and add the bourbon, cherry liqueur, and shrub. Top off with the sparkling water.

### Kombucha Sour

Ice cubes

3 ounces unflavored, Lemon Zing (page 189),
or Cherry Up (page 184) kombucha

1½ ounces bourbon

1½ ounces tart cherry juice

Splash of sparkling water

Fill a rocks glass with ice. Add the kombucha, bourbon, and cherry juice. Add sparkling water and stir.

### Pomegranate Pucker

Pomegranate arils (seeds)

4 ounces Lemon PomBucha (page 192)

2 ounces whiskey

Ice cubes

You can buy packages of pomegranate arils, but if you're working with a whole pomegranate, slice it in quarters and gently remove the arils from the white skin. Place the arils in a glass and add the Lemon kombucha and whiskey. Finish with a few ice cubes.

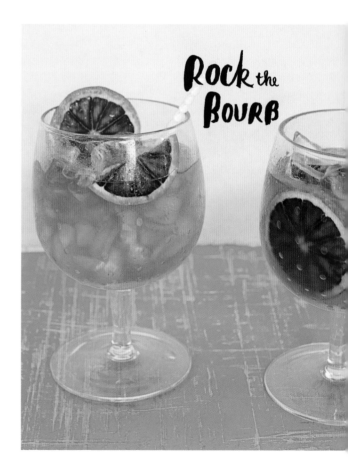

Rock the BOURB

# Gin Drinks

## Mint Fizz

    5 ounces gin
    4 ounces Apple Mint kombucha (page 202)
    1½ ounces simple syrup (page 246)
    1 egg white
    Splash of sparkling water
    Orange peel twist and mint sprig, for garnish

Pour the gin, kombucha, simple syrup, and egg white into a shaker and shake vigorously. Strain into a highball glass, top with sparkling water, and garnish with a twist of orange peel and the mint. The egg white will foam up when shaken, creating a beautiful pillow of "fizz."

## Porktini

    Ice cubes
    3 ounces Maple Pork Soda kombucha (page 211)
    2 ounces gin
    1 ounce sparkling water

Fill a glass with ice. Combine the kombucha, gin, and sparkling water in a shaker, shake well, and pour over the ice.

## Lavender Kollins

    Ice cubes
    2 ounces gin
    1 ounce Lavender Lemon kombucha shrub (page 239)
    3 ounces sparkling water
    Sprig of lavender, for garnish

Fill a glass with ice. Pour the gin and shrub over the ice, add the sparkling water, and stir gently. Garnish with lavender.

## Dakiri

    5 ounces rum
    2½ ounces Sour Mix Kombucha Shrub (page 246)
    1½ ounces simple syrup (page 246)
    Ice cubes

Combine the rum, sour mix, and simple syrup in a shaker with ice. Shake, then strain into a martini glass. If you prefer dark rum, cut back on the simple syrup for a balanced flavor.

# Rum Drinks

## R 'n' R

    Ice cubes
    4 ounces Rootbucha (page 145 or 203)
    2 ounces dark rum

Fill a rocks glass with ice. Pour the Rootbucha and rum into the glass.

## Kombujito

    2 fresh mint leaves
    1 ounce simple syrup (page 246)
    ⅛ teaspoon lime zest
    2 ounces light rum
    Ice cubes
    6 ounces Lime in the Coconut kombucha (page 189)

Muddle the mint leaves, simple syrup, and lime zest in a glass. Add the rum, stir, and strain into highball glass with ice. Top with the kombucha.

# BAR BASICS

Stocking the bar with kombucha shrubs in basic flavors makes it possible to whip up a delicious cocktail at a moment's notice. Store-bought counterparts are usually full of artificial preservatives and colorings that can yield an unappetizing flavor. These ones are made with real ingredients and kombucha, so they literally bring cocktails to life.

## Simple Syrup

As the name suggests, making this syrup is easy. Flavored simple syrups are simply shrubs without the vinegar! Just follow the shrub instructions on page 236, using 1 cup of water instead of 2 cups of vinegar.

*Yield: 1 cup*

> 1 cup sugar
> 1 cup water

Combine the sugar and water in a saucepan over medium heat. Stir until the sugar is fully dissolved. Cool and store in a jar in the fridge, where it will keep for up to 3 months.

## Sour Mix Kombucha Shrub

Sour mix adds flavor, tartness, and balance to cocktails and spawned its own category of beverages, appropriately termed "sours."

*Yield: 2 cups*

> 1 cup sugar
> 1 cup kombucha, kombucha vinegar, Citrus Mist (page 183) or other citrus-flavored kombucha
> ½ cup freshly squeezed lemon juice
> ½ cup freshly squeezed lime juice
> ½ teaspoon lemon zest
> ½ teaspoon lime zest

Add the sugar to a quart jar and pour in the kombucha, lemon juice, and lime juice. Shake to help the sugar dissolve, though it won't all dissolve at this point. Then add the zest. Store in the refrigerator, where the sour mix will keep for up to 3 months. Shake daily until all the sugar is dissolved.

## Grenadine Kombucha Shrub

This sweet syrup gives beautiful color and deep flavor to the likes of the Kurley Temple (page 233). Add a splash or two to any flavor of kombucha or soda water to create a quick and tasty drink.

*Yield: 2 cups*

> 1 cup sugar
> 1 cup unsweetened pomegranate juice
> 1 cup unflavored kombucha, kombucha vinegar, or Lemon PomBucha (page 192)

Combine the sugar and pomegranate juice in a saucepan over medium heat. Stir until all the sugar is dissolved. Remove from the heat. When cool, add the sweetened juice to a quart jar and top with the kombucha. Store in the fridge, where it will keep for up to 3 months.

# Tequila Drinks

## Klassic Kombucha-rita

    Sugar or salt, for rimming a glass
1½ ounces tequila
 1 ounce Lavender Lemon kombucha shrub
    (page 239)
 1 ounce triple sec
 ½ ounce freshly squeezed lime juice
    Ice cubes
    Lime slice, for garnish

Rim a rocks glass with sugar or salt. Combine the tequila, shrub, triple sec, and lime juice in a shaker with ice. Shake and strain into the rimmed glass. Garnish with a slice of lime.

## My Blue Rita

 5 blueberries
    Ice cubes
1½ ounces tequila
 1 ounce Holy Boly kombucha (page 184)
 1 ounce triple sec
 ½ ounce freshly squeezed lime juice
    Lime slice, for garnish

Muddle the blueberries in the bottom of a shaker. Add a handful of ice cubes; then pour in the tequila, kombucha, triple sec, and lime juice. Shake and strain into a rocks glass full of ice. Garnish with a lime slice.

## Mango Rita

12 ounces dark tequila
 8 ounces freshly squeezed orange juice
 1 cup diced mango (frozen or fresh)
 2 cups ice
 8 ounces Buddha's Delight kombucha
    (page 190)
    Sugar, for rimming glasses
    Orange wheels, for garnish

This makes a whole pitcher to share. Pour the tequila, orange juice, mango, and ice into a blender and pulse until slushy. Stir in the kombucha. Pour into rimmed rocks glasses and garnish with orange wheels.

# Vodka Drinks

## Basic Kombucha Kocktail

 1 part kombucha, any flavor
 1 part sparkling water
 1 part vodka
    Ice cubes

Combine the kombucha, sparkling water, and vodka in a rocks glass over ice. Use this as a base to create your own variations by combining different flavored vodkas with complementary flavored kombuchas.

## UnScrewd

 6 ounces freshly squeezed orange juice
 4 ounces Blood Orange Italian Soda (page 183)
    or Dreamy Orange (page 190)
 3 ounces vodka

Combine the juice, kombucha, and vodka in a high-ball glass. Or substitute champagne for the vodka to make a lovely mimosa.

## Kosmo

3 ounces Cran-bucha (page 184)

1 ounce vodka

Squeeze of fresh lemon juice

Ice cubes

2 ounces sparkling water

Lemon twist, for garnish

Combine the kombucha, vodka, and lemon juice in a shaker with ice. Shake lightly and strain into a martini glass. Top off with the sparkling water and garnish with a lemon twist.

## Healthy as a Mule

3 ounces Lemon Zing kombucha (page 189)

3 ounces sparkling water

2 ounces vodka

1 ounce Ginger kombucha shrub (page 239)

Ice cubes

Lime slice, for garnish

Pour the kombucha, sparkling water, vodka, and shrub over ice in a highball glass or copper mule mug. Stir and garnish with a slice of lime.

## Beet Kosmo

3 ounces Beet and Lemon kombucha shrub (page 239)

3 ounces sparkling water

2 ounces vodka

Ice cubes

Lemon wedge, for garnish

Combine the shrub, sparkling water, and vodka in a highball glass filled with ice. Garnish with a lemon wedge.

## Bloody Booch

2 ounces tomato juice

2 ounces Spicy Tomato kombucha (page 214)

1½ ounces vodka

½ ounce freshly squeezed lemon juice

Ice cubes

Dash of Worcestershire sauce

Celery salt

Freshly ground black pepper

Hot sauce

Horseradish (optional)

Celery stalk, for stirring

Lemon wedge, pickles, and olives, for garnish

Combine the tomato juice, kombucha, vodka, and lemon juice in a highball glass filled with ice. Add the Worcestershire, celery salt, black pepper, hot sauce, and horseradish (if using) to taste, and stir with a celery stalk. Garnish with a lemon wedge, pickles, and olives for a savory treat.

---

**KOMBUCHA MAMMA SEZ**

### Does the Hooch Kill the Good Stuff in the Booch?

"Alcohol can clean a wound, but does that mean it kills all the good stuff in our kombucha cocktails, too? No way! First of all, we mix and drink them pretty quickly (pace yourself, they're yummy!). It would take much longer to kill all the bacteria and yeast in that much booch, even if the alcohol were strong enough. Just as important, healthy acids, enzymes, and other goodies remain intact, providing liver support that mitigates the negative effects of alcohol and a better chance at avoiding a hangover. As the Chinese say, 'gān bēi' (Bottoms up!)."

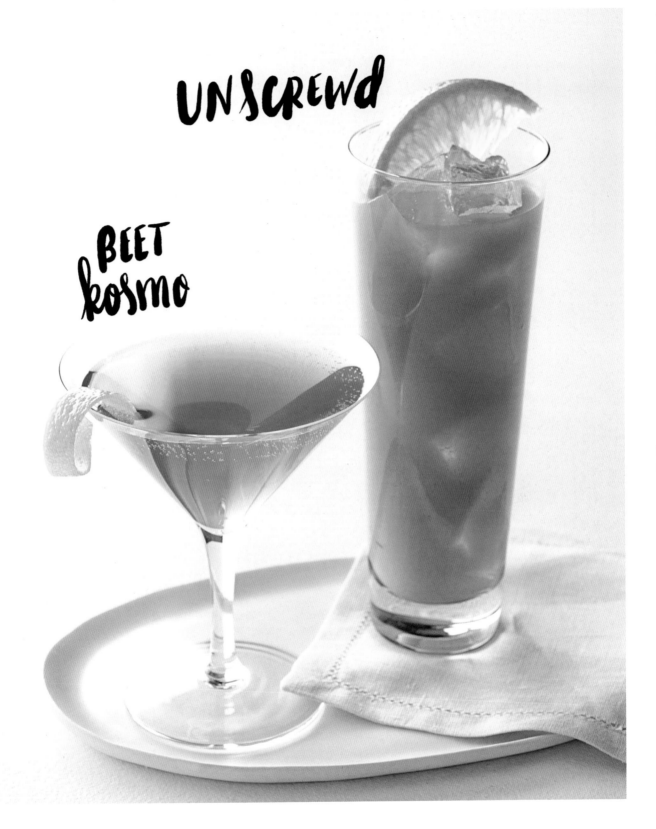

UNSCREWD

BEET
kosmo

## *Wine and Champagne Drinks*

### Le Vent d'Été

3 ounces champagne

3 ounces Summer Breeze kombucha (page 198)

2 ounces elderflower liqueur

Strawberry, for garnish

Elderflower petals, for garnish

Combine champagne, kombucha, and elderflower liqueur in a champagne flute. Garnish with a fresh strawberry and/or elderflower petals.

### Sparkling Kombucha Punch

16 ounces Summer Breeze kombucha (page 198) or Ginger Punch kombucha (page 201)

16 ounces sparkling wine

8 ounces sparkling water

Orange and lemon slices, for garnish

Chill the kombucha, sparkling wine, and sparkling water before combining in a pitcher or bowl. Float slices of orange and lemon on top.

### Kombuchagria

1 (750 mL) bottle fruity red wine

16 ounces Cold Fighter kombucha (page 185)

6 ounces pineapple juice

2 cups chopped fruit (a mix of peaches, lemons, limes, oranges, cherries, and/or strawberries)

Combine the wine, kombucha, pineapple juice, and fruit in a large pitcher. Let chill in the refrigerator overnight for best flavor.

## NEGUS – VICTORIAN CHILDREN'S PARTY WINE

During the Victorian era it was not uncommon to find children imbibing a nip here and there. Negus, as an example, is a mulled wine that was popular at special occasions such as children's birthday parties and was also doled out as wassail to Christmas carolers. We have our own favorite version made with lemon-flavored kombucha. Of course, you have to decide for yourself if this drink will be shared with the children or kept for the adults!

*Yield: 6 cups*

1 quart water

2 cups port wine

½ cup sugar

2 ounces Lemon Zing kombucha (page 189)

½ teaspoon grated lemon zest

¼ teaspoon ground nutmeg

Bring the water to a boil in a saucepan. In a pitcher, combine the port, sugar, kombucha, lemon zest, and nutmeg. When the water just comes to a boil, remove from the heat and pour over the sugared wine. Stir to warm thoroughly and ladle into mugs.

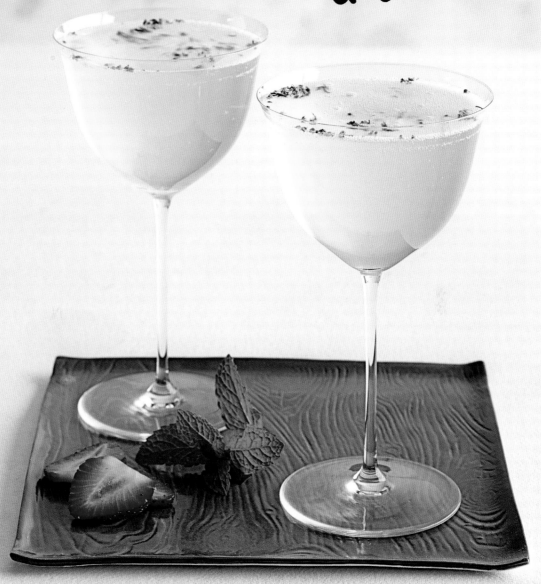

le vent d'été

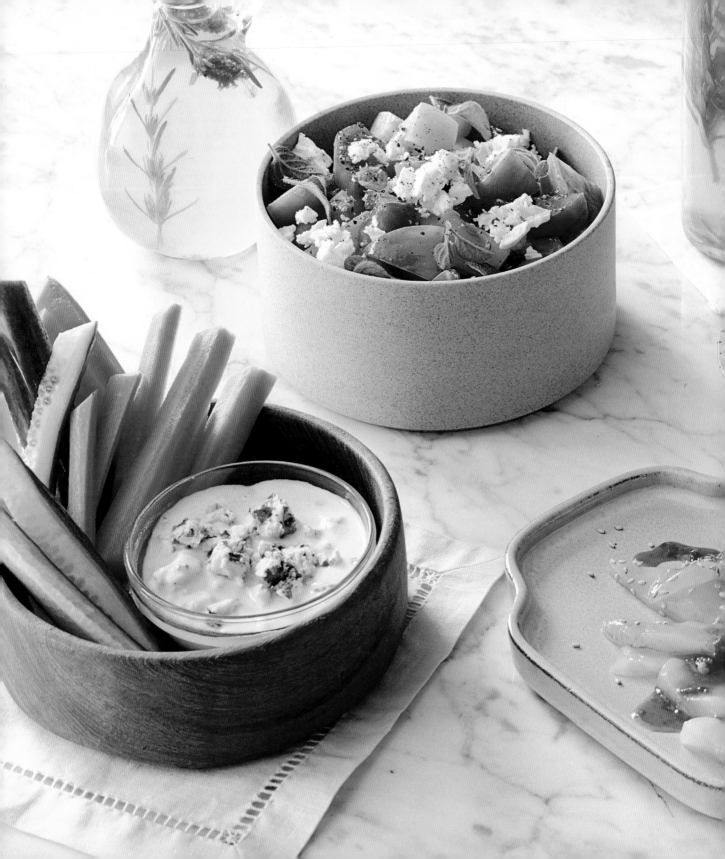

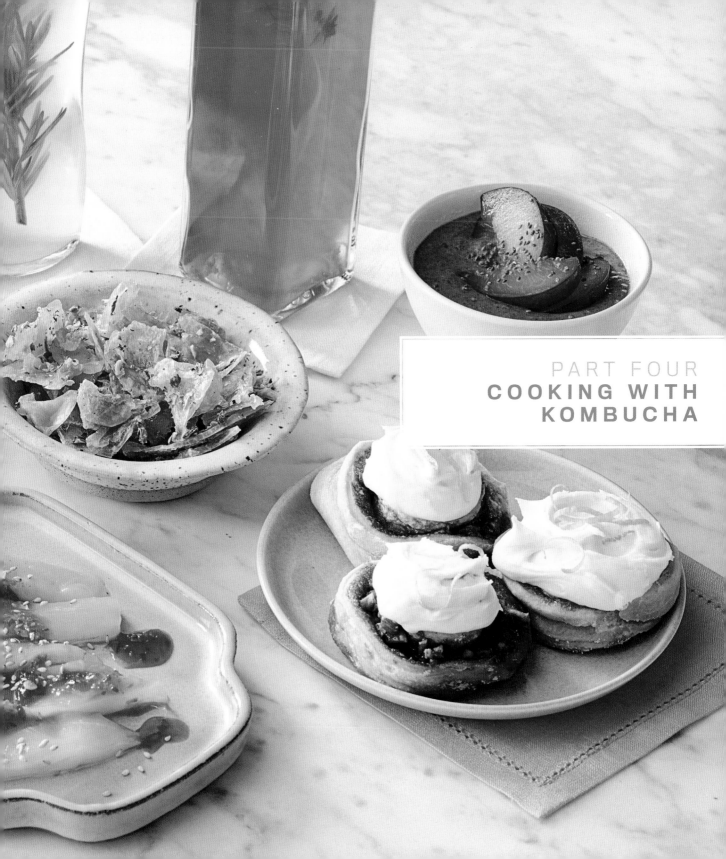

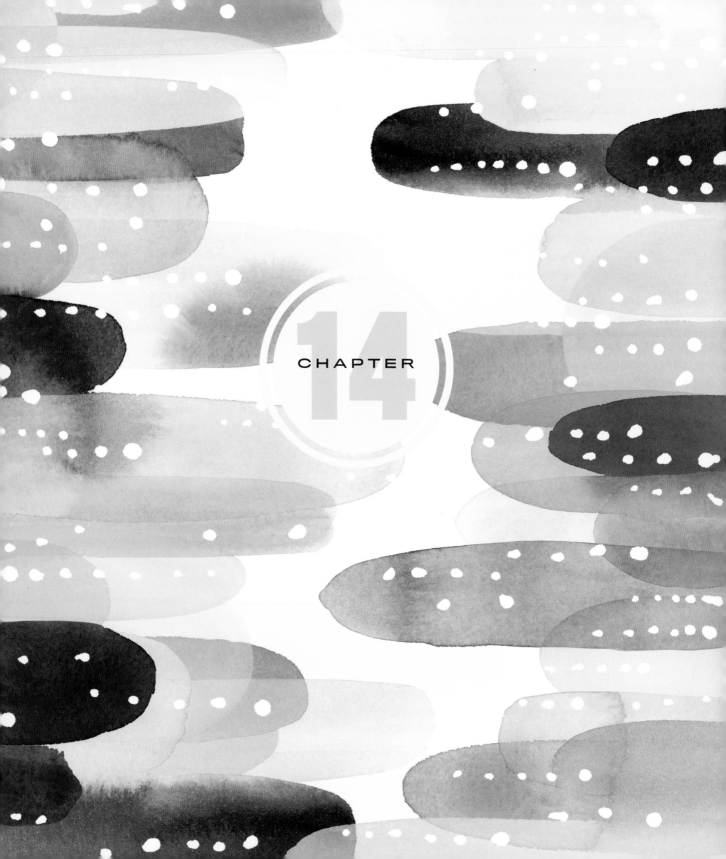

CHAPTER

14

# Pantry Staples

True confession: for most of my life, I have been afraid of cooking. Sure, I could throw a defrosted chicken breast in a pan with a jar of pasta sauce, but that was survival. My resistance was rooted in fear: fear of the unknown, fear of embarrassment, fear of failure. If a recipe didn't turn out perfectly, I never tried it again. I didn't enjoy being in the kitchen.

But after I discovered kombucha, something about the relationship between me and that strange brew eased my fears, built my confidence, and fueled a desire to branch out beyond the teakettle. I've embraced Julia Child's advice to "learn how to cook, try new recipes, learn from your mistakes, be fearless, and above all have fun."

After making kombucha part of our daily lives, we discovered that it can be used to enhance many recipes, particularly in the form of delicious, robust kombucha vinegar, which is as easy to make as kombucha itself. We use the vinegar to make healthful bone broth, and we combine it with yeast collected from our CB setup to create a tasty sourdough starter. We like to keep these three basics on hand as building blocks for delicious and nutritious meals.

# Invigorating Kombucha Vinegar

Kombucha vinegar is a snap to make: simply let a batch of kombucha tea ferment for longer than usual, anywhere from 4 to 10 weeks. As the sugar and other nutrients are consumed by the bacteria and yeast, the sourness of the kombucha tea increases. This means that the older the kombucha, the more potent the flavor and the higher the acetic-acid concentration. When the flavor is very sour, your kombucha tea is now kombucha vinegar. Keep a couple of bottles handy for cooking and general household use (see chapter 17).

Kombucha tastes vinegary because it is an acetic ferment, but unlike most commercial vinegars, which are 4 to 7 percent acetic acid, kombucha vinegar is about 2 percent. This gives it a somewhat milder flavor than other vinegars, though the tea base will also influence the flavor.

Our favorite kombucha vinegars are those we brew in oak barrels. Oak lends toasty and mellow notes that balance the tartness, and it creates yet another depth of flavor when used in vinaigrettes and marinades. (Learn about Barrel Brewing on page 127. )

## How to Make It

To make kombucha vinegar, start with a batch of kombucha (1 gallon or less) that is already at least four weeks old; it should have about 1 percent acidity at that point. To increase the acidity of the vinegar to 2 percent, add 2 teaspoons

## MAKING FLAVORED VINEGARS

Adding fresh herbs and spices to kombucha vinegar yields complex flavors and nutrients. Don't be shy about adding a couple of tablespoons of flavored vinegar to any of your favorite recipes for an extra jolt of flavor and nutrition. Here are some suggestions for flavors — mix and match them to create your own signature blends!

- **SAVORY:** garlic, onions, scallions, shallots, lemon zest
- **HERBAL:** thyme, oregano, mint, lemon balm, basil
- **FLORAL:** lavender, chamomile, rose, elderflower, hibiscus

Making flavored vinegars couldn't be simpler. Simply add 1 to 2 tablespoons of chopped fresh herbs and spices (1–2 teaspoons dried) to 1 quart of kombucha vinegar. Seal the bottle and allow the mixture to infuse for 2 to 3 weeks in a cool, dark location. Strain out the flavoring agents; then store at room temperature. The vinegar will keep indefinitely. If a SCOBY forms, compost it or feed it to some chickens.

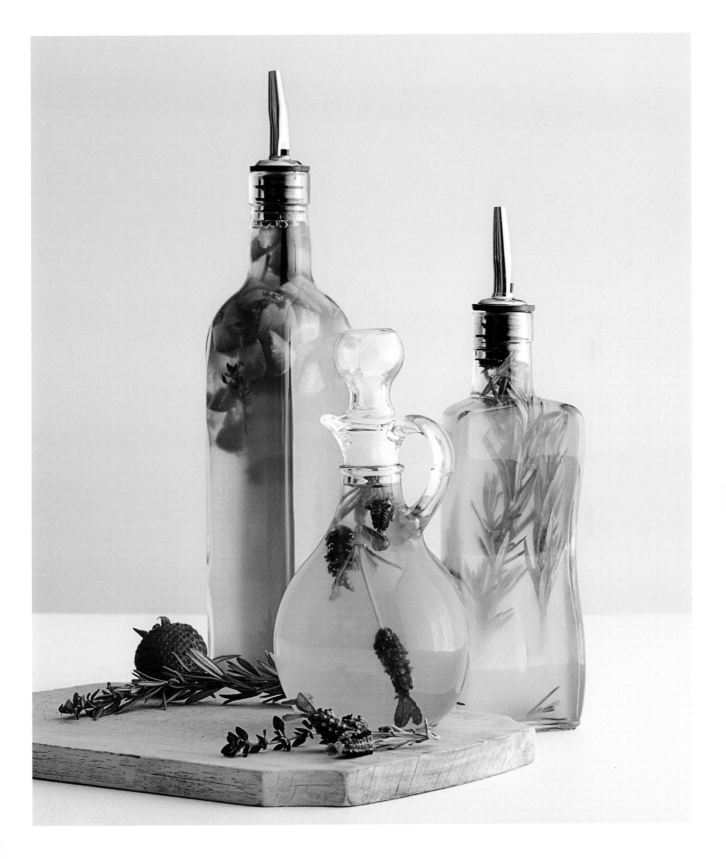

of sugar per pint of vinegar every two weeks for a period of six weeks (that's three rounds total). More rounds can be added as desired. Use immediately or flavor with herbs and ferment for up to six months, depending on how strong you like your vinegar. A SCOBY may form; you can either ignore it or remove it.

Because it has a relatively mild acetic-acid profile, kombucha vinegar tends to be less tart than other vinegars. When you're cooking with it, if you prefer a stronger vinegar flavor you can increase the amount of kombucha vinegar or supplement with another, tarter vinegar such as balsamic or apple cider.

## Pasteurizing Kombucha Vinegar

Kombucha vinegar is in itself a natural preservative due to its low pH, and it will keep indefinitely. However, it will continue to sour and ripen over time unless it is pasteurized, as even in the fridge kombucha continues to sour. In recipes that aren't cooked, such as condiments and dressings, kombucha vinegar can lead to off flavors over time due to continued fermentation. For these recipes, you may want to pasteurize the vinegar, effectively killing off the yeast and bacteria and putting a stop to fermentation.

*WORD NERD* **Vinegar**
*Combined from the French words* vin *(wine) and* aigre *(sour or bitter), vinegar is literally soured wine. In Chinese, the phrase "eat vinegar" means to be jealous — perhaps because the look on a jealous person's face is as if he or she had just drunk a big glass of vinegar!*

There are two methods for pasteurizing vinegar — heat and chemical. To pasteurize on the stove, heat the kombucha vinegar to 145°F (63°C) and hold it at that temperature for 30 minutes. To chemically pasteurize, crush 1 Campden tablet per gallon of vinegar and stir to dissolve. Cover the vessel and let it sit for 12 to 24 hours; then bottle.

Though the probiotics are sacrificed with pasteurization, the liquid retains its nutritional value, including healthy acids, and the flavor is unaffected. It is still an excellent preservative and will punch up the flavor of uncooked recipes. Pasteurized kombucha vinegar is a healthier, lower-acid alternative to distilled vinegar, much of which is made from genetically modified corn these days.

# Beautifying Bone Broth

We use homemade bone broth as a base for many meals because it is rich in nutrients and flavor. An excellent source of collagen (the protein found in connective tissues), it is also a good source of minerals and amino acids. Among other things, it contributes to healthy bones and joints, beautiful and supple skin, and immune health. It soothes and supports the health of the gut lining and stimulates the secretion of digestive acids, making it particularly beneficial for digestive health.

Adding kombucha vinegar to the pot acts as a solvent, extracting additional nutrients from the veggies and bones. It helps to free up the thick consistency of a proper gel that is one of the defining characteristics of a good bone broth.

The broth is a great substitute for water when you're making soups and rice or reheating leftovers in a pan. Low in sodium, it has a neutral flavor that can be adjusted according to the recipe and personal taste.

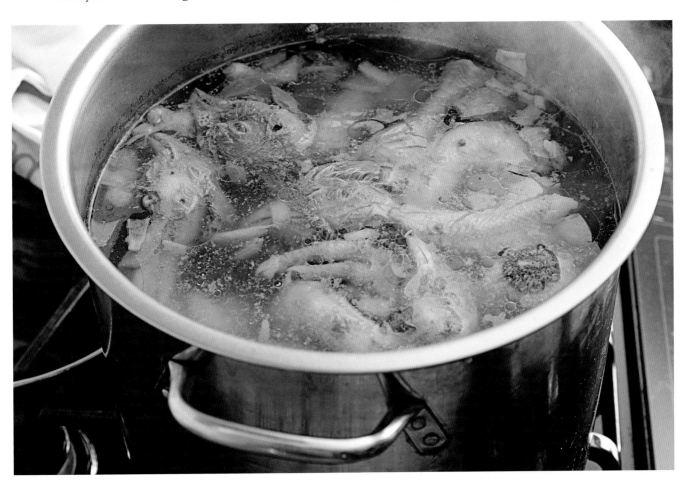

# Kombucha Bone Broth

This is our basic recipe for bone broth. We sometimes substitute 2 cups vegetable scraps — carrot peels, celery and onion ends, broccoli stalks, and other bits that we save in the freezer for just this purpose — for the chopped carrot and celery. Of course you can use whichever vegetables and herbs you prefer or even none at all.

If you prefer not to consume animals, simply omit the bones and include miso, seaweed, and lots of veggie scraps for flavor and additional nutrition.

*Yield: 7 quarts*

## INGREDIENTS

- 1–2 tablespoons fat: butter, coconut oil, or lard
- 2–6 garlic cloves, peeled and slightly crushed
- 1 onion, diced
- 2 sprigs fresh thyme or 1 teaspoon dried
- 2 sprigs fresh oregano or 1 teaspoon dried
- 2 sprigs fresh marjoram or 1 teaspoon dried
- 2 bay leaves
- 2–3 ribs celery, roughly chopped
- 2 carrots, roughly chopped
- 1–3 cups kombucha vinegar (page 256)
- 2 tablespoons sea salt
- ¼ cup miso paste or 1 (2-inch) piece dried seaweed (optional)
- 3–5 lb chicken heads and feet; or 4–6 lb beef knuckles and marrow bones; or 4–6 lb pork bones and ham hocks; or 3–5 lb fish heads and bones
- 2 gallons water

## INSTRUCTIONS

Melt 1 tablespoon of the fat in a large stockpot over medium heat. Add the garlic and onion and sauté until translucent, 3 to 5 minutes.

If the bottom of the pan looks dry, add another tablespoon of fat. Then add the thyme, oregano, marjoram, bay leaves, celery, and carrots to the pot, stir to coat, and sauté for a couple of minutes. Add the kombucha vinegar, salt, miso or seaweed, and bones. Pour in the water.

Bring to a boil, then cover and cook over low heat for 24 to 48 hours. The former is sufficient to create a nutritious broth, but I prefer to go 48 hours because it maximizes nutrient extraction from the ingredients.

As you notice foam forming on the surface, lightly skim it off, being careful not to remove the healthy fat. The broth should have a delightful aroma when you lift the lid.

Remove from the heat and strain out the solids.

Pour the broth into containers to cool. Store in the fridge, where the broth will keep for up to 1 week, or in the freezer, where it will keep indefinitely.

---

**KOMBUCHA MAMMA SEZ**

## Bone-Broth Dog Food

"We give Sydney the Kombucha Poocha the leftover heads and bones from the broth. The long boiling time coupled with the acidity of the kombucha causes the bones to be soft and easy to chew, even for our little chihuahua-terrier mix."

# Snappy Sourdough Starter

Soaking grain prior to consumption is a traditional practice that not only removes anti-nutrients such as phytic acid from grains but also allows wild yeast to populate the mix so that when the dough is baked, a natural rise occurs. San Francisco is famous for sourdough thanks to a unique strain of yeast that thrives in the local climate. Artisan bread makers continue these tasty traditions, and some are also making kombucha sourdoughs! The yeast in kombucha yields a denser bread with less rise and a richer flavor.

Starting a sourdough culture from scratch is a fun way to utilize excess yeast produced by the kombucha brewing process to create delicious, wholesome breadstuffs. (See page 109 for directions on collecting yeast.) One round of cleaning out a continuous brewer may not yield all the yeast you need; just capture as much as you can each time you clean the vessel, and store it in a container in the refrigerator with enough liquid kombucha to cover all the yeast.

Alternatively, the yeast can be dehydrated and powdered for future use. Simply place the yeast on a dehydrator tray, and put on the lowest setting, 95 to 110°F (35–43°C), until completely dry. Pulse the dried yeast in a coffee grinder to pulverize it, and store in an airtight vessel in a cool, dry location (the fridge works). You can also air-dry the yeast by spreading it out on a cookie sheet covered with a tea towel to allow air to flow but prevent bugs from getting into the yeast.

## Creating the Starter

This procedure makes about 3 cups of starter. You need the following:

   2 cups all-purpose flour
   1 cup sugar
¼–1 cup kombucha yeast
 1–2 cups kombucha or kombucha vinegar, at
       room temperature

Combine the flour, sugar, yeast, and kombucha in a medium nonreactive bowl and stir to form a lumpy mixture. Cover the bowl with a cloth, secured with a rubber band. Let sit at room temperature, stirring once a day, until small bubbles form in the mixture, which takes approximately 3 to 7 days.

## Feeding the Starter

The starter can be used for baking as soon as it becomes bubbly, but it is still weak at this point. Taking the time to feed it for a few days will ensure the best flavor and rising power.

For feeding and storing the starter, you'll want a nonreactive container that holds at least 3 quarts, has a tight-fitting lid, and fits on a refrigerator shelf. Add 1 cup of flour and 1 cup of kombucha or kombucha vinegar to the starter and stir until well combined.

Cover the container with a cloth, secured with a rubber band, and let sit at room temperature for one day. Feed the starter again each day for the next two days. At the end of the third day, the starter will be robust and ready for baking some bread!

## Using and Storing the Starter

This may seem like a lot of starter, but you will use 1 to 2 cups for most recipes. Every time you take some starter, replace that amount with an equal amount of flour and kombucha or kombucha vinegar, to maintain your supply. For example, if you take 2 cups of starter to make bread, stir back into the container 1 cup of flour and 1 cup of kombucha.

Between uses, store the starter tightly covered in the refrigerator. Because yeast are temperature-sensitive, the starter will work best when the amount needed for a recipe is brought to room temperature prior to use.

If you use your kombucha sourdough starter regularly — say, at least every week or two — the yeast will remain active, happily digesting the flour you add every time you take some starter and welcoming their compatriots with every replenishment of kombucha.

And you can ignore the starter for up to four to six months; it will remain viable, if slightly sluggish. However, if you haven't used and replenished the starter for longer than six months, you'll need to restart it before you can use it again. Keep 3 cups, discard the rest, and repeat the feeding process to rebuild its strength. Those wanting more lift from their kombucha sourdough may want to add a pinch of commercial yeast to hasten that process along.

# Kombucha Sourdough Cinnamon Rolls
## with Kefir Icing

These delightful breakfast (or anytime!) treats are best when enjoyed fresh from the oven and piping hot.

*Yield: 9 rolls*

DOUGH

- 1¾ cups unbleached all-purpose flour
- 2 tablespoons sugar
- ¼ teaspoon salt
- 1 cup kombucha sourdough starter (page 261), recently fed
- ½ cup whole milk
- 1 tablespoon butter, melted
- 1 teaspoon vanilla extract

FILLING

- ⅓ cup brown sugar
- ⅓ cup crushed nuts (optional; try pecans, walnuts, or almonds)
- 1½ teaspoons ground cinnamon
- 2 tablespoons butter, melted

FROSTING

- 1 cup confectioners' sugar
- 4 tablespoons (½ stick) butter, at room temperature
- 2 ounces kefir cheese (see page 271)
- ½ teaspoon vanilla extract
- ¼ teaspoon lemon oil (or ½ teaspoon grated lemon zest)

INSTRUCTIONS

To make the dough, combine the flour, sugar, and salt in a medium bowl and stir gently to mix. Make a

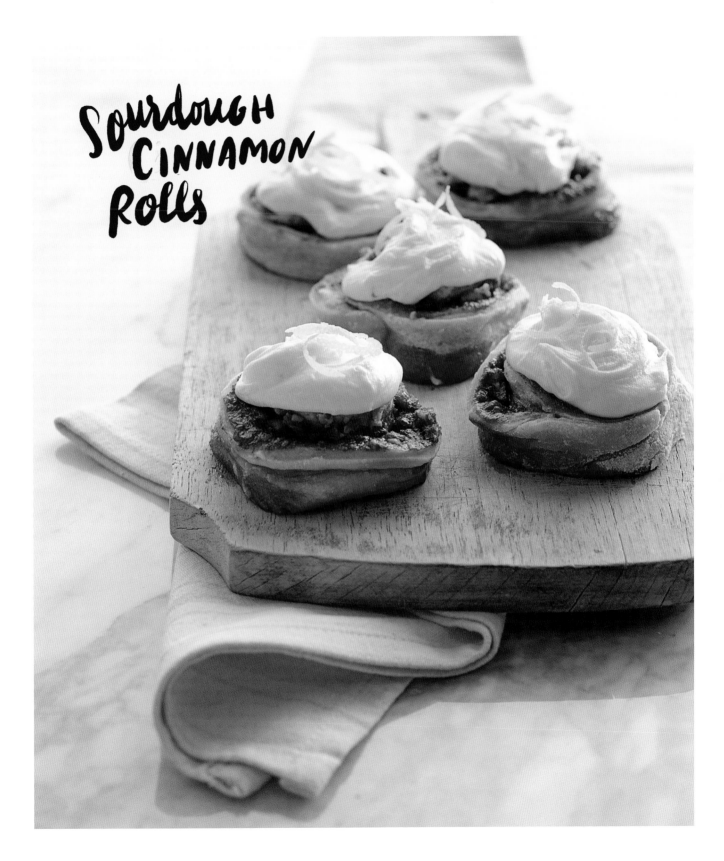

Sourdough
Cinnamon
Rolls

well in the middle of the flour mixture and pour in the sourdough starter, milk, butter, and vanilla. Using a wooden spoon or lightly greased hands, mix the ingredients to create a slightly sticky, pliable dough. Knead the dough for about 5 minutes. If it's too tacky, add more flour, 1 tablespoon at a time, while kneading to create a smooth, slightly sticky ball.

Place the dough in a greased bowl and put a warm, damp towel over the bowl. Set the bowl in a warm place and let rise for 3 to 5 hours. The longer it rises, the tangier the flavor will be. I sometimes let mine rise overnight.

While the dough is rising, make the filling: combine the brown sugar, crushed nuts, and cinnamon in a small bowl, mix well, and set aside.

After the first rise, turn the dough out onto a floured surface and use a rolling pin to flatten it into a rectangular shape. Spread the 2 tablespoons of melted butter over the flattened dough with a pastry brush. Sprinkle the filling mixture evenly over the butter.

Roll up the dough lengthwise into a log, firmly but not so tightly that it cracks. Use a sharp knife to cut the dough log into nine individual rolls. I cut it into thirds, then cut each third into three pieces.

Grease an 8-inch square pan with butter and place the cinnamon rolls into the pan. Cover with a warm, damp towel and let the dough rise, about 2 hours; the rolls may or may not fill the entire pan.

Preheat the oven to 350°F (175°C). Bake the rolls for about 25 minutes, until the tops are slightly brown. (If desired, brush the tops with additional butter to increase browning.) Let the rolls cool slightly before frosting them.

While the rolls are baking, make the frosting: Combine the confectioners' sugar, butter, kefir cheese, vanilla, and lemon oil in a medium bowl. Beat until fluffy, about 10 minutes. If you're doing this by hand, use a whisk and make sure your butter and kefir cheese are very soft.

Spread the frosting over the rolls. Serve immediately or store in the fridge, where they will keep for up to 1 week (if they last that long!).

# Fermented-Fruit Kombucha Sourdough Bread

When used to initiate a second fermentation, fruit becomes infused with good bacteria and yeast. The fermentation process does pull flavonoids, vitamins, and other nutritional constituents from the fruit, but not all of the nutrition is extracted in the 2 to 3 days of infusion. While we often compost the fruit or give it to the neighbor's chickens, we sometimes bake it into kombucha sourdough bread. Denser than other sourdoughs, it is delicious piping hot with a pat of butter.

*Yield: 2 loaves*

## INGREDIENTS

4–4½ cups unbleached all-purpose flour
2 cups kombucha sourdough starter (page 261), recently fed
1¼ cups water
1–2 cups fruit leftover from a secondary fermentation*
1 tablespoon salt

*Omit the fruit and add 1 tablespoon of sweetener (sugar or honey) to make a plain loaf.*

Combine 4 cups of the flour with the sourdough starter, water, fruit, and salt in a large bowl and mix well. You can knead the dough by hand on a lightly floured surface or with a food processor fitted with a dough hook. Knead until it comes together in a smooth, slightly sticky ball, 10 to 12 minutes by hand or 5 minutes in the mixer. If it's too tacky, add more flour, 1 tablespoon at a time.

Oil a large bowl. Set the dough ball in the bowl, and roll gently to coat all surfaces with oil. Cover the bowl with a warm, damp towel, set it in a warm spot, and let the dough rise until it has nearly doubled in size, 4 to 12 hours. For a tangier loaf, allow the dough to rise for 12 to 24 hours.

Separate the dough into two pieces and place each loaf in a greased bread pan. (To make a circular loaf, shape the dough into a ball and place it on a baking stone or in a Dutch oven.) Cover loosely with a warm, damp towel, and let rise until the dough just reaches the rim of the loaf pan, 1 to 1½ hours.

Preheat the oven to 450°F (230°C).

Use a sharp knife to score the top of the loaves with an X or slash marks. Bake for 10 minutes; then lower the temperature to 400°F (205°C). Bake another 25 to 30 minutes, until the tops of the loaves are golden. Turn out onto a wire rack and let cool completely.

# Condiments, Dressings, and Sauces

Condiments are the spice of (food) life, whether they sweeten, sour, or heat up our meals. And while zesty sauces and pickles have been livening up the flavor of food for thousands of years, originally they performed another function as well: digestive assistance.

That's right, the tangy ketchup on our fries, the spicy mustard on our hot dogs, and all the other traditional condiments are supposed to be alive(!) with beneficial bacteria and yeast that bolster both the digestive and the immune system. Classic examples include steak sauce on a rib-eye, sauerkraut on a Reuben, traditionally prepared salsas, and the classic chutneys of Indian cuisine.

Traditionally these condiments were made with ingredients that served as natural preservatives as well as fermentation starters — salt, sugar, lemon juice, and vinegar all assist in the culturing process.

Kombucha vinegar makes superior sauces that taste best when lightly fermented and consumed fresh. The longer they sit, the more the natural flavors may be altered. Some fermentation may improve the flavor, but at a certain point the yeast takes over.

For this reason, we recommend making small batches. Pasteurizing the kombucha vinegar prior to use allows for a longer storage time but kills off all the probiotics (see page 258). Freezing kills some of the probiotics, but not as many as in pasteurization, and it allows you to have smaller portions of your favorites readily available.

# Kombuchup

This thick, crimson ketchup is full of zip! Take it from "great" to "wowie-zowie" with curry, chipotle, or anchovy, à la the original "ketchup" (see History of Ketchup, below).

*Yield: 2½ cups*

### INGREDIENTS

- 12 ounces tomato paste
- ¼ cup sugar
- 2 teaspoons molasses
- ½ teaspoon sea salt
- ½–1 cup kombucha vinegar (page 256)

### FLAVORING SUGGESTIONS

*Mix and match to create your own favorite flavor.*

- 3 garlic cloves, minced, or ¼ teaspoon garlic powder
- 2 anchovy filets, chopped
- ¼ teaspoon chipotle powder
- ¼ teaspoon ground cinnamon
- ¼ teaspoon curry powder
- ¼ teaspoon ground mustard
- ⅛ teaspoon ground allspice
- ⅛ teaspoon cayenne
- ⅛ teaspoon ground cloves
- ⅛ teaspoon ground nutmeg

### INSTRUCTIONS

Mix the tomato paste, sugar, molasses, and salt with ½ cup of the vinegar in a medium bowl. If the ketchup is thicker than desired, slowly add more vinegar until it reaches your ideal consistency. For thicker ketchup, start with ¼ cup vinegar.

Add seasonings as desired. You can split the batch to make different flavors, but adjust the amounts accordingly.

Store in the refrigerator, where Kombuchup will maintain its flavor for about 2 weeks, or longer if you use pasteurized vinegar.

# HISTORY OF KETCHUP

Ketchup has been around for thousands of years, but it wasn't always made out of tomatoes. Originating in Asia as a fermented fish sauce called *kôechiap* or *kê-tsiap*, it dates back to 300 BCE. Easy to store on long voyages, the sauce made its way along trade routes to Indonesia and the Philippines. British traders who developed a hankering for the salty-sour fish flavor brought it back to England in the 1700s.

Over time, the base was made with a variety of ingredients, including oysters, mushrooms, and walnuts, but it remained extremely salty, making it a natural preservative. Colonists brought their traditional ketchup recipes with them to the New World. Though tomatoes were considered poisonous until the early 1800s, once that notion was dispelled they quickly gained popularity. By the time ketchup started showing up in American cookbooks of the mid-1800s, it was as a tomato-based sauce.

# Banana Ketchup

Responding to tomato rationing during World War II, a Filipino food scientist named Maria Orosa utilized the country's natural resources and invented banana ketchup! The bright orange color of the commercial product still sold in Filipino markets comes from adding annatto seeds. Since we left them out, this version has a more yellow-orange hue. We predict that kids and adults alike will go bananas for this delicious dipping sauce.

*Yield: 1½ cups*

## INGREDIENTS

2 tablespoons peanut oil

1 small yellow onion, chopped

2 garlic cloves, minced

1 tablespoon chili paste, or 1–2 fresh chiles (Thai, jalapeño, or serrano), chopped

1 cup mashed ripe bananas (2 medium bananas)

1 tablespoon tomato paste

½ cup kombucha vinegar (page 256), plus more as needed

¼ cup water

2 tablespoons dark brown sugar, plus more as needed

1 teaspoon soy sauce

## FLAVORING SUGGESTIONS

*Mix and match to create your own favorite flavor.*

2 teaspoons freshly grated ginger

1 bay leaf

½ teaspoon ground black pepper

½ teaspoon ground turmeric

¼ teaspoon ground allspice

⅛ teaspoon ground cloves

⅛ teaspoon sea salt

## INSTRUCTIONS

Heat the peanut oil in a medium saucepan over medium heat. Add the onion and sauté, stirring often, until soft and translucent, 5 to 7 minutes. Add the garlic and chili paste and cook for 1 to 2 minutes. Add the bananas, tomato paste, vinegar, water, sugar, soy sauce, and whatever spices you prefer, and stir well.

Bring to a boil; then reduce the heat and let simmer, partially covered, until the mixture thickens, 20 to 30 minutes. Remove from the heat and let cool for 10 minutes. If you used a bay leaf, take it out and discard.

Use a food processor or blender to purée the mixture. Taste. Add more kombucha vinegar to thin the consistency or add tartness, or add more sugar to sweeten. Store in a jar in the refrigerator, where it will keep for up to 3 weeks, or pasteurize to store for an extended period of time.

# Kombucha Mustard

Mustard has been spicing up hot dogs, egg salads, and Reuben sandwiches for centuries. Using whole mustard seeds creates a distinctive, flavorful mustard that trumps any store-bought processed fare. Anywhere you need some extra zing (and digestive help!), this mustard delivers bold flavor. It requires about a week to ferment, so plan accordingly.

*Yield: 2 cups*

## INGREDIENTS
½ cup yellow or brown mustard seeds
½–⅔ cup kombucha vinegar (page 256)
1 teaspoon sea salt

## FLAVORING SUGGESTIONS
*Mix and match to create your own favorite flavor.*
1 large garlic clove, minced
1 tablespoon diced onion
1 tablespoon honey
¼ teaspoon ground cumin
¼ teaspoon curry powder
⅛ teaspoon ground black pepper
⅛ teaspoon cayenne
⅛ teaspoon ground turmeric (for classic "mustard yellow" color)

## INSTRUCTIONS
Place the mustard seeds in a glass jar and add enough vinegar to cover the seeds. (They will plump up a lot as they ferment.) Add garlic and onion, if desired. Remember, a little bit goes a long way with the booch. Resist the temptation to add other spices at this stage or the mustard may become too bitter.

Cover with a tightly woven cloth, secured with a rubber band if needed, and let sit in a cool (65–74°F [18–23°C]), dark place for about 1 week. Check daily to ensure that the seeds remain fully submerged, topping off with additional kombucha vinegar as needed.

After about a week, the mustard seeds should be soft and break easily when lightly pressed. Pour the entire mixture into a food processor bowl, add the salt and whatever other spices you want to use, and pulse until the mixture reaches the desired consistency. Add more vinegar if needed.

# "Auntie Hannah's" Mayonnaise

Deviled eggs are an indulgence that not only pleases the palate but also provides an essential cholesterol imperative for healthy brain functioning. Get the best of both in this adaptation of the recipe that President Calvin Coolidge swore was the best in the world, that of his own Aunt Mary. Hand-beaten mayonnaise has a silkiness, elegance, and rich flavor that blow away the commercial stuff.

Crafting mayo by hand is neither difficult nor time-consuming, but it takes patience, constant whisking, and attention to detail to make an emulsion. A hand mixer, blender, or food processor makes the job easier. The butter base gives this mayo an extra richness and texture. The texture may be firmer than what you're used to, but it will soften up if left at room temperature or once it's spread on a sandwich.

*Yield: 2 cups*

## INGREDIENTS

- ½ cup (1 stick) butter, at room temperature
- 4 large egg yolks, at room temperature
- 1 teaspoon ground mustard
- 1 teaspoon salt, plus more to taste
- ½ cup extra virgin olive oil
- ½ cup kombucha vinegar (page 256)
- ½ cup freshly squeezed lemon juice
- ½ cup sunflower oil
- Freshly ground white pepper

## INSTRUCTIONS

Put the butter in a medium bowl, and lightly beat with a mixer or fork until it's creamy. In a separate bowl, whisk together the egg yolks, mustard, and salt; add the mixture to the butter and blend well. Slowly add the olive oil, drop by drop, whisking constantly until the mixture begins to thicken. Whisk in the kombucha vinegar and lemon juice; then add the sunflower oil in a very slow, thin stream, whisking constantly, until well blended.

If at any time it appears that the oil is not being incorporated, stop adding oil and whisk vigorously until the mixture is smooth, then continue adding oil.

Whisk in salt and white pepper to taste. Store the mayonnaise in an airtight container in the fridge, where it will keep for up to 3 weeks.

# HISTORY OF MAYONNAISE

Love it or hate it, mayonnaise has been an American sandwich staple for over one hundred years. German immigrant Richard Hellmann first featured his wife's version in their early twentieth-century New York deli. The sauce was so popular, and the jar it was packed in was so convenient for reuse by housewives, that he soon closed the deli and opened a mayonnaise factory, eventually distributing his product nationwide and dominating the market he helped create.

While Mr. Hellmann popularized the spread, at least here in the United States, the origins of the condiment itself are murkier and involve a dispute between well-acquainted food foes Spain and France. The French claim one of their own invented it as a substitute for cream at a dinner celebrating a military victory at Port Mahón, on the now-Spanish island of Minorca. Another French theory: the name derives from the Old French word for yolk, *moyeu*.

The Spanish agree that the condiment may have originated at Port Mahón but say it existed well before the arrival of any French forces and was known already as *salsa mahonesa* to the locals. Some food historians point to Mediterranean aiolis, whipped oil with garlic, as evidence for the Spanish claim. We may never know for sure, but the real question is, who was the Dutch genius who first decided to dip fries in it?!

# Kombucha Vinaigrette

A good vinaigrette must be easy to whip up with the ingredients on hand, so feel free to make substitutions to this basic recipe. We like to age our vinegar in oak, where it becomes imbued with tannins and other flavors from the wood, which adds complexity to any dish. If you don't have an oak barrel, you can add wood chips in the flavoring stage.

While classic vinaigrettes use a 3:1 oil-to-vinegar ratio, the reduced acidity of kombucha compared to other vinegars makes a 1:1 ratio perfect. Once we have a good mix going in our cruet, we simply top up as needed.

*Yield: 1 cup*

## INGREDIENTS

½ cup extra virgin olive oil
½ cup kombucha vinegar (page 256)
1 shallot, minced
2 garlic cloves, minced
⅛ teaspoon salt

## FLAVORING SUGGESTIONS

*Mix and match to create your own favorite flavor.*

1 teaspoon minced fresh herbs (thyme, rosemary, oregano, parsley, tarragon)
¼ teaspoon ground mustard
⅛ teaspoon ground allspice
⅛ teaspoon ground cloves
⅛ teaspoon ground cumin
Pinch of sugar (to balance flavors)

## INSTRUCTIONS

Combine the olive oil, vinegar, shallot, garlic, salt, and whatever seasonings you prefer in a small bowl and whisk together. Store at room temperature; it will keep nearly indefinitely.

# Blood Orange Kombucha Vinaigrette

Blood oranges owe their beautiful crimson color to being rich in anthocyanin, a powerful antioxidant. They are a personal favorite and as soon as they are in season, I stock up on 5-pound bags. When not squeezing them into Blood Orange Italian Soda kombucha (page 183), I'm whipping up this tangy dressing to complement summer greens.

*Yield: 1¼ cups*

## INGREDIENTS

½ cup freshly squeezed blood orange juice
½ cup extra virgin olive oil
½ cup kombucha vinegar (page 256)
2 garlic cloves, minced
⅛ teaspoon salt
2 sprigs fresh tarragon, chopped
2 sprigs fresh thyme, chopped
1 sprig fresh lavender, chopped

## INSTRUCTIONS

Combine the orange juice, olive oil, and vinegar in a small bowl and whisk together. Store at room temperature; it will keep nearly indefinitely.

# Buttermilk Ranch Dressing

This classic American salad dressing favorite was invented at the Hidden Valley Ranch in Santa Barbara in the 1950s. Pretty much universally loved since then, it is easy to prepare, goes great with salads and sandwiches, and makes a yummy dip for veggies and chips. This unexpectedly tangy, living version is sure to spark conversation and recipe requests at company picnics or family reunions. If you don't have buttermilk handy, make your own by blending ½ cup milk with 1 tablespoon kombucha vinegar.

*Yield: 1 cup*

### INGREDIENTS

- ½ cup buttermilk
- ¼ cup "Auntie Hannah's" Mayonnaise (page 268)
- ¼ cup sour cream or kefir cheese
- 1 garlic clove, finely minced or microplaned
- 1 tablespoon kombucha vinegar (page 256)
- 1 teaspoon finely chopped fresh tarragon, dill, parsley, scallions, or celery leaves
- ½ teaspoon Kombucha Mustard (page 268)
- A few dashes of Tabasco or another vinegar-based hot sauce

### INSTRUCTIONS

Combine the buttermilk, mayonnaise, sour cream, garlic, vinegar, tarragon, mustard, and Tabasco in a small bowl and whisk together. Cover and chill in the fridge for at least 30 minutes to allow the flavors to set.

## KOMBUCHA MAMMA SEZ

### Kefir Cheese

"Kefir, known colloquially as 'drinkable yogurt,' is another probiotic friend that has been with us for a long time. Originating in the Caucasus Mountains, its preparation was a closely guarded family secret passed down from generation to generation, often as part of a woman's dowry. In Turkish, *kef* means 'to feel good,' likely due to the positive effects of drinking kefir.

The kefir 'grain,' like a SCOBY, is a complex of yeast and bacteria. The culture ferments milk into a healthy, slightly fizzy drink, thereby preserving the milk and imbuing it with over 30 strains of healthy bacteria and yeast. Kefir cheese is made by straining kefir through cheesecloth to remove excess whey, yielding a creamy, thick 'cheese' that can be used in place of sour cream, cream cheese, or yogurt.

Kefir grains can be used to ferment a variety of 'milks,' including soy and nut milks for those seeking nondairy options."

To thicken the dressing, add equal amounts of sour cream and mayonnaise. To thin it, add more kombucha vinegar.

Store the dressing in the fridge, where it will keep for 1 week before the flavors start to change as the cultures age.

# Cultured Blue Cheese Dressing

Whenever we head back to Chicago, Alex and I enjoy an order of piping-hot buffalo wings and huge waffle-cut fries from a local wing joint, a favorite from childhood. At home, we've done our best to replicate that taste from our youth, but we traded out the original blue cheese dressing for this probiotic-rich version, which adds a pleasant tang and loads of bacterial buddies to help with digestion. Bring on the heat!

*Yield: 1 cup*

### INGREDIENTS

6–8 ounces blue cheese, crumbled
  ½ cup kefir cheese (see page 271) (or substitute sour cream)
  ½ cup plain whole-milk yogurt
  ¼ cup kombucha vinegar (page 256)
  ½ teaspoon freshly ground black pepper
  ½ teaspoon salt
  ¼ teaspoon garlic powder or 1 garlic clove, minced

### INSTRUCTIONS

Combine the blue cheese, kefir cheese, yogurt, vinegar, pepper, salt, and garlic powder in a small bowl and whisk together. Cover and chill in the fridge for at least 30 minutes to allow the flavors to set. Store in the fridge, where it will keep for 1 week before the flavors begin to change as the cultures in the vinegar and kefir cheese age.

# Kombuchup BBQ Sauce

Want to win the barbecue sauce contest at the county fair? With Kombuchup as your secret ingredient, that blue ribbon may be within reach! At the very least, vegetables and meats are sure to take first prize with your family when you slather on this tangy, mouthwatering sauce. We also use it to make our famous SCOBY jerky (page 298).

*Yield: 2½ cups*

### INGREDIENTS

2 cups Kombuchup (page 266)
2 tablespoons kombucha vinegar (page 256)
2 tablespoons Worcestershire sauce
1 tablespoon brown sugar
1 tablespoon granulated sugar or to taste
1 tablespoon freshly squeezed lemon juice
2 teaspoons freshly ground black pepper
2 teaspoons ground mustard or 2 teaspoons Kombucha Mustard (page 268)
2 teaspoons onion powder

### INSTRUCTIONS

Combine the Kombuchup, vinegar, Worcestershire sauce, brown sugar, granulated sugar, lemon juice, black pepper, mustard, and onion powder in a small bowl and whisk together. Store the sauce in the fridge, where it will keep for up to 2 weeks before the flavors start to change as the cultures age.

# CULTURED Blue Cheese DRESSING

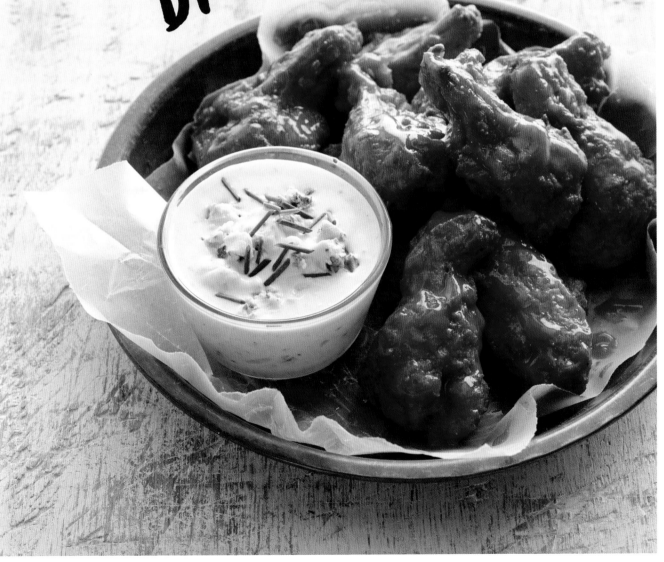

# Kombucha Dipping Sauces and Marinades

Big and little dippers will love these bold sauces for everything from dumplings and egg rolls to chicken nuggets and french fries. Whip up a selection of these dips to enjoy with SCOBY "Squid" Sashimi (page 300). Simply whisk the ingredients together and dip away!

## Phuket Style

    1 tablespoon chili paste
    1 tablespoon kombucha vinegar (page 256)
    1 teaspoon freshly squeezed lime juice
    1 teaspoon soy sauce
    ½ teaspoon sugar
    2 sprigs fresh mint, chopped

## Dim Sum

    1 tablespoon soy sauce
    1 tablespoon kombucha vinegar (page 256)
    1 teaspoon sesame or peanut oil
    Chili paste, to taste
    Salt, to taste
    Freshly ground white pepper, to taste

## Spicy Curry

    3 tablespoons "Auntie Hannah's" Mayonnaise (page 268)
    1 teaspoon curry powder
    1 teaspoon kombucha vinegar (page 256)

## Curry Mustard

    3 tablespoons Kombucha Mustard (page 268)
    1 teaspoon curry powder
    1 teaspoon kombucha vinegar (page 256)

# Teriyaki Sauce

This flavorful sauce has its humble roots in Japan as a simple soy glaze. However, when Japanese immigrants landed in Hawaii to work the pineapple plantations, they couldn't resist adding the sweet fruit to their sauce, making this a true Asian-American collaboration that has become a "traditional" American flavoring for chicken and steak.

Pineapple is a terrific addition to any marinade; in addition to balancing the salt, it is rich in bromelain, a naturally occurring enzyme that tenderizes meat. This version is also great with vegetables and burgers of any kind, whether meat, mushroom, or grain-based.

*Yield: 2 cups*

INGREDIENTS

    ⅔ cup mirin, or sherry with a pinch of sugar added
    ½ cup Beautifying Bone Broth (page 259) or other broth
    ½ cup pineapple juice
    ¼ cup brown sugar or 2 tablespoons honey
    ¼ cup soy sauce
    ¼ cup kombucha vinegar (page 256)
    2 teaspoons sesame oil
2-5 garlic cloves, minced or pressed
    1 (1-inch) piece fresh ginger, minced or grated
    Dash of red pepper flakes (optional)

## INSTRUCTIONS

Combine the mirin, broth, pineapple juice, brown sugar, soy sauce, vinegar, sesame oil, garlic, ginger, and red pepper flakes in a small saucepan over medium-high heat. Bring the mixture to a boil, and then reduce the heat and let simmer for 10 minutes. Taste and adjust the sugar and spices as desired. Allow to cool for 15 minutes before using.

*WORD NERD:* **Teriyaki**

*The word* teriyaki *comes from the Japanese* teri, *referring to the shine created by the sugar in the sauce, and* yaki, *the cooking method of grilling or broiling. Traditionally the meat is dipped in or brushed with sauce several times during cooking, creating a glazed look.*

---

**A KOMBUCHA LEGEND:** The Samurai

According to some legends, Japan's elite warrior sect, the samurai, carried kombucha to battle in skin flasks around 1200 CE. The brew was said to lend them energy and stamina, and as their supply dwindled, they refreshed it with sweet tea, creating a kind of personal CB as they journeyed to battle.

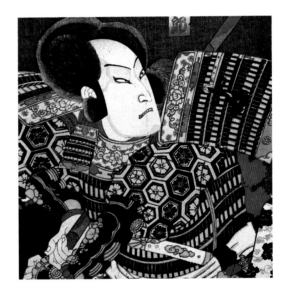

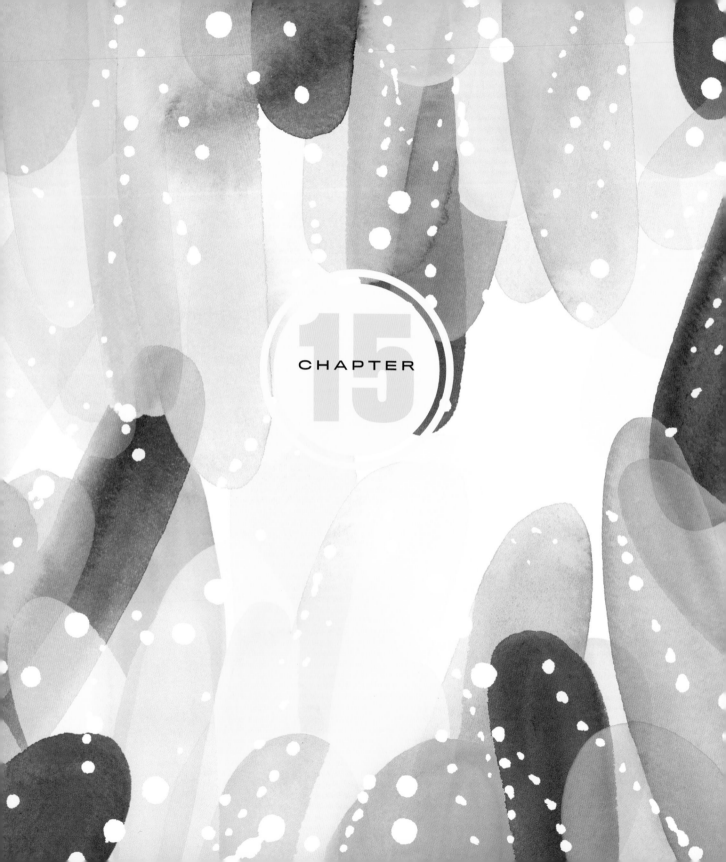

CHAPTER

15

# Snacks, Salads, Sides, and Sweets

Swap traditional snacks, sides, and sweets for fermented treats that not only deliver loads of flavor but also keep your engine moving by assisting with digestion. We include a dab of sauerkraut, fermented veggies, and/or yogurt with just about every meal to make sure we're getting our daily dose of the "good guys."

These recipes are ones that you may have made many times. But with the probiotic and nutritional power of kombucha, they are elevated from ho-hum to hubba-hubba. Watch as family and friends return for more without a clue about the secret to their savory delight. And although regular consumption of kombucha often shifts the palate away from overly sweet foods, we all enjoy a treat now and then. The sweets included here use kombucha in old favorites such as cake, sorbet, and even gummy candies, giving a healthier twist that everyone can feel good about enjoying.

Many of these foods will keep indefinitely, but as we mentioned in the condiments section, even in the fridge the flavor may change and become more bitter over time as the culture develops. Eating fermented foods fresh will ensure the best taste and most enjoyment.

# Snacks

## Mom's Kombucha Fridge Pickles

Mom kept us stocked up on these easy pickles as they reminded her of childhood summers in Southern California. The cold cucumber slices were refreshing on muggy days, and the faintest whiff of tart vinegar has me instantly salivating like Pavlov's dog. Like a good daughter culture, I've evolved Mom's classic recipe by adding kombucha vinegar and fresh herbs to capture the flavors of our local season.

*Yield: 1 cup*

### INGREDIENTS

- 1 cup sliced cucumbers (2–3 cucumbers; Persian, English, and pickling cukes work best)
- 2 garlic cloves, minced
- 1 cup kombucha vinegar (page 256)
- ⅛ teaspoon salt
- Pinch of sugar
- Water, to top off

### FLAVORING SUGGESTIONS

*Mix and match to create your own favorites.*

- 1 or 2 lemon slices
  - Several sprigs of fresh dill, thyme, or oregano
- 2 or 3 onion slices
  - ¼ jalapeño, seeded and diced
  - 1 carrot, julienned or shaved into thin rounds with a vegetable peeler

### INSTRUCTIONS

Combine cucumbers, garlic, vinegar, salt, sugar, and any flavorings in a medium bowl. Add enough water to submerge all the ingredients. Toss to combine; then cover and let chill in the refrigerator for at least 24 hours. The longer they sit, the more garlicky they get!

## BREAD-AND-BUTTER PICKLES

How did these sweet-and-sour cucumbers end up being named after bread and butter? Many claim the name came about during the Great Depression. It's said that a man was so poor that he turned to selling his pickled cucumbers by the side of the road to make money to buy bread and butter. Another Depression-era story claims that to stretch the bread and butter, sugared cucumber slices were put in sandwiches.

The most likely answer, however, relates to the cucumber sandwiches that are common fare in England. According to the *Oxford English Dictionary*, *bread and butter* is a phrase that means "a type of everyday food; the means of living." Bread and butter were (and still are for many) staples found in every household, as were pickled vegetables. Since there were always pickles on hand, they were as common as bread and butter.

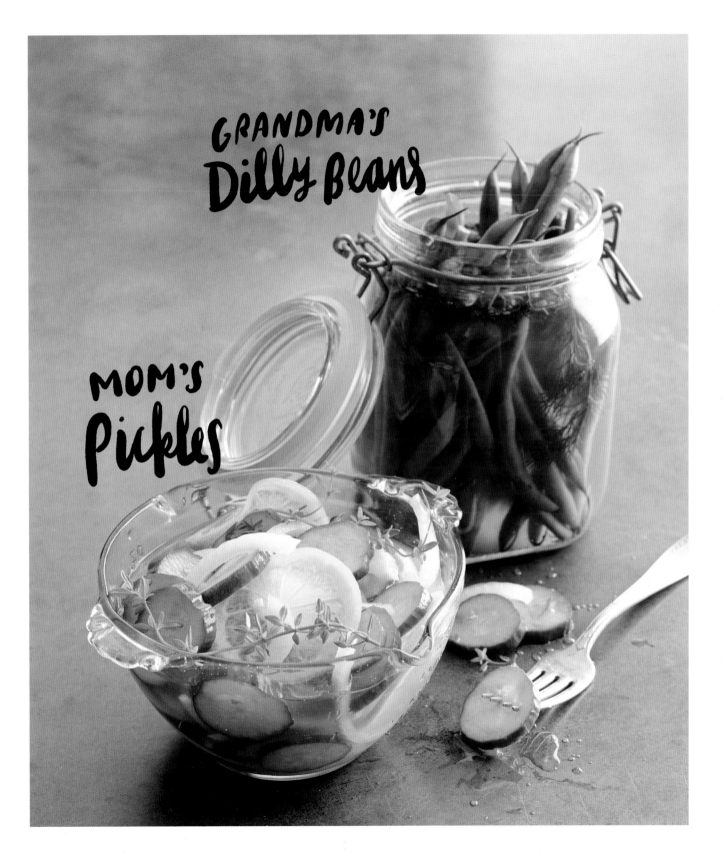

GRANDMA'S
Dilly Beans

MOM'S
Pickles

# Sugar 'n' Spice Kombucha Pickles

These pickles really take off if lightly fermented at room temperature for up to a week. To make a sweeter bread-and-butter-style pickle, increase the sugar to ¼ cup and refrigerate immediately.

*Yield: 1 pint*

### INGREDIENTS

2 or 3 pickling cucumbers, sliced or cut into spears
⅛ cup sugar
2 teaspoons mustard seeds
½ teaspoon red pepper flakes
¼ teaspoon freshly squeezed lemon juice
¼ teaspoon ground turmeric
⅛ teaspoon ground allspice
⅛ teaspoon ground cinnamon
½ cup kombucha vinegar (page 256)

### INSTRUCTIONS

Combine the cucumbers, sugar, mustard seeds, red pepper flakes, lemon juice, turmeric, allspice, and cinnamon in a pint jar or glass container. Pour in enough vinegar to cover the ingredients. Stir to combine; then cover and leave in dark, cool spot for 3 to 7 days. Taste frequently. When the flavors have melded to your liking, move the pickles to the fridge and enjoy.

# Grandma Crum's Dilly Beans

Grandma Crum loved that my siblings and I spent two weeks every summer with her up at the farm in Minnesota, but being city kids, we were bored to tears. Looking back now, though, those are some of the best memories from my childhood: climbing on tractors at the John Deere dealer across the gravel road, swinging on the branches of the giant willow tree, and sitting on the porch with a big pile of green beans in our laps, snapping the ends and pulling out the strings. Grandma may not have known a thing about kombucha, but she sure knew how to "dilly" a green bean!

*Yield: 1 quart*

### INGREDIENTS

1 pound green beans, topped and stringed
2 garlic cloves, slightly crushed
2 teaspoons dill seeds
1 teaspoon black peppercorns
1 teaspoon Celtic sea salt
1 dill head or sprig of dill leaves
½ cup kombucha vinegar (page 256)
Water, to top off

### INSTRUCTIONS

Stand the green beans up in a 1-quart glass jar. Add the garlic, peppercorns, salt, and dill. Pour in the kombucha vinegar. Add enough water to fill the jar, leaving ½ inch of headspace. Seal tightly and let sit in a cool, dark place for 3 to 5 days, until the beans mellow. When they reach your preferred flavor, move the dilly beans to the fridge.

# Salads

## *Hot Potato Salad* with *Kombucha Mustard Dressing*

This homage to my German ancestry is updated with heirloom potatoes for color and nutrition, while the kombucha adds extra zip. The longer the flavors mingle, the tastier it gets. We know from experience that this sweet, salty, sour salad disappears fast at gatherings. Garnish with sour cream or kefir cheese (see page 271) for a knockout finish.

*Yield: 1 quart*

### INGREDIENTS

- 2 pounds heirloom potatoes, peeled and diced (mix purple Peruvian, Yukon Gold, and Ruby Crescent for varied color and flavor)
- 1 teaspoon sea salt
- ½ pound sliced bacon
- ¾ cup chopped onion
- ¾ cup kombucha vinegar (page 256)
- ¼ cup sugar
- 1½ tablespoons spicy mustard or Kombucha Mustard (page 268)
- Salt and freshly ground black pepper
- 2 tablespoons chopped scallions or chives, for garnish
- Kefir cheese or sour cream, for garnish

### INSTRUCTIONS

Put the potatoes in a large pot. Cover with cold water and add the salt. Bring to a boil and cook for 15 to 20 minutes, until the potatoes are tender and easily pierced with a fork. Remove from the heat and run under cold water.

While the potatoes are boiling, cook the bacon in a cast-iron skillet over medium heat until crisp. Remove with a slotted spoon and drain on paper towels.

Pour off all but ¼ cup of the rendered bacon fat and add the onion to the skillet. Sauté over medium heat for about 5 minutes, until the onion turns translucent. Whisk in the kombucha vinegar, sugar, mustard, and salt and pepper to taste. Continue cooking, stirring the mixture from time to time, until thick and bubbly, about 7 minutes. Turn off the heat and let cool for a few minutes.

Put the potatoes in a large bowl. Crumble in the bacon, then add the warm dressing and toss to combine. Garnish with scallions and a dollop of kefir cheese. Serve warm or at room temperature; refrigerate any leftovers.

# Herbed Tomato and Feta Salad *with Scallions*

This salad may have been my first-ever attempt at cooking with kombucha, and it remains one of our favorites because it tastes better and better each day. It's a joyous balance of salty, sour, and savory with a snap of scallion tying it all together! We love the juice the tomatoes create, but if you want to reduce the liquid, remove the seeds from half the tomatoes before chopping them.

*Yield: 2 servings*

### INGREDIENTS

- 2 cups diced tomatoes (about 3 medium tomatoes)
- ½ cup crumbled feta cheese
- ⅓ cup kombucha vinegar (page 256)
- 1 scallion, chopped
- 1 teaspoon fresh herbs (thyme, oregano, chervil, tarragon, etc.)
- 1 teaspoon salt
- 1 teaspoon freshly ground black pepper

### INSTRUCTIONS

Combine the tomatoes, feta, vinegar, scallion, herbs, salt, and pepper in a large bowl and stir gently. Taste and adjust the seasonings, if necessary. To deepen the flavor, chill the salad in the fridge for a few hours before serving.

# Deep Green Salad *with Blood-Orange Vinaigrette*

Hearty greens pack a nutritional punch, but they can sometimes be tough to swallow and digest. The kombucha vinegar and citric acid from the oranges in this recipe help the body get the most out of the savory greens while balancing the sweet notes from the freshly squeezed oranges, fresh mint, and cranberries.

*Yield: 2 servings*

### INGREDIENTS

- 1 bunch Swiss chard, kale, or other dense leafy greens
- 1 tablespoon chopped fresh mint
- 1 tablespoon dried cranberries
- 1 cup Blood Orange Kombucha Vinaigrette (page 270)
- ½ cup kombucha vinegar (page 256)
- 1 tablespoon olive oil
- 1 teaspoon honey (optional)
- Salt and freshly ground black pepper
- 2 tablespoons sliced almonds

### INSTRUCTIONS

Remove the tough stalks from the greens. The secret to making this salad easy to chew comes not only from the acidic dressing but also from a food processor. Combine the greens and the mint in a food processor fitted with the chopping blade; pulse until the leaves turn to confetti, about 30 seconds.

Whisk the orange juice, vinegar, olive oil, and honey together in a small bowl. Season with salt and pepper to taste.

Toss the greens with the vinaigrette in a large bowl. Add the cranberries and almonds; then cover and chill for at least 20 minutes in the fridge to allow the greens to soften.

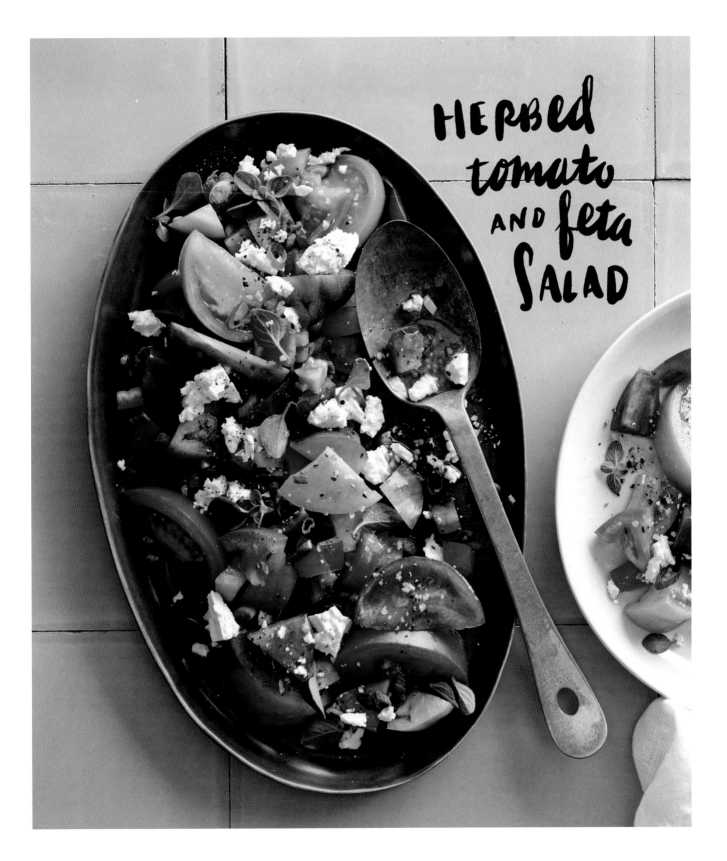

HERBED tomato AND feta SALAD

# Sides

## *Kombucha Kraut — Three Ways*

As a kid, the pungent odor of sauerkraut reminded me of sweaty feet and sent me running in the opposite direction! Alex, on the other hand, grew up munching kraut-covered brats in Cincinnati, a town with a rich German heritage. He challenged me early on in our relationship to reconsider my revulsion, and now I not only enjoy kraut with nearly every meal, but I also love kraut juice shots!

Salt has been critical to food preservation since ancient times, prized for its ability to keep pathogens at bay. The salt pulls water molecules from the raw food, creating brine. Bacteria already present on the skin of fruits and veggies, primarily lactobacilli, work in concert with the salty brine to break down the material. Fermented food is easy to digest, tastily sour, and full of probiotics — and, as an extra benefit, keeps for a long, long time.

Tools of the trade that will help with these recipes include a kraut pounder or tamper and a weight. The kraut pounder is typically a wooden implement with rounded ends that releases liquid from the fibers of the cabbage. It usually has a smaller end that is useful for tamping down the sauerkraut into the jar. The fewer air pockets, the better the fermentation.

To prevent the cabbage from being exposed to oxygen and contracting mold, a weight is placed on the brined matter to keep it submerged. Kraut weights are usually ceramic disks with a hole in the center to allow carbon dioxide to dissipate naturally, but a clean stone or a plastic baggie filled with water

## HISTORY OF SAUERKRAUT

The practice of pickling cabbage originated over two thousand years ago with Chinese laborers building the Great Wall. Unlike German kraut, Chinese sauerkraut was preserved using rice wine. Like many great Chinese inventions, this tasty dish was carried from the East to Europe a thousand years later by Genghis Khan — that story sounds familiar! (See Genghis Khan's Soldiers, page 174.)

Not surprisingly, *sauerkraut* is German for "sour cabbage." Cabbage is dry-cured with salt, which draws out the liquid to create a tasty, useful brine. Curing kraut preserves the vegetable's nutrition — very helpful for the deep winter, when fresh vegetables were not an option.

Many stores now carry raw, locally produced sauerkraut in a variety of both classic and modern flavors. But it is very easy to make at home and is another great "gateway food" to better choices, so consider starting a crock of kraut today!

does the trick also. Alternatively, a jar with an airlock can be used.

These three recipes are just examples — add ingredients that inspire you to find your own favorite!

### INSTRUCTIONS FOR 1 QUART OF KRAUT

Add shredded cabbage and salt to a medium bowl and toss to combine. Cover with a towel and let sit at room temperature for 2 to 4 hours. After having time to sweat, the cabbage will release some liquid into the bowl. Use your hands to pound or squeeze the cabbage to release even more liquid. When it seems like you've extracted as much liquid as possible, add the spices, fruit, or herbs, and toss to combine.

Pack a quart jar tightly with half of the cabbage mixture. Pour the liquid from the bowl into the jar, followed by the kombucha vinegar. Fill the jar with the remaining mixture of ingredients, pressing down with a tamper or wooden spoon as you go to create a layer of liquid across the top. Use a kraut weight to hold the cabbage under the liquid. Cover the jar with a towel and let sit in a cool, dark place for 5 to 14 days. Taste frequently. When the kraut has the right balance of tart and salty, store in the refrigerator.

**Note:** So long as the food remains submerged in the brine, it is protected against unwanted bacteria and mold. Sometimes bubbles push some material out of the liquid, leading to mold. Traditionally, the moldy layer would be scraped off and the properly fermented kraut below the surface would be enjoyed. However, now that many people have compromised immune systems, most recommend tossing a moldy batch into the compost pile. Others with more robust immunity might consider removing the moldy layer and digging in anyway — trust *your* gut!

## Klassic Kraut

This is the foundation recipe for creating whatever variety of kraut appeals to you. Caraway seeds make for a clean and classic flavor.

### INGREDIENTS

    1 head green cabbage, shredded
    1 tablespoon salt
    1 teaspoon caraway seeds
    1 cup kombucha vinegar (page 256)

## Apple-Ginger Kraut

Crispy apple and pungent ginger pack a flavorful punch in this dynamo kraut. Crunchy, spicy, and delicious, it's the perfect topping for a gourmet burger and adds pep to any plate.

### INGREDIENTS

    1 head green cabbage, shredded
    1 tablespoon salt
    1 apple, diced or thinly sliced
    1 (1-inch) piece fresh ginger, peeled and
        thinly sliced
    1 cup kombucha vinegar (page 256)

## Blood-Orange Juniper-Berry Kraut

I admit to having a slight obsession with blood oranges. The deeply hued flesh contrasting with the orange peel ignites my imagination and taste buds. In this recipe, the sweet and tangy flavor of the orange pairs perfectly with the piney juniper berry, and the slices of fruit add colorful pizzazz.

### INGREDIENTS

    1 head cabbage, shredded
    1 tablespoon salt
    1 medium blood orange, sliced thinly, with rind
    1 teaspoon dried juniper berries
    1 cup kombucha vinegar (page 256)

# Kombucha Koleslaw

Shredded cabbage with dressing has been a side salad since Roman times. Usually not much more than greens, herbs, and seasoning, the addition of mayonnaise elevates humble cabbage to an American classic. Though likely imported by European ancestors (*koolsla* is Dutch for "cabbage salad"), it has earned a place at many a picnic and gathering.

Although this slaw gets better the longer the flavors mingle, all too often it is eaten before anyone else has a chance to make that discovery. Make a double batch so everyone clamoring for coleslaw gets a scoop!

*Yield: 3½ cups*

## INGREDIENTS

3 cups shredded red or green cabbage
½ cup shredded carrot
½ cup "Auntie Hannah's" Mayonnaise (page 268)
½ teaspoon celery seed
⅛ cup kombucha vinegar
Salt and freshly ground black pepper

## FLAVORING SUGGESTIONS

*Mix and match these optional ingredients as desired.*

¼ cup raisins
¼ cup diced apple
¼ cup dried cranberries
⅛ cup slivered almonds

Combine the cabbage, carrot, mayo, celery seed, vinegar, and any other flavorings in a large bowl. Season to taste with salt and pepper. Toss thoroughly. Let the slaw chill in the fridge for at least 30 minutes to allow flavors to merge before serving.

# Kombucha Red Slaw

Southerners love tangy flavors, so the fact that they put ketchup in coleslaw makes perfect sense. Traditional red slaw hails from North Carolina, where it forms part of any Lexington-style barbecue plate. Adding Kombuchup to the mix imparts a rich tomato flavor, while the extra vinegar gives it a crisp bite. Together, they meld into a unique side dish that adds color and pizzazz to any barbecue. For extra heat, use Kombuchup BBQ Sauce (page 272) instead of plain Kombuchup.

*Yield: 2 cups*

## INGREDIENTS

2 cups shredded green cabbage
⅓ cup Kombuchup (page 266)
⅓ cup kombucha vinegar (page 256)
2 teaspoons red pepper flakes, or hot sauce to taste
1 teaspoon salt
1 teaspoon freshly ground black pepper

## INSTRUCTIONS

Combine the cabbage, Kombuchup, vinegar, red pepper flakes, salt, and pepper in a large bowl. Toss well to coat the cabbage. Let chill in the fridge for 30 minutes to allow flavors to meld before serving.

# Kimbuchi

Kimchi is the Korean counterpart to sauerkraut. A catchall term for any number of fermented vegetable combinations, nowadays it is most closely associated with Napa cabbage, spicy red pepper, and sometimes fermented fish. This version is mild; check out Spicy Fishy Kimbuchi (page 288) for more fire.

*Yield: 1 quart*

### INGREDIENTS

- 1 head Napa cabbage, cut into bite-size pieces
- 1 cup julienned carrots
- 1 cup julienned daikon radish
- 1 scallion, trimmed and cut lengthwise
- ¼ teaspoon red pepper flakes
- 2 tablespoons kombucha vinegar (page 256)
- 1 tablespoon soy sauce

### INSTRUCTIONS

Combine the cabbage, carrots, daikon, scallion, red pepper flakes, vinegar, and soy sauce in a large bowl and toss to coat evenly. Use a kraut pounder or wooden spoon to tamp the cabbage mixture into a quart jar. This should cause a layer of liquid to rise to the top.

Use a kraut weight to keep the cabbage submerged in the brine. Cover the jar with a towel and let sit in a cool, dark place for 3 to 5 days, tasting frequently. When you like the flavor, move the kimchi to the refrigerator, where it will keep for up to 3 months, depending on your personal preferences for sour.

## KIMCHI, KRAUT'S KOREAN COUSIN

The spicy-hot kimchi that most of us are familiar with has come a long way from its humble beginnings as a dish of salted radishes. Traditionally, ancient Koreans prepared salted vegetables to help them digest grains like barley and millet — before rice became the dominant grain of Asia. References to Korea's fermentation prowess can be found in the third-century Chinese historical annals known as the *Records of the Three Kingdoms*; the first written record of kimchi was made in the eleventh century.

Unlike sauerkraut, a dish specific to cabbage, Korean kimchi can include any number of vegetables — radishes, bamboo shoots, leeks, and mushrooms were common. Food historians cannot pinpoint when chile peppers were introduced to the region, though many claim it was in the 1600s, when Japan invaded Korea. Hot peppers caught on like wildfire and radically changed the flavor, appearance, and fermentation techniques associated with kimchi.

Nature loves diversity, and Korea loves kimchi. Today there are hundreds of traditional varieties!

# Spicy Fishy Kimbuchi

Spicy cuisine is a point of pride for many Koreans, and as such traditional kimchis pack a fiery wallop. This recipe also includes nutrient-dense fish, which ferments as the kimbuchi ages. A little bit goes a long way — adjust the fire and fishiness to your family's preference.

*Yield: 1 quart*

## INGREDIENTS

    1 head Napa cabbage, cut into bite-size pieces
    1 cup julienned carrots
    1 cup julienned daikon radish
    4 garlic cloves, crushed
    1 (1-inch) piece fresh ginger, peeled and diced
    1 scallion, cut into ¼-inch pieces
    ½ jalapeño, seeded and diced
    2 sardines, mashed, or 1 tablespoon
        anchovy paste
    2 tablespoons kombucha vinegar (page 256)
    2 teaspoons sugar

## INSTRUCTIONS

Combine the cabbage, carrots, daikon, garlic, ginger, scallion, jalapeño, sardines, vinegar, and sugar in a large bowl and toss to coat evenly. Use a kraut pounder or wooden spoon to tamp the cabbage mixture into a quart jar. This should cause a layer of liquid to rise to the top.

Use a kraut weight to keep the cabbage submerged in the brine. Cover the jar with a towel and let sit in a cool, dark place for 3 to 5 days, tasting frequently. When you like the flavor, move the kimchi to the refrigerator, where it will keep for up to 3 months, depending on your personal preferences for sour.

# Kombucha Viche

In Quechua, a native South American language, *siwichi* refers to a traditional dish of the Peruvian coast. The fish is "cooked" by the acids of the citrus fruits, which denature the proteins in the fish, causing them to turn opaque without heat. Kombucha, being naturally acidic, lends depth and subtle flavor to the dish.

The key to a delicious and safe ceviche is using the freshest seafood possible. Semifirm white fish is the best choice; options include snapper, sea bass, striped bass, grouper, or flounder. Octopus, scallops, and shrimp also respond well to this treatment.

*Yield: 6 servings*

## INGREDIENTS

    2 pounds firm, fresh red snapper fillets (or
        other firm-fleshed fish), deboned and
        cut into ½-inch pieces
    1 cup seeded, chopped tomatoes
    ½ cup kombucha vinegar (page 256)
    ¼ cup freshly squeezed lemon juice
    ¼ cup freshly squeezed lime juice
    ½ red onion, finely diced
    1 serrano chile, seeded and finely diced
    2 teaspoons salt
      Pinch of ground oregano
      Dash of Tabasco or pinch of cayenne
      Chopped cilantro, sliced avocado, and
        tortillas or tortilla chips, for serving

## INSTRUCTIONS

Combine the fish and tomatoes in a large bowl.

Whisk together the vinegar, lemon and lime juices, onion, serrano, salt, oregano, and Tabasco in a small bowl. Pour the vinegar mixture over the fish and tomatoes and toss gently to coat.

Cover tightly with a lid or plastic wrap. Let sit, covered, in the refrigerator for at least 1 hour. Stir at least once during this time to ensure that all of the fish is thoroughly covered with the vinegar mixture. The longer it sits, the more the flavors will meld.

Serve chilled with cilantro, avocado slices, and tortillas or tortilla chips.

# Watermelon–Blackberry Salsa

Watermelons originated in southern Africa. Salsas and *tomatls* (Aztec for tomato) originated in South America. Mix and match, and presto! A cool, refreshing twist on the classic pico de gallo. Use ½ cup of this salsa to spice up your next batch of Gazboocho (page 303).

*Yield: 4 cups*

## INGREDIENTS

1½ cups seeded, cubed watermelon
1 cup hulled, sliced blackberries
½ cup peeled, seeded, diced cucumber
½ cup peeled, diced jicama
½ cup diced mango
⅛ cup freshly squeezed lime juice (about 2 medium limes)
⅛ cup kombucha vinegar (page 256) or Peño Cucumber kombucha (page 214)
2 garlic cloves, minced
1 jalapeño, seeded and minced (omit if you're using jalapeño-flavored kombucha)
½ small red onion, finely chopped
6–8 fresh basil leaves, finely chopped
1 tablespoon sugar
1½ teaspoons grated lime zest (about 1 lime)
1 teaspoon salt
Freshly ground black pepper

## INSTRUCTIONS

Combine the watermelon, blackberries, cucumber, jicama, and mango in a medium bowl.

Whisk the lime juice, vinegar, garlic, jalapeño, onion, basil, sugar, lime zest, salt, and pepper to taste in a small bowl.

Pour the dressing over the fruit mixture and toss to coat thoroughly. Chill in the fridge for 30 minutes to allow flavors to set before serving.

# Sweets

## Kombucha Chai Spice Cake *with Ginger Frosting*

This is a deliciously different holiday or special-occasion cake! Use Chai Spice kombucha (page 197) in place of the kombucha vinegar for more intense chai flavor.

*Yield: 1 double-layer 8- or 9-inch cake*

### CAKE

- 10 chai tea bags
- 1 cup boiling water
- 1⅔ cups all-purpose unbleached flour
- 1¼ teaspoons baking powder
- 2 teaspoons ground cinnamon
- 1 teaspoon ground cardamom
- 1 teaspoon ground cloves
- 1 teaspoon fennel seeds
- 1 teaspoon ground ginger
- Zest of half an orange (optional)
- ¼ cup (½ stick) butter, at room temperature
- 1 cup sugar
- 2 eggs
- ⅛ cup kombucha vinegar (page 256)

### CHAI SPICE FROSTING

- 3 ounces cream cheese or kefir cheese (page 271), at room temperature
- ¼ cup (½ stick) butter, at room temperature
- 1 teaspoon ground cinnamon
- ½ teaspoon ground cardamom
- ½ teaspoon ground cloves
- ½ teaspoon ground ginger
- 2 cups confectioners' sugar

### INSTRUCTIONS

**Make the cake.** Steep the tea bags in the boiling water for 5 minutes. Remove the tea bags, squeezing out as much liquid as possible. Let the tea cool in the refrigerator for 30 minutes.

Preheat the oven to 375°F (190°C). Butter and lightly flour two 8- or 9-inch round cake pans.

In a medium bowl, whisk together the flour, baking powder, cinnamon, cardamom, cloves, fennel, and ginger. Set aside.

Combine the orange zest and butter in a large bowl and beat for 30 seconds. Add the sugar and beat until well combined. Add the eggs one at a time, beating for 1 minute after each egg. Add the cooled tea and mix well.

Add half the dry ingredients to the butter mixture, then the vinegar; then add the other half of the dry ingredients, beating well after each addition.

Divide the batter evenly between the cake pans. Bake for 30 to 35 minutes or until a toothpick inserted in the center of the cakes comes out clean.

Let the cakes cool on wire racks for 10 minutes, and then remove them from the pans. Let cool completely before frosting.

**Make the frosting.** Beat the cream cheese, butter, cinnamon, cardamom, cloves, and ginger in a medium bowl until light and fluffy. Gradually add the confectioners' sugar, beating until smooth.

Spread the frosting evenly over one cake layer, and then top with the second layer and finish frosting.

## A Volcano in Your Cake!

"The baking-soda-and-vinegar volcano is science-fair cliché, but using vinegar in cake? Yes! That good old experiment illustrates perfectly why adding vinegar to baked goods improves the texture and adds lift: the acid reacts with the dry base ingredients to create air bubbles. Moreover, the vinegar flavor doesn't come through (unless you accidentally use the garlic-flavored variety!)."

# *Kombuchello*

Grandma Crum always served Jell-O for dessert. Mandarin orange slices suspended in cool lime gelatin and topped with fresh whipped cream made the hot summer nights of southern Minnesota a lot more delicious. This is an easy treat to make using fruit left over from a secondary fermentation.

*Yield: 4 servings*

### INGREDIENTS

½ cup cold water

2 tablespoons beef gelatin or powdered agar
(use 1–2 tablespoons more for a firmer set)

½ cup sugar

4 cups flavored kombucha

¼ cup chopped fruit, in bite-size pieces
(optional)*

Whipped cream, for serving (optional)

*If you're using fresh pineapple, papaya, ginger, figs, guava, or kiwi, chop them, toss them in a saucepan, and cook for at least 10 minutes over high heat before adding them to the gelatin. They contain bromelain, an enzyme that breaks down gelatin and causes it to lose its thickening properties. Bromelain is deactivated by heating, so canned versions may be used without heating.*

### INSTRUCTIONS

Pour the cold water into a small saucepan. Sprinkle the gelatin over the water and let rest for 5 minutes. Gelatin can be tricky to work with at first as it has a tendency to clump. Breaking up the powder as best you can while sprinkling it over the water will help to reduce clumping. Stir gently with a fork so that clumps are broken up immediately.

Add the sugar to the saucepan. Stir gently over low heat until the water is slightly warmed and both the sugar and gelatin are dissolved. Remove from the heat and add the kombucha.

Pour into a gelatin mold, ramekins, or an 8-inch square pan. Add the fruit. Place in the refrigerator and let chill for 2 to 4 hours, until set. Cover the gelatin once it has cooled.

Cut into finger-size squares or cubes and serve with a dollop of whipped cream or layer with whipped cream to make a gelatin parfait.

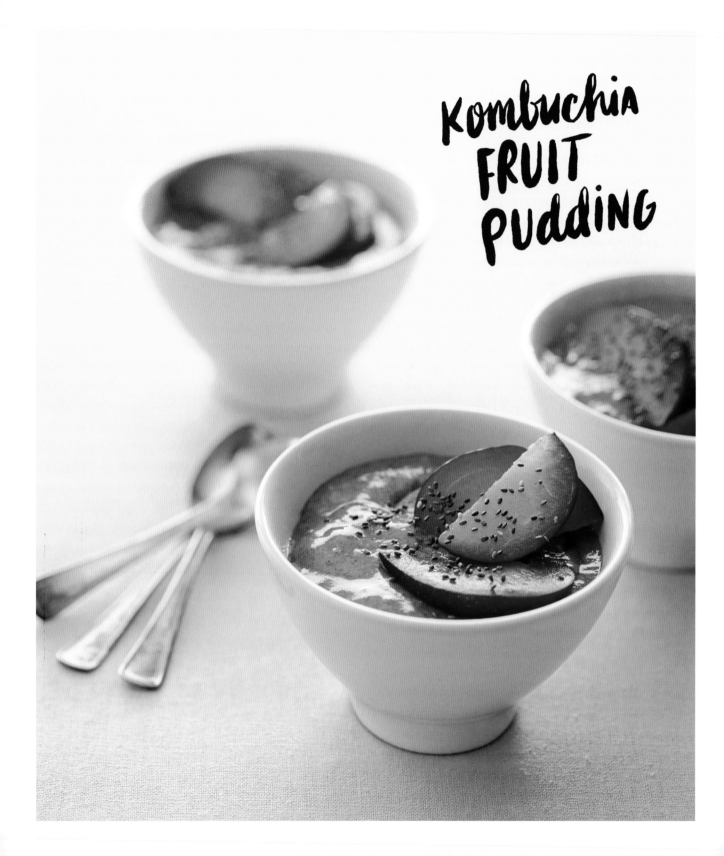

Kombuchia
FRUIT
PUDDING

# Kombuchia Fruit Pudding

This tasty treat packs a nutritious one-two punch — first from the kombucha and second from the chia seeds, a virtual superfood. Using more chia creates a stiffer gel that can be eaten like pudding. Use less to make a topper for ice cream or yogurt, and more to create a spreadable version. The fun, slippery texture is a nice complement to the sweet-sour flavor. Mix in some fruit left over from a secondary fermentation for additional probiotic benefit and flavor.

*Yield: 4 servings*

## INGREDIENTS

2 cups fresh or frozen fruit (berries, peaches, plums), chopped as needed
½ cup kombucha
3 tablespoons chia seeds
2–3 tablespoons honey
¼ teaspoon salt

## FLAVORING SUGGESTIONS

*Mix and match to create your own favorite flavor.*

2 sprigs fresh mint
¼ jalapeño, seeded and diced
¼ teaspoon ground cinnamon
¼ teaspoon ground ginger
⅛ teaspoon ground allspice
⅛ teaspoon ground cloves

## INSTRUCTIONS

Combine the fruit, kombucha, chia seeds, honey, and salt in a blender, along with any other seasonings you might want. Purée until the mixture reaches the desired consistency. The more the chia seeds are ground up, the stiffer the gel.

Allow the mixture to sit for a few minutes before using, as it will continue to gel. If you want a firmer consistency, add more chia seeds and pulse. Store in the fridge, where the purée will keep for up to 2 weeks.

# Gum-boocha Bears

Gummy bears are one of our favorite candies, but most commercial versions are loaded with ingredients we can't even pronounce. This recipe uses more gelatin than the Kombuchello to create a candylike treat. Sneaking in veggies or fruit is a great way to boost the nutrition. Since these candies are sweetened, they can be a tasty way to use up kombucha that is too sour to drink.

*Yield: 2 cups*

## INGREDIENTS

2 cups mixed diced fruit and veggies (e.g., half strawberries/half beets or half carrots/half mangoes)
1¼ cups fruit-flavored kombucha
6 tablespoons beef gelatin or 1 tablespoon powdered agar
¼ cup honey

## INSTRUCTIONS

Purée the fruit and veggies with ½ cup of the kombucha in a blender until smooth.

Pour an additional ½ cup of kombucha into a small bowl, sprinkle in the gelatin, and let sit for 5 minutes. To prevent clumping, sprinkle the gelatin granules evenly across the surface.

Heat the remaining ¼ cup kombucha in a medium saucepan over low heat until it is just warm to the touch. Add the honey and stir until it is completely dissolved. Pour the warm kombucha over the gelatin mixture. Add the puréed fruit and stir to combine.

Pour the mixture into a silicone candy mold, onto lightly oiled ice cube trays, or onto a sheet pan lined with parchment paper, spreading it to make a ¼-inch-thick layer.

Place the gelatin in the fridge and let chill for about 30 minutes to set. Then remove from the mold or trays or cut into bite-size pieces. Store the candy in an airtight container in the fridge, where it will keep for up to 2 weeks.

## Fruity Kombucha Coconut Sorbet

Melt away the heat of summer nights with this tasty dairy-free treat, in which the creamy coconut milk complements the tart kombucha and sweet fruit. Using fresh fruit heightens the flavor and seasonality of the dish. Make a kombucha parfait by layering this sorbet with Kombuchello (page 291) and Kombuchia Fruit Pudding (page 293), topped with a dollop of fresh whipped cream.

*Yield: 1 pint*

### INGREDIENTS

1 cup coconut milk
1 cup kombucha
2 teaspoons vanilla extract
¼ cup honey
1 cup sliced fruit

### INSTRUCTIONS

Combine the coconut milk, kombucha, vanilla, and honey in a blender. Add the sliced fruit and purée. For a colder, creamy sorbet, add a few ice cubes. Pour the purée into a container and freeze until set, about 30 minutes.

## Love Potion Sorbet

Love Potion 99 (see page 184) is the Kombucha Mamma's signature flavor. This sorbet starts with blueberries, which give a deep purple hue, and uses lavender and rose for a floral hint. Using Love Potion 99 kombucha instead of plain will add greater depth to the fruity flavor.

*Yield: 1 pint*

### INGREDIENTS

2 cups (about 1 pound) fresh or frozen blueberries, puréed
⅔ cup sugar
⅓ cup simple syrup (page 246)
1½ cups kombucha
1 tablespoon rose water
2 drops lavender essential oil

### INSTRUCTIONS

Combine the blueberry purée, sugar, and simple syrup in a saucepan over medium heat. Bring to a simmer, and then remove from the heat and refrigerate for at least 2 hours.

Stir the kombucha into the blueberry mixture.

Pour the mixture into an ice cream maker and add the rose water and lavender oil. Churn for 20 to 30 minutes, then freeze for a few hours until set.

**Note:** No ice cream maker? No problem! Make this recipe with a food processor instead by pouring the mixture into a freezer-safe plastic bag and freezing flat until solid. Crumble the frozen mixture into a food processor and purée until smooth. Pour into a container and freeze again until solid. This process yields a fine-textured, gelato-like sorbet.

## Try Kombuch-icles!!

"These fun and easy treats are full of electrolytes and probiotics, so you can feel good refueling with them on a hot day. Simply fill a Popsicle tray or ice cube tray with flavored kombucha. Add chopped fruit for extra flavor. If you're using an ice cube tray, cover it with plastic wrap and insert toothpicks for sticks, or use the cubes in a drink. Freeze until solid, about 30 minutes.

This is a good way to use up some sour kombucha — just combine it with sugar or honey to taste, stir until the sweetener is dissolved, then freeze!"

### A KOMBUCHA LEGEND:
## It Came from Outer Space

Pyramids, crop circles, and . . . SCOBYs? It is natural for new enthusiasts to wonder at some point: is the kombucha culture a strange and wonderful gift from our alien friends? Modern-day kombucha legends such as Betsy Pryor and Laraine Dave have expressed the idea without irony. Others may simply be uncomfortable with the sight of an ugly mother and make the accusation after one too many stiff kocktails. No matter the reason, more than one first-time SCOBY experience has left a person wondering if the culture is from outer space!

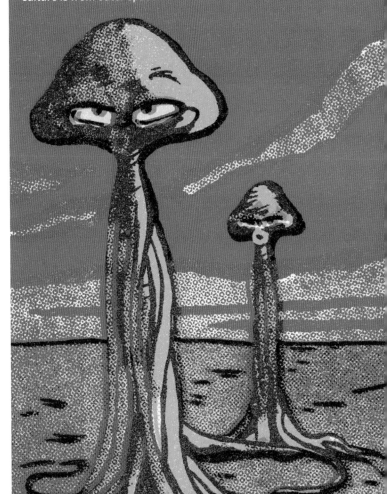

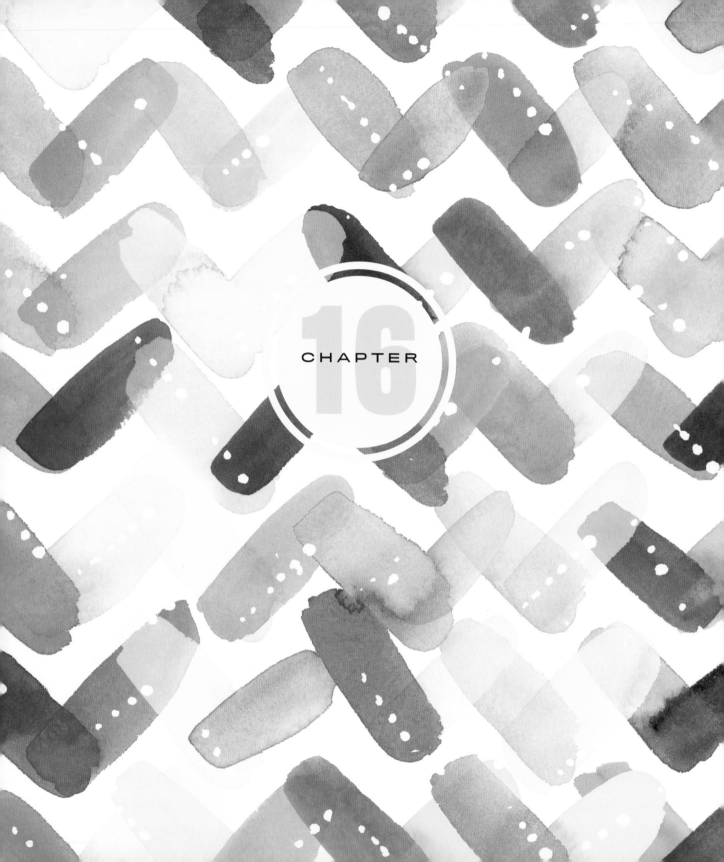

CHAPTER

16

# Consuming Your Cultures

Since the kombucha culture is so prolific, we often end up with more SCOBYs than we need. So what can we do with all those extras? In chapter 17 we talk about some other uses, but since this is the recipe section, we're going to talk about eating them! They make a tasty snack, or you can use them in stir-fries with fresh veggies, or chop them finely as a savory garnish for salads, or add them to smoothies and other blender drinks.

A kombucha culture looks so weird that you probably can't begin to fathom what it might be like to chomp on one. Well, there's only one way to find out, and that's to give it a try. The firm texture of the cellulose makes for a chewy mouthful, while the healthy acids and yeast strands provide a mild tang.

There is a good reason to eat the cultures: they are made of cellulose, or long strands of linked glucose, which we know more commonly as fiber. While animals such as ruminants are able to digest cellulose, humans lack the enzymes needed to break down these long chains of glucose. For us, the SCOBY is a good source of *insoluble* fiber. Insoluble fiber passes through the digestive tract like a broom, sweeping out waste along the way.

Here are some of cellulose's other benefits:

- Contains no calories
- Absorbs water, making it easier to pass stool
- Aids in waste removal, including metabolic waste normally excreted in bile
- Lowers cholesterol levels by absorbing excess cholesterol from the bloodstream
- Slows the absorption of sugar and helps normalize blood sugar levels

# Preparing the SCOBY

The tastiest "meat" comes from young, white SCOBY that is about ¼ inch thick. To remove some of the naturally tangy flavor prior to using it in a recipe, chop the SCOBY into bite-size pieces and soak them in a covered bowl of fresh water for 30 minutes. Repeat the soaking cycle as desired.

If the sour flavor is stubborn, try soaking the SCOBY in milk instead. Of course if tang is part of the recipe then soaking is not needed.

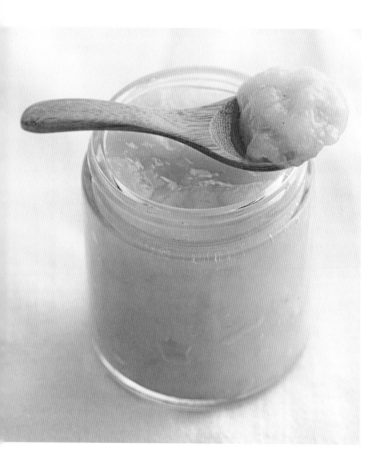

# Making SCOBY Jerky

Brewing as much as we do, we often end up with extra SCOBYs, so we came up with a way to put that good probiotic cellulose to work with these unique and flavorful jerkies. SCOBY snacks have a habit of disappearing quickly, so make a big batch to keep plenty on hand!

There are two ways to turn the SCOBY into jerky — cut it into strips, marinate, and dehydrate, or purée it, combine it with the marinade, and dehydrate. The strips soften in the mouth but require a bit of chewing, whereas the purée is more like a fruit roll-up in consistency.

*To make jerky strips,* cut the SCOBY into bite-size pieces using a knife or sturdy kitchen scissors. Because of the chewiness, keep the pieces on the small side. Pour the marinade over the SCOBY strips, and either toss or stir to coat all the pieces. Let marinate for 12 to 24 hours at room temperature to hasten the absorption of flavor. The SCOBY will take on the color of the marinade.

*To make a purée,* place as much SCOBY as you like in a blender. Add just enough kombucha to cream the culture and prevent motor burnout; generally you will need about ⅛ cup of kombucha per cup of SCOBY. Purée at high speed until the mixture reaches a creamy yet fluffy texture.

If necessary, use a spatula to liberate larger pieces from the blades throughout the process. (Using a food processor results in a stringier texture as well as less consistent flavor and mouthfeel, so stick to a blender for this one.)

## Marinating the SCOBY

If you're working with SCOBY strips, use about ½ cup liquid marinade per cup of chopped SCOBY. Go easy on the salt, as the flavor becomes concentrated once absorbed by the SCOBY. We like to include a good yeast glob or two in the marinade for additional benefits. Marinate for 12 to 24 hours at room temperature before moving on to dehydrating.

If you're working with a SCOBY purée, simply combine the purée with the marinade, mixing well. Let the mixture sit at room temperature for 12 to 24 hours. Then drain off the excess liquid and move on to dehydrating.

## Dehydrating the SCOBY

Dehydrating SCOBY jerky using a dehydrator is easy. If you have strips, simply spread them on dehydrator trays lined with wax paper, and place in the dehydrator on the lowest setting (95–110°F [35–43°C]). For a purée, use the trays designed for use with fruit leathers, or shape the purée into a long, ¼-inch-thick rectangle on a dehydrator tray lined with wax paper.

Dehydrate the jerky for 12 to 36 hours, depending on how stiff you like it. If the jerky sticks to the wax paper, stick it in the freezer for 15 minutes before peeling it off.

If you don't have a dehydrator, use your oven instead at the lowest setting and prop the oven door open slightly. Check on the jerky every few hours to see if it's done. Or go solar! Place the tray out in the sun, covered with a light cloth to keep bugs away. To prevent the material from sticking, use toothpicks or skewers to create a tent. Sun-drying may take longer depending on the amount of exposure to direct sunlight.

### Teriyaki Jerky

"This recipe uses the teriyaki sauce on page 274 to achieve that classic 'beef jerky' flavor without the beef. Cut the jerky into very small pieces to make vegan-friendly 'SCOBacon bits.'

Combine 2 cups of chopped or puréed SCOBY with 1 cup of teriyaki sauce in a bowl. Toss or stir to mix evenly. Cover and let marinate for 12 to 24 hours. Drain off the excess liquid; then dehydrate, following the instructions below."

## Flavor Suggestions

The great thing about SCOBY jerky is that it lends itself to endless experimentation with many different flavors. Here are some sample marinade combos, or you can use any of the dipping sauces on page 274.

- *Asian:* soy sauce with chopped scallions and grated ginger
- *Latin:* salsa with chopped jalapeño and a dash of cumin
- *Southeast Asian:* coconut milk with curry powder and minced lemongrass
- *Mediterranean:* olive oil with chopped garlic and herbs (e.g., rosemary, oregano, parsley, thyme)
- *BBQ:* Kombuchup BBQ Sauce (page 272)

# SCOBY: The Other White "Meat"

Fresh SCOBYs can be used as a substitute for meat or mushrooms or as a healthful enhancement to your own favorites. Closely monitor this delicacy to prevent overcooking. Left unattended, it will turn rubbery, but when sautéed just right, it has a pleasantly chewy yet yielding texture similar to well-prepared octopus or squid. Here are a few of our favorite ways to enjoy this other "other white meat."

## SCOBY "Squid" Sashimi

No kombucha recipe collection would be complete without a sashimi recipe using SCOBY "squid." The trick is to lightly poach the SCOBY to break down the cellulose and make it easier to chew without overcooking it, which will make it even tougher. Pair it with a dipping sauce (page 274) or serve it on a bed of Kimbuchi (page 287).

*Yield: 2 servings*

INGREDIENTS

    2 cups kombucha vinegar (page 256)
    2 tablespoons seaweed, fresh or dried
8-10 (1-inch) pieces SCOBY, ⅛ to ¼ inch thick

INSTRUCTIONS

Combine the vinegar and seaweed in a shallow pan. Cover and bring to a light simmer over medium heat. Add the SCOBY pieces to the liquid. Cover and poach until the pieces become opaque, 2 to 3 minutes.

Remove the pan from the heat. Fish out the SCOBY pieces and chill thoroughly, covered, before serving.

For sushi, lay the SCOBY "squid" pieces on a bed of sushi rice. Add a small dab of wasabi for extra fire.

## SCOBY "Squid" Teriyaki Stir-Fry

Meaty morsels of SCOBY "squid" shine in a tantalizing ginger-scallion soy sauce. Even the carnivores at the table will ask what kind of meat this is!

*Yield: 2 servings*

INGREDIENTS

    1 cup chopped SCOBY, in bite-size pieces
¼–½ cup teriyaki sauce (page 274)
    ¼ cup peanut oil
    1 cup sliced mushrooms
    ½ cup julienned bell pepper
    ¼ onion, sliced
    ¼ cup vegetable broth
    ½ cup sliced green veggies (bok choy, broccoli, asparagus, or whatever you prefer)
    Cooked jasmine rice, for serving

INSTRUCTIONS

Cover the SCOBY pieces with teriyaki sauce in a medium bowl. Toss to coat and let marinate in the fridge for 24 to 48 hours.

Heat the oil in a skillet over medium-high heat. Add the mushrooms, bell pepper, and onion, and sauté until the onion is translucent, 3 to 5 minutes. Add the broth and swirl to deglaze the pan. Add the veggies and cook until tender, 5 to 10 minutes.

Add the marinated SCOBY "squid" pieces, including the teriyaki marinade. Cook until SCOBY pieces are slightly opaque and tender, 3 to 5 minutes. Serve over jasmine rice.

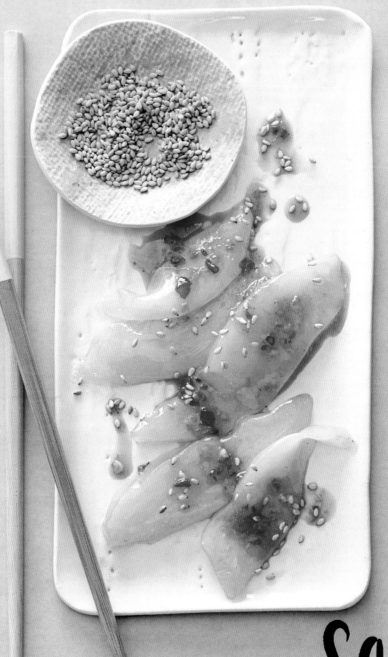
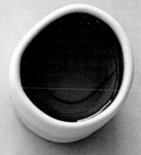

SCOBY
"SQUID"
Sashimi

# SCOBY "Squid" Tom Kha Gai
## (Thai Coconut Soup)

This savory and sweet soup warms the soul. The ginger helps ward off colds and improve circulation, making it a terrific winter soup. SCOBY meat has a natural tang that I find pleasing in this recipe, so I skip the soaking step.

*Yield: 4 servings*

## INGREDIENTS

- 1 (14-ounce) can coconut milk
- 1 (1-inch) piece fresh ginger, peeled and sliced
- 3 (1-inch) pieces fresh lemongrass
- 1 teaspoon Thai chili paste or 2 Thai chiles, chopped
- 1 cup chopped SCOBY, bite-size pieces
- 2 cups Beautifying Bone Broth (page 259) or other broth
- 1 cup sliced mushrooms
- 1 tablespoon Thai or Vietnamese fish sauce
- 1 tablespoon freshly squeezed lime juice
- 1 teaspoon sugar
- ¼ cup chopped fresh basil
- ¼ cup chopped fresh cilantro

## INSTRUCTIONS

Combine the coconut milk, ginger, lemongrass, and chili paste in a large bowl and stir well. Add the SCOBY pieces and toss to coat. Cover and let marinate in the refrigerator for 24 to 48 hours. The longer it sits, the deeper the flavor.

Remove the SCOBY pieces, reserving the marinade.

Combine the remaining marinade with the broth in a medium saucepan. Bring to a boil over high heat. Add the SCOBY pieces, mushrooms, fish sauce, lime juice, and sugar. Reduce the heat and let simmer until the SCOBY pieces are slightly opaque and tender, 5 to 10 minutes.

Remove and discard the lemongrass. Garnish with the basil and cilantro before serving.

### KOMBUCHA MAMMA SEZ

"Do not overcook the SCOBY, as it gets chewier the longer it is cooked. As soon as you notice the SCOBY change color, taste it to see if it is ready to eat."

# Gazboocho

Tomatoes traveled from South America to Spain, where gazpacho became the beloved cold tomato soup of Andalucía. Traditionally the ingredients were pounded with a mortar and pestle, but these days a few quick pulses of the food processor does the trick. This soup only gets better after some time in the fridge and tastes great with a slice of Fermented-Fruit Kombucha Sourdough Bread (page 264) slathered in butter.

*Yield: 4 servings*

## INGREDIENTS

  3 cups chopped fresh tomatoes (about
      2 medium tomatoes)*
  1 cup diced cucumber
  ½ cup chopped red bell pepper
  ¼ cup diced celery
  ¼ cup diced red onion
  2 cups tomato juice
  ½ cup kombucha vinegar (page 256)
  ¼ cup extra virgin olive oil
  ¼ cup puréed SCOBY
  2 teaspoons sugar
  6 dashes Frank's Red Hot, Tabasco, or other
      hot sauce, or to taste
  2 garlic cloves, minced
    Salt and freshly ground black pepper
    Sliced avocado, sour cream (or kefir cheese
      [see page 271] or yogurt), and chopped
      cilantro, for serving

*Frozen or home-canned tomatoes would work,
      but we don't recommend using commercial
      canned tomatoes here.*

## INSTRUCTIONS

In a food processor or blender, combine half of the tomatoes, cucumber, bell pepper, celery, and onion. Add 1 cup of the tomato juice, along with the vinegar, olive oil, SCOBY, sugar, hot sauce, and garlic. Season to taste with salt and pepper. Pulse until all the ingredients are blended into a colorful mixture resembling salsa.

Pour the mixture into a large bowl. Add the remaining 1 cup tomato juice and the remaining tomatoes, cucumbers, bell pepper, celery, and onion. Stir the mixture and taste, adding more salt, pepper, and hot sauce as desired. Chill the soup in the refrigerator for 1 to 2 hours, until cold.

Remove the soup from the fridge and stir. Ladle into bowls and garnish with a few slivers of fresh avocado, a dollop of sour cream, and chopped cilantro.

# Let Them Eat SCOBY

While the tangy flavor and chewy texture of a SCOBY might seem better suited for a salad or main course, a little sugar or fruit can turn the culture into a delectable postmeal treat or a snack for any time of day. These snacks and sweet treats not only quell cravings but provide nutrition as well.

Kombucha vinegar (page 256) adds volume to cakes and cookies, while SCOBYs can be candied or turned into fruit leathers, and kombucha itself adds zing to traditionally sugar-laden gelatin snacks. Feel good serving up these treats knowing that the small amount of sugar is what helps the medicine go down.

## *SCOBY Fruit Leather*

We find that everyone goes gaga for this tasty treat, and when they find out it's made from a kombucha SCOBY, they are incredulous that something that looks so inedible can become something so delicious. When dehydrated at a low temperature, the culture maintains its healthy acids and bacterial activity, secretly making this leather a terrific probiotic-rich snack.

*Yield: 10-12 pieces*

### INGREDIENTS

- 2 cups diced fruit (strawberries, peaches, pears)
- ¼ cup sugar
- 2 cups puréed SCOBY
- 1-2 teaspoons spices or herbs (optional, but some of our favorites are basil, cinnamon, cloves, nutmeg, and thyme)

### INSTRUCTIONS

Combine the fruit and sugar in a medium saucepan over medium heat. Cook, stirring frequently, until the fruit and sugar are thoroughly broken down and combined, about 10 minutes. Add the fruit mixture and SCOBY purée to a blender, along with the spices, and pulse until the mixture has the texture of applesauce and all the ingredients are combined.

Spread the mixture onto wax paper or silicone dehydrator sheets in a layer about ¼ inch thick. Dehydrate for 12 to 36 hours. If you're using a dehydrator, use the lowest setting (95–110°F [35–43°C]). If you're dehydrating in an oven, set it to its lowest temperature and prop the door open.

Once the mixture is dried and no longer sticky, gently remove from the wax paper. If the leather is difficult to remove from the wax paper, stick it in the freezer for 10 to 15 minutes; then peel off. Cut the leather into strips. These can be rolled up or cut into bite-size pieces. Store in an airtight container at room temperature; they will keep indefinitely but might dry out over time.

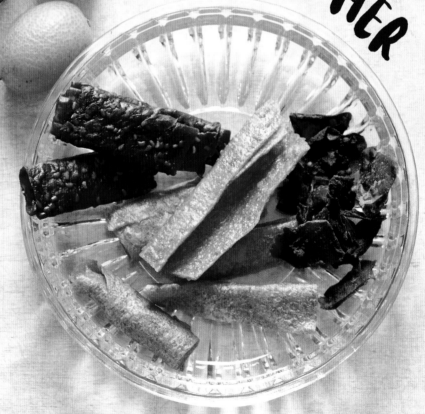

Fruit LEATHER

# Candied SCOBY

As we've seen, the SCOBY is a versatile medium. Here it is candied in sugar syrup, then dehydrated at a low temperature to preserve the probiotic benefit. The culture will continue to ferment the sugar, but the yummy taste will ensure that these candies don't sit around for too long! For a sweeter flavor, soak the SCOBY before candying it (page 298).

*Yield: 1 cup*

## INGREDIENTS

> 2 cups diced SCOBY
> 2 tablespoons sugar
> 2 cups simple syrup (page 246)

## FLAVORING SUGGESTIONS

*Mix and match to create your own favorite flavor.*
> 1 tablespoon ginger syrup or minced fresh ginger
> 1 tablespoon crushed rose petals
> 1 tablespoon crushed lavender
> 1-2 drops edible essential oil

## INSTRUCTIONS

Spread the SCOBY pieces in a wide shallow dish and sprinkle with the sugar. Add the simple syrup; there should be enough to fully submerge all the pieces. Dust with flavorings, if desired.

Cover tightly and marinate at room temperature for 24 hours.

Drain any extra liquid from the pan. Sprinkle with extra petals, spices, or other garnishes. Use a dehydrator at the lowest setting (95–110°F [35–43°C]) or bake the SCOBY pieces in an oven set to its lowest temperature, with the door propped open. Dehydrate for 12 to 36 hours, until the SCOBY has a jellylike consistency and the pieces are easy to chew.

Store in an airtight container at room temperature. The candy will keep indefinitely due to the low pH of the culture (a natural preservative), but it tastes better when it is fresh.

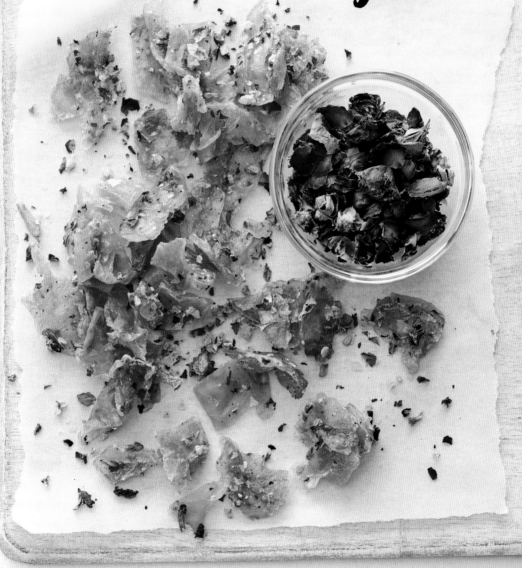

CANDIED
SCOBY

CHAPTER

17

# Beyond the Beverage

## OTHER USES FOR KOMBUCHA

Kombucha's versatility makes it useful in many ways other than simply being a beverage. Its low pH means it's naturally antiseptic, which affords a host of practical applications from general household cleaning to wound treatment. Kombucha vinegar can be substituted for distilled or cider vinegar not only in any recipe, but also for any household application such as cleaning floors, disinfecting kitchen and bathroom surfaces, and shining windows.

The SCOBY itself can be used to slough away dead skin cells, fed to chickens, and made into nutritious dog chews. The cellulose is durable enough that researchers are studying ways to use it as healing bandages, and crafters have turned it into jewelry and coin purses. Some people even think SCOBYs could be developed into a sustainable fabric.

Kombucha's numerous applications make it a natural component of "closed-loop" systems, in which its waste products can be converted into toxin-free commodities. Whether as compost or foodstuff, there is some way to turn every by-product of the kombucha brewing process into something useful.

# Kitchen Uses

Forgo that collection of special cleaning solutions rife with harsh ingredients; all you need is a spray bottle of kombucha vinegar. Numerous studies have shown kombucha's efficacy in eradicating pathogenic organisms such as *E. coli*, salmonella, and listeria, so in addition to drinking up, use booch to clean, disinfect, and add sparkle to your home, while cutting down on toxic ingredients. Kombucha vinegar (page 256) can be used in any household application that calls for distilled or cider vinegar; here are a few that you may not have thought of.

## Fruit-Fly Trap

Mix a drop or two of dish soap with ¼ to ½ cup of kombucha vinegar in a shallow dish. (You can also use flavored kombucha that's too sour.) Place the dish on a counter or shelf. Refresh whenever you find several fruit flies floating in the liquid.

## Laundry Booster

Life is dirty — it's how you deal with the aftermath that makes all the difference. Grease stains are a normal part of cooking or dealing with food. With swift attention and an extra boost from kombucha, grease stains quickly disappear. Rub a little dish soap directly on the stain. (Scrub with a brush to help release older

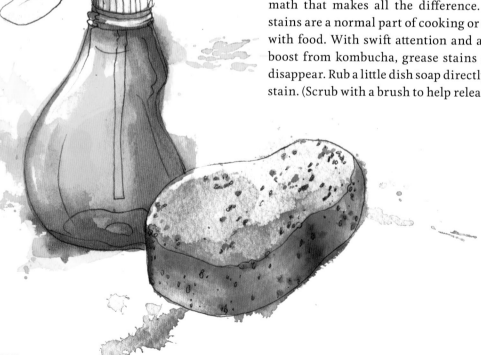

stains.) Rinse the soap off with kombucha vinegar, strained first to avoid getting any yeast strands on clothing. Launder as usual.

Another tip is to add a cup of kombucha vinegar to the wash cycle (put it in the bleach cup). It'll leave fabric fibers naturally soft and remove stale odors.

## Kitchen Patrol

Kombucha is a natural disinfectant, and a drop of tea tree or lemon essential oil boosts the antiseptic effect and offers a lovely smell. Combine 1 cup of kombucha vinegar with a drop or two of essential oil in a small spray bottle and shake to combine. Spray the surface of cutting board or countertops, let sit for a few minutes, and wipe clean with a cloth. It also makes cleaning up around the stove a snap.

## High Shine

Acetic acid is a solvent that can be used to remove buildup and water spots from stainless steel and chrome. Simply dip a cloth in kombucha vinegar or spray it directly on any lackluster surface. Rub gently until the stain disappears. Some elbow grease may be required for tough stains (maybe a genie will appear to grant your wishes!).

# Home Spa

Beauty may only be skin deep, but when it comes to dealing with issues like acne, psoriasis, or eczema, many feel frustrated by the lack of quality options that don't merely cover up symptoms. While drinking kombucha may help beautify skin from the inside out, both the beverage and the culture have topical applications that can contribute to a glowing complexion.

Kombucha's mild astringency balances the pH of the skin and kills bacteria that may cause pimples or other blemishes. Kombucha vinegar has a tonifying effect, inspiring cellular regeneration by stimulating the small capillaries under the skin to bring more blood flow and oxygen to the surface, thus generating new skin cells. Plus the low pH creates a mild acid peel that gently exfoliates by breaking the bonds of dead skin while the nanofibers of the cellulose gradually fill in fine lines and wrinkles. Because kombucha vinegar is less concentrated than regular vinegar, it can be used daily as a toner without being overly drying.

Cosmetics companies are catching on, and kombucha is a hot ingredient popping up in everything from cleansers and toners to facial masks made of bacterial cellulose. Save big bucks and turn your extra SCOBYs and kombucha vinegar into instant beauty boosters. Note that nearly all of the beauty products made with kombucha vinegar or SCOBY will keep for an extended period of time, though their potency will eventually deteriorate, so it's best to make small batches and replenish them often.

The recipes below make terrific pampering gifts for friends, neighbors, and family. Grab a kombucha kocktail, light a candle, play some peaceful music, and let the self-care begin!

# Simple SCOBY Face Mask

In Japan, drugstores offer facial-care products that are essentially bacteria cellulose grown into thin sheets and packaged as single-use, disposable face masks. Rather than fork over a load of cash for a cosmetics company to grow your mask, use an extra SCOBY to detox your skin. This could be part of a weekly or biweekly antiwrinkle routine.

For a single treatment, use one ¼-inch-thick SCOBY, large enough to cover your face (about 4 to 6 inches across), and a towel to catch drips.

Rinse your face, and then find a comfortable place to recline — a couch, bed, or mat on the floor works best. Wrap the folded towel around your neck, leaving enough handy to wipe up drips from the SCOBY. With clean hands, lay the SCOBY on your face. Gently press the culture onto your skin so that it touches every part, leaving enough space to breathe comfortably.

Now take a deep breath and imagine nanofibers of cellulose filling in your wrinkles. **Note:** Avoid getting kombucha in your eyes; it may sting. If it does, rinse with cool water.

Rest in a comfortable position for 5 to 15 minutes; then remove the SCOBY and return it to a special hotel for topical SCOBYs only so as not to mix with brewing SCOBYs. Rinse your face with cool water and gently pat dry. Any red splotches are the result of increase circulation and will quickly fade.

# Facial Toner

Facial toners are intended to make pores look smaller, giving skin a healthy, vibrant glow. This gentle, refreshing version can be used morning and evening as part of your regular skin-cleansing routine.

*Yield: 2 cups*

INGREDIENTS

1½ cups distilled or purified water

½ cup kombucha vinegar (page 256)

5–10 drops essential oil or 1 tablespoon fresh herbs (try lavender, rose, or chamomile)

*Note: To use fresh herbs in place of the essential oil, combine the herbs with the vinegar and let steep for 1 to 3 weeks. Then strain out the herbs and combine the infused vinegar with the water.*

## INSTRUCTIONS

Combine the water, vinegar, and essential oil in a bottle, and shake to distribute the essential oil evenly. To use, shake well, and then apply to face and neck with a clean cotton ball, using upward strokes.

You can also store this toner in a small spray bottle and mist it onto your skin. If a SCOBY forms and clogs the pump, unscrew the top and run the pump under warm water to dislodge it. Storing the toner with a closed cap and inserting the spray pump only when you're applying the toner will prevent that problem, as will using an older vinegar — the older the vinegar, the less likely it is to create a new SCOBY.

# Kombu-Klay Mask

Clays contain nourishing, soothing minerals and work to detoxify the body by drawing out impurities through the skin. When combined with the power of kombucha, this mask does double duty to detoxify and stimulate new skin cell growth. This mask is best made fresh for each application. Try it up to once a week if you enjoy the effects. Cosmetic-grade clays are available online and at health food stores.

*Yield: 1 treatment*

## INGREDIENTS

    1 tablespoon clay (kaolin, green, red, white, or bentonite are all good choices)
    1–2 teaspoons kombucha or kombucha vinegar (page 256)
    1–2 drops skin-safe essential oil (optional)

## INSTRUCTIONS

Mix the clay and the kombucha in a small bowl to create a smooth, spreadable paste. Add the essential oils, and mix thoroughly.

Smooth onto your clean face (or any acne-prone areas). Let dry completely (about 20 minutes); then remove with a warm, wet washcloth.

Rinse with cool water and pat dry with a soft towel. Follow with your favorite nongreasy moisturizer.

# SCOBY SENSITIVITY

Some reddening of the skin after application of a SCOBY is normal. As the culture pulls toxins through the dermis, it also increases circulation, causing skin cells to regenerate while sloughing away the dead skin cells. If the redness doesn't subside within a few minutes, reduce the amount of time that the SCOBY is in contact with the skin.

For creams and similar products made with SCOBYs, test for sensitivity by applying a small portion of the cream inside the upper arm. Check after 5 minutes to see how it is working. Some tingling may occur, which is normal. If the tingling becomes uncomfortable, wipe away the SCOBY with a clean damp cloth.

# Kombucha Yeast Mask

Yeast, which are rich in B vitamins and trace minerals, stimulate circulation to create a rosy glow. Since yeast bodies are by-products of the brewing process, put them to work in your beauty routine! (See page 109 for how to harvest yeast.) This mask works wonders on acne and acne-prone areas. Use as often as desired.

*Yield: 1 treatment*

## INGREDIENTS

- 1 tablespoon raw honey
- 1 teaspoon kombucha yeast (in solid or liquid form)

## INSTRUCTIONS

Mix the honey and yeast in a small bowl to create a spreadable paste. Smooth onto your face. Leave on for 15 to 20 minutes; then wash off with warm water. The yeast may cause a tingling sensation that most people find pleasurable. If it becomes uncomfortable, wash the mask off immediately.

# Soothing SCOBY Cream

SCOBY cream has myriad uses — as a facial mask, to calm eczema or psoriasis flare-ups, as an emollient to soften dry skin, as a wound poultice, and more. Start with this basic recipe and then mix in skin conditioners or essential oils if desired. The texture is similar to that of applesauce — other oils may help bind the cream better — but using it while it's a bit goopy also works great.

*Yield: 1 cup*

## INGREDIENTS

4–6 ounces SCOBY
⅛ cup unflavored kombucha or kombucha vinegar (page 256)
1–2 drops essential oil, for fragrance (optional)

## EMOLLIENT SUGGESTIONS

Leave your cream plain or choose one or two of these options:

- 1 ounce olive oil
- 1 ounce almond oil
- 1 ounce vitamin E oil
- 1 ounce rose-hip oil

## INSTRUCTIONS

Combine the SCOBY and half of the kombucha in a blender. Pulse a few times; then purée, adding more kombucha as necessary to achieve the texture of applesauce. The cellulose won't break down completely unless you have a very powerful blender, so the cream may be a bit chunky.

**KOMBUCHA MAMMA SEZ**

## Culture Tips

- Thin SCOBY babies, ⅛ to ¼ inch thick, have the most comfortable feel on the skin.
- It's easy to breathe through the SCOBY, but for extra comfort, cut eye, nose, and mouth holes with a clean pair of scissors.
- You can use a single culture four to six times as a facial mask. For maximum potency, store them in strong liquid between uses.
- Store cosmetic SCOBYs in a separate hotel so they don't get mixed up with your brewing SCOBYs.

If you're using one of the emollient oils, stir it in with a whisk after the cream is blended. If you like, add a drop or two of your favorite cosmetic-grade essential oil for a lovely fragrance.

Apply to the affected area and leave on until it dries out completely. As it dries, which takes 10 to 20 minutes, the cream will become a solid layer that easily peels off.

Store the cream in a glass jar with a plastic lid in a cool place out of direct sunlight. It will remain viable for months. Over time it may grow a skin on the top to prevent evaporation; if this happens, simply break up the skin with your fingers and mix it back into the cream prior to use. If the cream is left unattended for too long it may develop mold — in this case, dispose of it and whip up a fresh batch.

# Dry-Skin Cream

Dry weather and cold winds often leave skin feeling about as smooth as an alligator's tail. A lack of healthy fats in the diet also contributes to dry, chapped skin. So whether you eat them or slather them directly onto ravaged skin, this cream will soothe while simultaneously locking in deep, long-lasting moisture.

*Yield: About ⅔ cup*

## INGREDIENTS

¼ cup Soothing SCOBY Cream (facing page)
⅛ cup coconut oil

## INSTRUCTIONS

Mix the SCOBY cream and coconut oil into a paste. Smooth the paste onto the affected area. Let it dry (10–20 minutes), then rinse off with warm water and pat dry. No other moisturizer is needed.

If you have extra cream, store it in a sealed container in a cool, dark location; it will keep for up to 2 months.

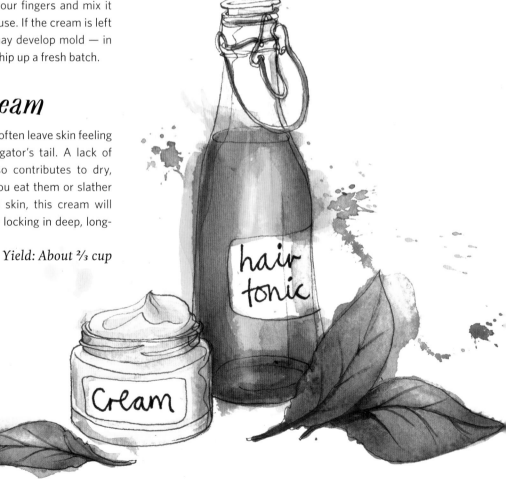

# Wrinkle/Scar Cream

Aging is a normal process, and the damaging effects of this toxic world only hasten the wrinkles. Nourishing the skin protects against damage and may undo some of the effects wrought by exposure to the sun, toxic beauty products, and chlorine. This formula also helps reduce the appearance of scars and liver spots.

*Yield: About ⅔ cup*

## INGREDIENTS

- 2 tablespoons coconut oil
- 1 tablespoon shea butter
- ½ teaspoon vitamin E oil
- ½ cup Soothing SCOBY Cream (page 314)
- 1 tablespoon rose-hip oil

## INSTRUCTIONS

Combine the coconut oil, shea butter, and vitamin E oil in the top of a double boiler over medium heat. Warm, stirring occasionally, until thoroughly melted and mixed. Remove from the heat and let cool for 10 to 15 minutes. Stir in the SCOBY cream and rose-hip oil.

To use, gently massage the cream into the skin. Let dry (10–20 minutes); then rinse off with a warm washcloth, and pat skin dry.

Store extra cream in a sealed container at room temperature; it will keep for up to a month.

# Calming Skin Lotion

Hot, itchy skin never feels good, but the cooling effects of yogurt and oatmeal combined with the softening properties of the SCOBY bring quick relief to calm and soothe. Turmeric is naturally anti-inflammatory and has a long history of use for skin ailments. Follow with a little coconut oil to moisturize the affected area. This formula is gentle enough for use with eczema and psoriasis.

*Yield: About ⅓ cup*

## INGREDIENTS

- 1 teaspoon oats
- ¼ cup Soothing SCOBY Cream (page 314)
- ⅛ cup plain Greek yogurt or kefir cheese (page 271)
- ¼ teaspoon ground turmeric

## INSTRUCTIONS

Grind the oats to a fine powder in a coffee or spice grinder. Combine the ground oats with the SCOBY cream, yogurt, and turmeric in a small bowl and stir into a paste; the turmeric will give it a pleasant yellow tinge.

Smooth thickly onto the affected area. Leave the cream on until it is dry, about 20 minutes. Then rinse off with warm water.

Extra cream can be stored in the fridge in a sealed container for up to 1 week. In fact, chilling it first makes it feel extra soothing!

# Foot Detox

Pamper your pooped piggies with this relaxing foot soak. The soles of the feet are an important detoxification point, which means soaking is more than just a way to soothe jangled nerve endings. Those with toenail fungus or chapped skin may benefit from daily soakings.

We like to use vinegar infused with peppermint (to stimulate circulation) and/or thyme (to kill bacteria that cause odor). After a relaxing footbath, dry your feet thoroughly with a soft towel, rub in some coconut oil or shea butter, and put on a comfy pair of socks for deep moisturization.

*Yield: 1 treatment*

## INGREDIENTS

1 cup Epsom, mineral, or Himalayan pink salt
¼ cup kombucha vinegar (page 256) mixed with 2 to 3 drops of peppermint and/or thyme essential oil or infused with 1 tablespoon of fresh herbs, chopped

## INSTRUCTIONS

Fill a basin large enough for both feet with warm water. Add the salt and vinegar and stir to dissolve the salt. Put your feet in the basin, and relax for 20 minutes or until the water feels cold. If the footbath has loosened any dry skin, promptly exfoliate with a pumice stone or exfoliating mitt. Dry thoroughly with a soft towel.

---

**KOMBUCHA MAMMA SEZ**

## Bath Soak

"In a world full of quick showers, taking a bath is a downright luxury. Taking some time to unwind at home is a great way to treat yourself without breaking the bank. In the bathwater, kombucha vinegar softens the skin and gently draws out toxins.

Draw a warm or hot bath, adding 1 cup of kombucha vinegar and ½ cup oats, ground into powder or whole oats tied into a sock and secured with a rubber band. For an extrarelaxing treat, use vinegar infused with your favorite herbs or essential oils."

---

# Hair Tonic

Shampoos contain harsh surfactants that create a lovely lather but strip hair of natural oils that protect it from the elements. Many find that reapplying those oils with conditioner creates a cycle of chemical addiction that can also disrupt the immune system. Others exhort "no 'poo" but go too far with harsher vinegars and baking soda mixtures that leave hair feeling like straw. Kombucha is gentle enough to soften the hair while leaving enough natural oil intact to give hair a healthy sheen. Simply apply to wet hair, work in with fingers, and rinse.

Using this "no 'poo" tonic, Alex has been shampoo-free for many years. For those with oily hair, this tonic works better if you don't rinse; I leave it in after shampooing and my hair is soft and shiny by the time it dries.

# HAIR TONIC HERBS

If using fresh herbs use ¼ to ⅓ cup of each herb. If using dried use ⅛ to ¼ cup of each herb. Shake the bottle to combine ingredients at regular intervals (at least once a week over a period of 3 to 6 weeks); then strain the herbs. If using essential oils, add 5 to 10 drops of each.

| HERB | Normal | Dry | Oily | Sensitive | Hair Loss |
|---|:---:|:---:|:---:|:---:|:---:|
| Basil | x | | | | x |
| Bay leaf | | | x | | |
| Black tea ● | | | | | |
| Burdock root | | x | x | x | x |
| Calendula ◉ ● | x | x | x | x | |
| Chamomile ◉ | x | x | x | | |
| Comfrey ● | | x | | x | |
| Elderflower | | x | | | |
| Hibiscus ● | | | | | |
| Horsetail | x | x | x | x | |
| Lavender | x | x | x | x | |
| Lemon balm/Lemon grass/ Lemon peel ◉ | | | x | | |
| Nettle ● | x | x | x | x | x |
| Parsley | x | x | | | |
| Peppermint | | | x | x | |
| Rose petals/rose hips ● | | | | | |
| Rosemary ● | x | | x | x | x |
| Sage ● | x | x | | x | x |
| Thyme | | | x | x | |

**HAIR TYPE** (column group header over Normal, Dry, Oily, Sensitive, Hair Loss)

◉ Golden highlights

● Dark highlights

● Red highlights

We age our hair tonic with the herbs for at least 3 months to ensure that all of the sugar is gone from the kombucha (no one wants sticky hair!). This also prevents cultures from growing in the bottle. Kombucha vinegar is less acidic than other vinegars and is easier on the hair follicles.

*Yield: 2 cups*

### INGREDIENTS

2 cups kombucha vinegar (page 256)
Herbs or essential oils (see chart on facing page)

### INSTRUCTIONS

Combine the vinegar with the herbs in a jar with a lid. Let age at room temperature for 2 to 4 weeks and up to 3 months. Then strain out the herbs, if necessary, and transfer to a plastic or other shatterproof container for use in the shower. It will keep indefinitely.

**KOMBUCHA MAMMA SEZ**

## Fighting Bacteria with Bacteria

"Sweat itself does not have an odor, but once exposed to certain types of bacteria, it can become pretty stinky. We have found that splashing some facial toner or hair tonic (page 317) on our clean armpits kills the bacteria that cause smells and leaves us fresh and chemical-free without deodorant! For pits that are already stinky, pour some toner or tonic on a washcloth and scrub them well."

# Home First Aid

When applied topically, kombucha's low pH and unique cellulose structure speed healing and prevent infection. Many people have reported swifter healing after applying a SCOBY or kombucha vinegar to a minor wound. Clean the wound thoroughly, and then place a thin SCOBY over the wound or dip a clean bandage in kombucha vinegar and apply directly to the wound.

It may sting a little, just like iodine, but that feeling will fade and eventually the pain of the injury itself will ease. Use gauze or a clean cloth to secure the SCOBY, and refresh it once the culture has dried out. Kombucha vinegar and cultures can also soothe the sting of sunburn and other minor burns, as well as treat fungal infections.

Use the culture to treat seborrheic dermatitis, which refers to any of several types of fungal infections that occur on the surface of the skin. Though most often associated with infants (cradle cap), it can afflict children into adulthood, though it may be called dandruff in older sufferers. Often due to toxic overload in the body, this condition can be treated by using the kombucha culture topically to help reset the pH of the scalp and inhibit the growth of microbes.

Characterized by red or yellow flaky skin that may turn into welts when scratched, the irritation can often be calmed with the cool tingle of a SCOBY or an application of Soothing SCOBY Cream (page 314). Apply the kombucha culture to the affected area. Secure with a bandana or gauze. Leave in contact with the skin for at least 10 to 15 minutes and up to 24 hours or until it dries out. If the skin feels too sensitive, remove immediately and rinse with cool water. It may need a few applications before it completely heals. These can be spaced out every few days or every few hours depending on how your body reacts.

Here are a few easy concoctions to add to your medicine cabinet or have on hand in the kitchen.

## MEDICAL APPLICATIONS

Beyond home uses, the cellulose created by the *Komatagaeibacter xylinum* (formerly *Acetobacter*) bacteria is being cultivated for pharmaceutical applications such as living bandages, internal repair structures (e.g., heart stents), and temporary skin substitutes in the treatment of burns, grafts, dermal abrasions, and ulcers.

### Living Bandages

A Brazilian company, Fibrocel, has developed a living bandage under the name of Dermafill (*xylinum* cellulose). The bacteria responsible for "spinning" the cellulose are the same as those in kombucha — *K. xylinum*. The open structure of the microbial cellulose allows it to absorb water up to one hundred times its weight while retaining flexibility. The bacteria in the "living" bandage adhere to the skin and create a "scab" that allows oxygen exchange while moving with the skin, speeding healing below the surface of the skin and requiring fewer changes than nonporous bandages.

Using the kombucha culture in this capacity adds benefits of healthy acids to speed the healing process. These can include hyaluronic acid, which helps the skin retain moisture; usnic acid, which acts as an analgesic; and catechins, which decrease inflammation.

### Blood Vessels

Another biotech company is using bacterial cellulose to create blood vessels for microsurgery. Termed BASYC, which stands for **BA**cterial **SY**nthesized **C**ellulose, this "biomaterial" has demonstrated a close resemblance to human tissue, minimizing the risk of rejection and adverse effects. Similar technologies are being developed in labs around the world.

# Sunburn-Relief Spray

Spritz this cooling concoction wherever it's needed to cool sunburned skin, or soak a washcloth in the solution and lay it across the affected area. Be careful not to get the solution into your eyes or nasal passages, as it could sting.

*Yield: About 1 cup*

INGREDIENTS

    1 cup kombucha vinegar (page 256)
    ¼ cup aloe vera gel
    1 tablespoon vitamin E oil
    1–2 drops camphor essential oil

INSTRUCTIONS

Combine the vinegar with the aloe, vitamin E oil, and camphor in a spray bottle and shake well. Spray directly on affected areas, shaking before each use. Repeat as needed. No refrigeration is needed, but chilling the mixture prior to use boosts the cooling effect.

# Four Thieves Kombucha Spray

The war on bacteria using antibacterial products has been shown to be a failure, often leading to "superbugs" — pathogenic bacteria that are resistant to bactericides. Instead of making an antibacterial concoction, use kombucha vinegar to create "probacterial" sprays that kill pathogenic organisms on contact while establishing healthy bacterial colonies on the skin.

This formula is perfect for cold season. Keep germs at bay by spraying it on hands, keyboards, doorknobs, or wherever a little extra protection is needed. Fresh herbs work best (make it in the summer so it is ready for winter), but you can substitute half as much in dried herbs.

*Yield: 2 cups*

INGREDIENTS

    2 cups kombucha vinegar (page 256)
    2 teaspoons fresh rosemary
    ½ teaspoon fresh sage leaf (¼ leaf)
    ¼ teaspoon minced garlic
    ¼ teaspoon fresh lavender
    ¼ teaspoon fresh mint
    ¼ teaspoon fresh oregano

INSTRUCTIONS

Combine the vinegar with the rosemary, sage, garlic, lavender, mint, and oregano in a glass jar with a lid. Let steep at room temperature, out of direct sun, for at least 2 weeks and up to 2 months. The longer it steeps the more potent the mixture.

Strain out the herbs and store the vinegar in a spray bottle. Spritz generously, being careful to avoid the eyes and other sensitive areas.

## KOMBUCHA MAMMA SEZ

### Kombucha Drops

"Putting pieces of fresh SCOBY through a press extracts a liquid with a high concentration of bacteria and yeast cells. These 'drops' are then preserved with alcohol in a ratio of 1:1 (e.g., 1 tablespoon of liquid to 1 tablespoon of alcohol). Use alcohol that is at least 80 to 100 proof for best results; plain vodka is fine. Take 15 drops, 1 to 3 times per day, when traveling or when no kombucha is available."

# Flea and Tick Repellent

This spray is safe to use on humans, as well as dogs and cats, to ward off fleas and ticks. Avoid sensitive areas, like the eyes, as it could sting. To apply to your pet's face, spray the repellent onto your own hands and gently fluff into your pet's fur, avoiding the eyes and snout.

*Yield: About 3 cups*

## INGREDIENTS

2 cups kombucha vinegar (page 256)

¼ cup distilled vinegar

2 tablespoons sweet almond oil

2 tablespoons lemon juice

1 teaspoon minced garlic

## INSTRUCTIONS

Combine the kombucha vinegar, distilled vinegar, almond oil, lemon juice, and garlic in a glass jar with a lid. Let steep at room temperature for 1 week; then strain out the garlic.

Store in a spray bottle. Lightly spritz your clothes or skin and your pet's fur before walking in the woods to prevent ticks and fleas from hitching a ride!

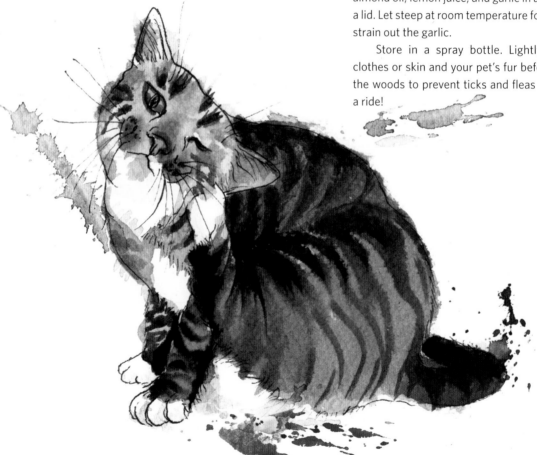

# Uses in Crafts

The SCOBY is so durable that some people have taken to tanning extra cultures into a leatherlike material to create unique crafts. Being hydrophilic, an untreated SCOBY will absorb up to one hundred times its weight in water, so once it's dried, keep any SCOBY-leather items out of water. Most people who dabble in this craft prefer to use natural tanning methods such as oiling the dried SCOBY with jojoba or some other natural oil to create a more water-resistant material.

## *SCOBY Earrings*

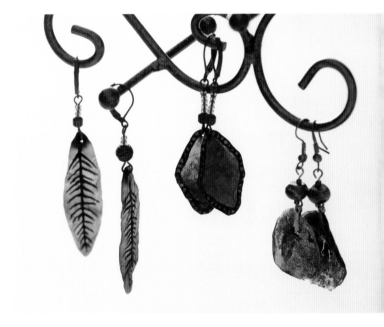

MATERIALS

> 1 SCOBY, at least ½ inch thick
> Leather punch
> Jewelry pliers
> Earring hooks
> Scissors
> Paint, feathers, and beads, for decoration
> (optional)

INSTRUCTIONS

Dehydrate the SCOBY until it is leathery but still somewhat pliable. Cut into whatever shapes you want; simple shapes such as rectangles, ovals, and circles will hold together best. Punch a hole in the top of the shape, and use the pliers to attach the earring hooks. Decorate with paint, feathers, or beads for a unique look.

# Coin Purse

## MATERIALS

- 1 SCOBY, at least ½ inch thick
- Natural dye (optional)
- Oil (jojoba, beeswax, coconut, or lanolin), to maintain flexibility and prevent tearing
- Waxed linen cord
- Leather needle

## INSTRUCTIONS

Dry the SCOBY until it is leathery but still somewhat pliable. If desired, use a natural dye to create a design on the SCOBY. Let the dye set completely before oiling to prevent any bleeding.

Rub the oil generously and evenly into the dried culture, rubbing it in and wiping off any excess. Once the pieces have achieved the desired luster, use waxed cord and a leather-working needle to affix a drawstring around the edge, inserting it about ¼ inch from the edges of the SCOBY. Double-knot the ends of the cord to prevent it from slipping out.

While it should not be exposed to significant amounts of rain or water, it can be cleaned by lightly wiping it with a damp cloth.

## HOW TO DRY A SCOBY

There is no wrong way to dehydrate a SCOBY, so use whatever method is available to you. Dehydrators are great, obviously, but the sun is free and does as good a job. In most climates a SCOBY simply left indoors at room temperature will dehydrate just fine over a few days (the only consideration might be attracting fruit flies!). Turning it every 12 or 24 hours will speed the drying process and ensure that it is even on both sides.

When the SCOBY becomes very thin, perhaps a quarter inch thick if it started at an inch, it may be ready to use, but keep in mind that the SCOBY will continue to shrink as it dehydrates. Cut pieces slightly larger than needed to accommodate this. Experiment with various stages of drying to find out how dry a SCOBY needs to be to work best for your project.

Oiling the cultures from time to time with olive oil will help to preserve the shape and luster of the SCOBY "leather."

# Spent Tea Potpourri

One thing that is not in short supply for kombucha brewers is spent tea leaves. While they make lovely compost (particularly because they are nitrogen-rich), they can also be used to create potpourri. Tea leaves absorb odors much as baking soda does. Adding essential oils to your spent tea potpourri creates a distinct fragrance and mood.

## MATERIALS

1–2 tablespoons spent tea leaves
1–2 drops essential oil

## INSTRUCTIONS

Dry the tea leaves by spreading them out on a baking sheet and leaving them in a warm, sunny spot. Once they're dried, gather the leaves in a small bowl or muslin cloth bag. Sprinkle with a drop or two of essential oil, and place wherever you desire a fresh scent. Refresh from time to time by stirring the leaves and adding another drop of essential oil. Compost when the leaves seem to be completely spent.

# Bacteria-Powered Planet

## SCOBY Fashion (Really!)

From beverage to bandage to bracelet, the kombucha culture is incredibly flexible. Artists, fashion designers, and medical researchers are continually amazed at the number of ways in which bacterial cellulose can be utilized as a sustainable resource. The material caught the eye of sci-fi fan and fashion graduate Suzanne Lee, who stumbled upon the concept of biofabrics at an art installation while researching her book, *Fashioning the Future*.

Sustainability has been slow to arrive in the fashion and textile industry, so when Suzanne learned that she could possibly "grow a dress," she decided to try it herself. She was invited to speak at a TED Conference in 2011. The video of her talk, which featured several pieces, including shoes, a jacket, and a skirt, went viral, and suddenly Suzanne found herself serving as a consultant to other companies hoping to create novel fabrics.

The biggest challenge has been preserving the fabric once the garment is complete, preventing it from soaking up water or sustaining damage, while also maintaining the biodegradability of the clothing, which is part of the point of the project. Undeterred by these obstacles, other artists have picked up on the trend by making their own clothing, "vegan leather," and SCOBY-based jewelry — all from bacterial cellulose!

# Good Bugs in the Garden

SCOBYs are good for all beings, including the ones that live in the dirt. Adding old SCOBYs to a compost bin will speed the decomposition process and adding SCOBY purée to the soil will help acidic-pH-loving plants thrive. To use SCOBY purée in the garden, simply whip some up in the blender, and then dig a hole or trench ½ to 1 inch deep about 3 to 6 inches from the base of the plant. Pour in ½ cup of SCOBY purée, and then cover with dirt. Burying the SCOBY in the dirt masks the odor and prevents fruit flies from finding it.

Add SCOBY to the soil when putting in new plants to boost the available nutrition. We compost cultures and tea year-round and then add to the garden in spring and fall to help Mother Nature prosper.

# Pets Are People, Too

Pets are cherished additions to our families and, like us, are powered by bacteria. Bred to cohabitate with humans, many pets suffer from similar health ailments due to subpar food and overexposure to toxins. Though not all will take to the flavor right away, cats, dogs, horses, pigs, chickens, and many other animals enjoy a kombucha snack. We know firsthand that many dogs love dried SCOBYS, which make a much healthier chew toy than bleached cowhide or subpar "cookie" treats.

Dogs may also benefit from a little kombucha mixed into their food or water to populate their guts with good bacteria. Small dogs do well with 1 to 2 ounces, whereas bigger dogs can consume up to 4 ounces a day. It need not be included with every meal, so monitor how your pet responds. Many owners observe that their dogs experience improved gut health as evidenced by regular and well-formed bowel movements and softer fur when small amounts of kombucha are included in their meals. Nearly any kind of pet will benefit if they feel instinctually compelled to try it. It will be obvious if they don't like it as they will simply refuse to consume it.

Diluted kombucha vinegar can be used as a natural cleaning spray to remove dirt and oils from your dog's coat, avoiding the chemicals in pet shampoos. The acids soften skin and fur, and if the brew is sour enough, it can deter fleas. Blend a 50/50 mix of kombucha vinegar (page 256) and water in a bottle, add a drop or two of tea tree or neem oil for deterring pests, spray it on, and let air-dry.

## SCOBY Dog Treats

For a natural chew toy with probiotic punch, lightly dehydrate a SCOBY until it is no longer moist but not thoroughly dry; then toss to your pooch. Size the treat to your dog — smaller dogs might eat too much, which can upset their stomachs. No matter what the size of the dog, offer small pieces at first to make sure his digestive system will accept this new occasional treat. Many dogs will munch it right down, but try smearing it with peanut butter at first if your dog is hesitant.

# Farm Animal Fuel

One thing that is empirically obvious is that chickens love SCOBYs. Whenever we bring extras to our neighbors' pen, the birds scramble over each other like mad, fighting for the coveted cultures. Many studies have demonstrated that adding SCOBY or kombucha to chickens' diet, at a rate of as little as 0.75 percent of the total feed, can result in larger eggs with sturdier shells. High in lysine and other amino acids, kombucha aids in digestion, allowing the hens to more easily absorb nutrients from their feed. Additional studies have indicated that chickens fed kombucha grew larger and their ability to digest protein increased. (See studies cited on page 370.)

Pigs, cows, and horses all gravitate to kombucha in their water supply or SCOBYs in their feed. One study in sheep demonstrated reduced numbers of parasites and elimination of respiratory issues in immunocompromised sheep who were given kombucha as an oral supplement (Manuel, R. C., et al. [2014]). These studies, though preliminary, suggest that kombucha has a net beneficial effect on all types of organisms, especially when it comes to alleviating issues associated with digestion and immunity.

If viable natural alternatives can demonstrate real results, the reduction of toxins in our food supply and our bodies from eliminating mass pharmaceutical use in raising livestock could be tremendous. And while only a few producers are currently using them, we anticipate that as more learn about the inexpensive benefits that can arise from feeding animals bacterial cellulose, usage of these by-products is sure to rise.

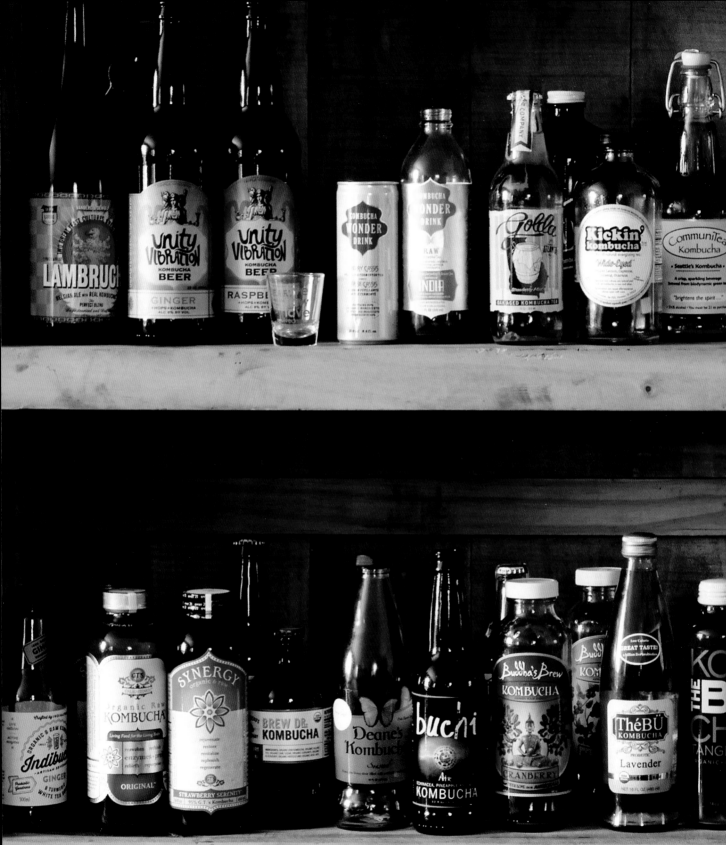

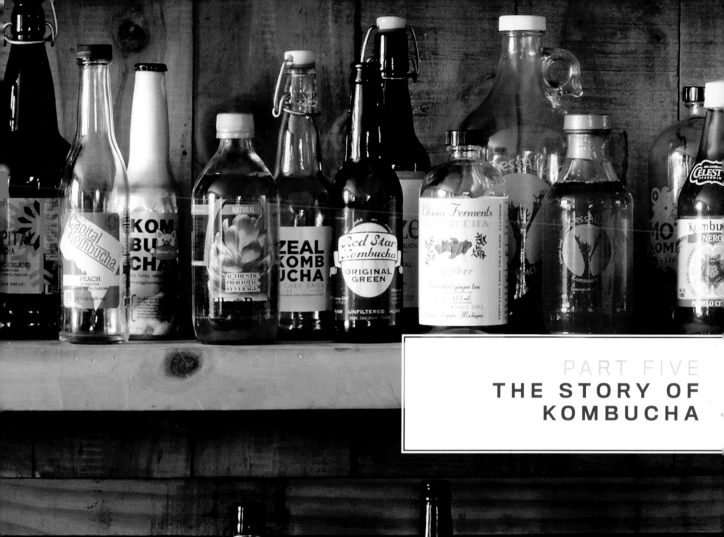

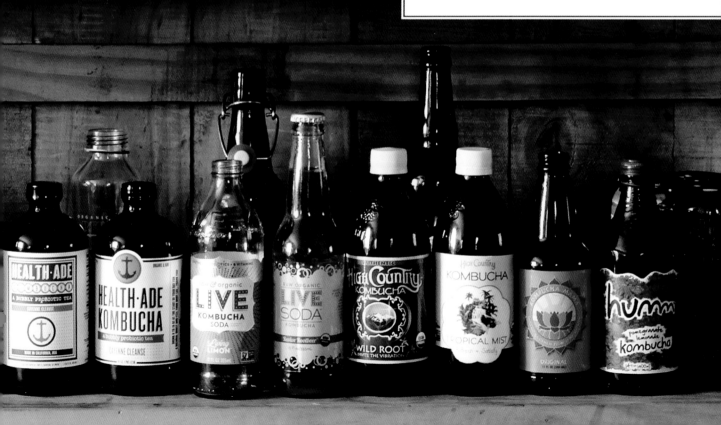

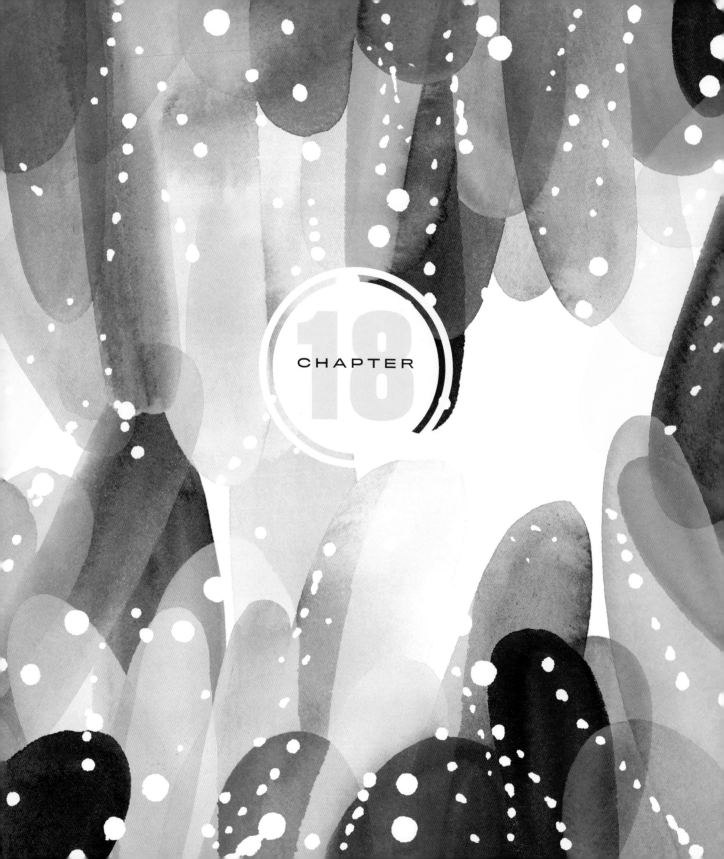

CHAPTER **18**

# The History and Science of Kombucha

CONDENSED

Because kombucha's various ancient origin stories are passed around among homebrewers as freely as SCOBYs, many people assume that our knowledge of kombucha's history is all folklore and no substance. Nothing could be further from the truth! In fact, kombucha has been studied for more than a hundred years by scientists around the world, with a recent boom in interest since around the year 2000. Here we examine the facts and fiction that surround this "magical mushroom."

# Kombucha Is Here to Stay

Whether the many legends surrounding kombucha's origin are literally true or more symbolic and mythical is shrouded in the mists of time. While some of the legends seem unlikely, there is a kernel of truth at the heart of each one — the power of kombucha, with its healing properties and "otherness," has always been palpable to those who brew it, drink it, and pass it on to friends.

When we peel back the mythology and look at the written evidence, the history of kombucha's origins may not be as distant as we might like to think. This in no way changes what it is; rather, it simply puts the ferment into historical perspective.

The legend that anoints kombucha with the oldest origins has it arising in China around 221 BCE (see page 96). China remains the most likely candidate; after all, tea originated there, and the Chinese have practiced fermentation for thousands of years, so it is an easy jump from fermenting one thing to another.

But is kombucha more than two thousand years old? Realistically, the most likely answer is no. In that earliest kombucha origin story, the first emperor of China, Qin Shi Huang, supposedly consumed *lingzhi* — the elixir of immortality. The common Chinese name for kombucha, however, is *haibao* (sea treasure); *lingzhi* refers to reishi mushrooms, not kombucha. As one of the common names for kombucha is "mushroom tea," perhaps the meaning was lost in translation or misapplied, given the resemblance of the SCOBY to a mushroom cap.

It should also be noted that tea was not commonly consumed in China until the Tang dynasty (618–907 CE), nearly a thousand years after the time of Qin Shi Huang. In all our research on ancient fermentation practices of China, we have been unable to find any references to fermenting tea. The same is true when we investigated the fermented foods of Tibet — while Tibetans drink plenty of tea with yak milk and butter and they brew barley beer, there is no mention of fermenting tea with a culture or vinegar mother.

Perhaps naturally, the consensus among the Chinese people we interviewed was that kombucha is native to China, though whether its origins lie in Manchuria, Shandong province, or the Bohai Sea district (where the Legend of the Sea Treasure takes place; see page 121), there is little concrete evidence. Manchuria is just north of Korea, and Shandong is across the East China Sea from Korea. If kombucha began in either of these areas, it is easy to see how it may have spread into the southern Korean kingdom of Silla before 414 CE, which is when the Korean doctor Komu-ha is said to have brought his "special remedy" for the ailing Japanese emperor In-giyō (see page 140). Perhaps through a historical game of "telephone," the name of the doctor was changed to Dr. Kombu.

## What about Japan?

The main confounding factor in the Japanese origin legends again is the absence of tea consumption until some five hundred years after Komu-ha (sometimes referred to as "Dr. Kombu") is said to have cured the emperor around 414 BCE, according to Buddhist texts. Another potential reason for the confusion is that the samurai traditionally consumed *kombu-cha*, a tisane made by steeping seaweed in water (*kombu* — seaweed, *cha* — tea). It is easy to imagine how this translation may have been misconstrued by early researchers.

Japan is often credited with kombucha's origin in Russian stories, since it was brought back to Russia after the Russo-Japanese War (1904-1905). However, the war was fought not in Japan but in southern Manchuria and Korea, around the Liaodong Peninsula, just a short hop across the Bohai Sea and not too far from Beijing. So while there is not a definitive origin story, nearly all of the stories center in this region of northern China around the Bohai Sea.

Frankly, we find a number of kombucha origin stories, and those of other fermented drinks such as kefir or jun, to be unsupported by much logic or weight. In many cases, they involve overly specific details of what most certainly is a cultural phenomenon — the sharing of food and drink — that would be exceedingly difficult to trace to any concrete "beginning."

No matter which country claims it as their own — China, Russia, Korea, or Japan — kombucha is here to stay. Fermentation may seem magical, but it's just the hard work of billions of little buddies making the food better for us. Whether kombucha is thousands of years old or only a few hundred, the fact is that humans and fermentation evolved together, and fermentation continues to expand our consciousness and existence as we delve into the science of what it means to live in a bacterial world.

**KOMBUCHA MAMMA SEZ**

## Our Best Guess

"After all our research, what we think happened is that centuries ago, someone left out a cup of sweetened tea or sweet wine. An insect or two landed in the cup, leaving behind *Acetobacter* that colonized with some local yeast and began the very first kombucha ferment.

The person who discovered the fermented tea relied on his or her own senses — a practice we have nearly lost — to detect a delicious brew. This lucky discoverer then threw the whole thing into another batch of sweet tea, and thus the "culture of kombucha" was born.

The fact that the SCOBY can be a host to several different types of bacteria and yeast indicates that it likely can thrive in a variety of locations. The warmer temperatures preferred by the culture certainly hint at more tropical origins; however, as the technology of fermentation was already strong within all of the ancient cultures, it is not a far stretch to imagine that once they discovered it, the peoples of that time would know how to nurture a ferment."

# The Kombucha Timeline

Here we present the highlights of historical research, mysterious myths, and important figures in the story of the "wonder mushroom" and "miracle tea" that has fascinated so many around the globe. (For more research, see page 342–43 and appendixes 1 and 2.)

Everyone along this path has contributed to the kombucha story in some important way. The work of some of these pioneers helped lay the foundation for the fields of bacteriotherapy and microbiome research.

## 414
Komu-ha, a Korean doctor summoned to heal the Japanese emperor In-giyō, uses kombucha tea in treatments (see A Kombucha Legend, page 140).

## ~600
According to the Legend of the Sea Treasure (see page 121), kombucha originates around this time.

## BEFORE THE COMMON ERA

## COMMON ERA

## ~6000
Jars in Mesopotamia from this era show signs of having been used for fermenting vegetables, the first record of fermentation.

## ~1300
In the Bible, Boaz encourages Ruth to drink her vinegar beverage (Ruth 2:14).

## 221
Qin Shi Huang, the first Chinese emperor, supposedly drinks kombucha as an elixir for long life (see A Kombucha Legend, page 96).

## ~1200
Genghis Khan's soldiers and Japanese samurai perhaps carry kombucha in flasks (see A Kombucha Legend, pages 174 and 275).

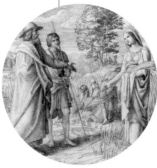

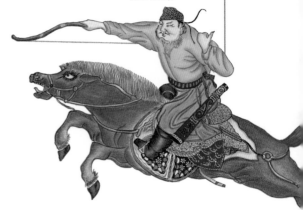

## 1805

Russian intellectual I. Ryadovsky writes about drinking "vinegar" (perhaps kombucha?) and consuming fermented Chinese peas while traveling in Mongolia.

## 1880s

Chinese laborers brought in to build railroads in northern Mexico may have brought SCOBYs with them, marking the first kombucha in the New World. Still called *hongo chino* (Chinese mushroom) or simply *hongo* (mushroom), it is most often cultivated using local herbal tisanes and fermented similar to *tepache* (see "Kompache," page 147).

## 1890s

Dr. Nikolay Vasil'evich Kirilov, Russian ethnographer and student of Tibetan medicine, conducts trials in Siberia that involve the regular consumption of kombucha by elderly people. He notes a reduction of symptoms from arteriosclerosis, benefits to digestion, and assistance in battling gastrointestinal issues.

## 1800s

## 1852

German chemist Robert D. Thomson presents the earliest known scientific paper about fermentation and the production of bacterial cellulose before the Royal Philosophical Society of Glasgow, marking the first experiments and documentation of what would later be named the Acetobacteraceae family.

Though clearly discussing vinegar rather than kombucha, his experiments specifically identify not only the production of the SCOBY-like "vinegar plant," as he called it, and the accompanying sour liquid, but also the creation of carbon dioxide and small amounts of alcohol, based on taste and smell.

## 1886

Adrian J. Brown, fellow of the Royal Society (Great Britain), first isolates and identifies *Bacteria xylinum,* which he uses to produce a new batch of red wine vinegar that grows a culture across its top. One of about 30 cellulose producers in the *Acetobacter* genus, it is eventually renamed *Gluconacetobacter xylinus.*

## 1896

Dr. Rudolf Kobert, professor and respected chair of multiple departments, including pharmacology, at the University of Rostock in Germany, takes special interest in the efficacy of traditional Russian folk remedies. He publishes a 32-page guide, *About Kvass and Its Preparation*, followed in 1913 by *The Kvass: Safe, Inexpensive and Popular National Drink.* These writings may have referred more to traditional Russian kvass made with bread or the "tea kvass" we know as kombucha.

## 1910-1914

Dr. A. A. Bachinskaya, a Russian biologist at the Women's Botanical Laboratory Medical Institute in St. Petersburg, conducts experiments on kombucha cultures collected from all over the country. She publishes four articles featuring the first ever morphology and biology of the culture, which comprises acetic-acid-producing *Bacteria xylinum* and torula yeast, and describing the widespread usage and beneficial results of the beverage where her samples were collected.

Bachinskaya theorizes that as *B. xylinum* was found throughout Europe, Asia, and Africa, it could have been spread by insects to suitable media (such as sweetened tea), where the bacteria colonized with whatever wild yeast were present in the environment.

## 1913

Dr. Gustav Lindau, a German mycologist and botanist deeply involved in the study of lichens, publishes a paper that includes the first widely accepted scientific name for the kombucha culture itself, *Medusomyces gisevii* Lindau. He bases the name on the culture's similarity in appearance to a jellyfish and the incorrect theory that it is a yeast culture only.

Later that year, German researcher Dr. P. Linder refutes Lindau and confirms Bachinskaya by identifying the presence of both yeast and acetic bacteria organisms in kombucha, though he recognizes greater variation in the cultures.

## EARLY 1900s

## 1910s

## 1904-1905

Some sources claim that kombucha is introduced to Russia by soldiers returning home from the Russo-Japanese War, fought over control of Manchuria and Korea. Since the war was fought on Asian soil, the Russian soldiers likely brought the culture back from those places, though they attributed its origin to Japan. Perhaps Japanese prison camps were supplying wounded soldiers with kombucha? Most likely kombucha had already made its way to Russia by this time, and the soldiers merely hastened a spreading phenomenon.

The practice of brewing kombucha is now common enough that images of fermenting jars of tea and SCOBYs slip into the backgrounds of paintings. Many Russians of the time hold a special place in their hearts for the *gribok,* or "little mushroom," that keeps them healthy and strong.

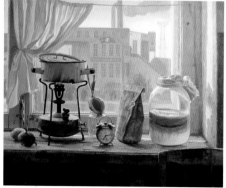

Philip Kubarev,
*Morning*

## 1915

Professor Stephan Bazarewski reports in the *Korrespondenzblatt Naturforscher-Vereins zu Riga* (Correspondence of the Nature Researchers Society in Riga) that a Latvian folk remedy known as *brinum-ssene* (wonder mushroom) is credited with considerable healing capabilities. For the next 40 years, Russian scientists investigate the properties of the culture and its effects on a number of ailments and diseases.

## 1926-1935

More than one hundred research papers, scientific articles, and surveys of medical research, the majority from Germany but also from Russia and other countries, discuss the benefits of kombucha. Collectively, these papers recommend it for the treatment or alleviation of conditions such as constipation, arteriosclerosis, high blood pressure, anxiety, irritability, pain, headaches, vertigo, gout, angina, diabetes, hemorrhoids, dysentery, dyspepsia, typhus, tonsillitis, stomatitis, poor digestion, and even aging. (For more detail, see German and Russian Research, 1920s to 1960s, page 342.)

## 1927

Dr. H. Waldeck publishes a firsthand account of his introduction to kombucha in 1915 Russia by a chemist who helped cure Waldeck's constipation by brewing up a batch. The chemist proudly stated that this sour "wonderdrink" was good for antiaging as well as combating "all kinds of ailments." He claimed that it was the Russian secret weapon for healing injured soldiers during World War I.

Waldeck, who served in Russia during the war, returned home to Germany with his own *wunderpilz* ("wondrous mushroom") and began brewing and testing, specifically targeting kombucha's interaction with the digestive system.

## 1920s

## 1916

Polish chemist Josef Bolshich proves that kombucha cultures and kefir grains are different, each with its own structure, morphology, and inherent healing properties.

## 1917

Dr. Rudolf Kobert releases his findings in the scientific journal *Mikrokosmos*, reporting that kombucha is helpful for intestinal disorders, hemorrhoids, and joint rheumatism.

In a later volume of *Mikrokosmos*, Dr. P. Linder echoes Kobert's findings, especially in regard to kombucha's relief of intestinal issues and hemorrhoids.

## 1928

Dr. W. Wiechowski, a board member of the Institute of Pharmacology and Pharmacognosy Institute at the German University of Prague, publishes a paper titled "What Position Should a Doctor Take on the Kombucha Question?"

He not only recommends kombucha for severe angina, mild constipation, and even diabetes, but he also offers perhaps the most levelheaded and robust defense of kombucha's role in health to date:

"Because kombucha contains completely harmless elements, there is no reason to warn against its use, which is primarily for diet, not therapy. The fact that often distressing symptoms could be eliminated by the regular use of kombucha justifies making it available to as many people as possible whether science can explain it or not."

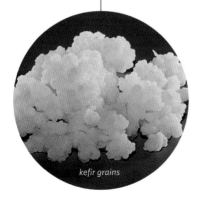

*kefir grains*

## 1931

Dr. D. Scherbachov rekindles Russian interest in kombucha with an article in *Soviet Pharmacy* recounting international research that shows it to be helpful in reducing blood pressure and inhibiting atherosclerosis. (For more detail, see German and Russian Research, 1920s to 1960s, page 342.)

## 1940s

Dr. Rudolf Sklenar, a German stationed in Russia during World War II, works with local farmers who introduce him to their "miracle tea," which he brings home and uses for over 40 years to treat patients, including many with cancer.

## 1950s

Italians have a brief, torrid romance with kombucha, which may have been brought back by soldiers after World War II. The elixir is revered for its "magical" powers. A new tradition evolves: SCOBYs can be passed to friends only on Tuesdays; if done successfully, the reward is three wishes granted by St. Antonio.

The tea is featured on magazine covers and in articles throughout Italy and memorialized in Sicilian pop-star Renato Carosone's hit "Stu fungo cinese," about this strange "Chinese fungus."

## 1953-1957

Studies detail kombucha's effectiveness in healing wounds and relieving symptoms of intestinal diseases and typhus. Russian studies show relief in cases of atherosclerosis, high blood pressure, acute tonsillitis, severe stomatitis (mouth sores or inflammation), and dysentery, among other ailments.

---

**1930s**   **1940s**   **1950s**

---

## 1938

Published studies establish kombucha's therapeutic effect on digestion-related issues as well as dysentery and dyspepsia. These writings also affirm the safety of kombucha for children.

## 1942-1959

More advanced methods for investigating kombucha are developed (see following entries) and a great deal of research, primarily conducted in Russia, centers on kombucha's antimicrobial properties and its efficacy in treating or alleviating a number of conditions, including intestinal disorders, inflammation, and infections.

## 1950

Three doctors at a hospital in Omsk develop an outpatient observation program with local residents who drink the popular homebrew. Results indicate that those who begin consuming kombucha regularly subsequently find relief from a variety of ailments, including acute inflammation, angina, and digestive problems.

## 1951

Joseph Stalin orders an investigation into kombucha's potential anti-cancer properties (see Stalin Seeks Cure for Cancer, page 344).

## 1959

Studies confirm kombucha's beneficial effects on dysentery in infants. Other studies show that adding SCOBYs to chicken feed increases growth 15 percent.

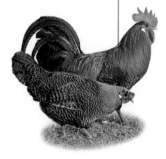

## 1960s

San Francisco's hippie counterculture is rumored to have been home to an early kombucha revival in this decade.

## 1970s

Chinese scientific papers describe the SCOBY's cellulose structure and identify the components of the ferment.

## 1980s

Ronald Reagan is rumored to have heard of Aleksandr Solzhenitsyn's supposed experience with kombucha during the author's long imprisonment in labor camps. The story was that Solzhenitsyn combated cancer by drinking kombucha, but in his novel *The Cancer Ward*, he refers to "birch tree cancer" or "birch tree fungus," a name for the *chaga* (*Inonotus obliquus*). *Chaga,* which was proven to be an efficacious adaptogen by Soviet scientists in the 1950s, is in fact a mushroom and not at all related to kombucha.

Nonetheless, Reagan's aides reportedly acquired a culture for the president when he developed cancer, and he supposedly consumed as much as a liter of kombucha a day until his death many years later — a "true kombucha story," among many others, that is still active online.

**1960s**   **1970s**   **1980s**

## 1960

The Cold War brings research on kombucha to a halt in Russia and Eastern Europe.

## 1964

Dr. Rudolf Sklenar of Germany publishes his findings on the use of kombucha to treat cancer patients.

## 1983

Noted American food scientist Keith Steinkraus, who studies the chemical and nutritional changes that occur during microbial fermentation, lists kombucha in his comprehensive tome *Handbook of Indigenous Fermented Foods*.

## 1985

Dr. Rudolf Sklenar, in collaboration with his niece, Rosina Fasching, publishes *Tea Fungus Kombucha, The Natural Remedy and Its Significance in Cases of Cancer and Other Metabolic Diseases*. The slim volume includes his treatment protocol as well as many testimonials from patients with a variety of ailments.

## 1987

Dr. Veronica Carstens, former First Lady of Germany, publishes a magazine article "Help from Nature — My Remedies against Cancer" that specifically mentions her use of kombucha in treatment protocols as it "detoxifies," "enhances metabolism," and "improves immunity."

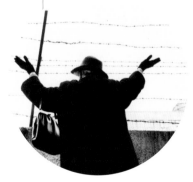

## 1991

Günther Frank, a passionate and experienced German homebrewer and contributor to the original kombucha listserv (see page 351), publishes *Kombucha: Healthy Beverage and Natural Remedy from the Far East*. The book, which highlights the research published since the late nineteenth century, particularly in Germany, Russia, and Eastern Europe, becomes a highly respected resource.

## 1996

Len Porzio names the SCOBY — the symbiotic culture of bacteria and yeast — to differentiate the culture from the tea. (For more on Len Porzio, see page 353.)

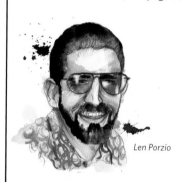

*Len Porzio*

## 1990s

## 1993

Betsy Pryor receives a kombucha culture from a nun at a Los Angeles meditation center. She starts selling cultures from her business, Laurel Farms, and two years later publishes her book *Kombucha Phenomenon*.

## 1995

- Two women in Iowa who happened to be brewing kombucha at home fall ill and one passes away. A myth that blames the kombucha takes hold and still persists on the Internet. (See The Kombucha Bogeymen, page 25.)
- Michael Roussin publishes the results of lab analysis of the components of kombucha, based on more than 1,100 samples from around the country.
- GT Dave begins brewing kombucha in his mother's kitchen, launching the brand that would build the modern commercial kombucha empire. (For more on GT Dave, see page 354.)

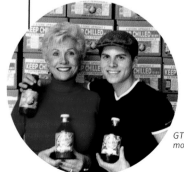

*GT Dave and his mother, Laraine*

## 2000-PRESENT

Academic interest in researching kombucha's properties picks up with a study by Cornell University. Researchers around the world, from the United States to Serbia to India, take up the cause (see The Modern Research Movement, page 344).

## 2010

The commercial kombucha industry experiences a temporary setback when bottles are pulled from shelves due to concerns about alcohol levels (see page 349).

## 2000-PRESENT

### 2001

Kombucha Wonder Drink is founded, followed by High Country Kombucha in 2003. The first two nationally available bottled brands after GT, they mark the beginning of kombucha's expansion from a single offering to a category with hundreds of brands.

### 2003

Fermentation revivalist Sandor Katz includes kombucha in his seminal work *Wild Fermentation.*

### 2004

Hannah Crum creates Kombucha Kamp as a home-based brewing class, then establishes the Kombucha Kamp website in 2007.

### 2011

The modern kombucha boom begins as the number of commercial brands explodes from a few dozen to hundreds, with more coming on board every month.

### 2014

Hannah Crum and Alex LaGory found Kombucha Brewers International (see page 354).

### 2015

The commercial kombucha industry in the United States generates between $500 and $600 million in sales.

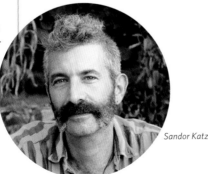

*Sandor Katz*

# GERMAN AND RUSSIAN RESEARCH, 1920s TO 1960s

Some highlights of the following discussion are included on The Kombucha Timeline, page 334.

## German Research Boom

A decade of significant German research focused on the benefits of kombucha, beginning in 1926 with Dr. Wilhelm Henneberg's substantial tome *Handbook of Fermentation Bacteriology (Mycology Specialty, with Special Reference to Yeast, Acetic and Lactic Acid Bacteria)*. Henneberg's work was notable because he had written about vinegar-making bacteria in a 1907 article for the *Central Journal of Bacteriology* without mentioning kombucha. In his later work, he discusses "Teakwass" as a widespread Russian remedy "against all sorts of diseases, especially against constipation." This type of finding was reinforced and built upon by many others.

In 1927, Dr. Gerhard Madaus wrote in his magazine *Art of Healing* (issued as a three-volume text *Biologische Heilkunst* [Biological Healing Arts] in 1938) that kombucha helps cell walls regenerate and therefore may help with arteriosclerosis. In the same year, E. Dinslage and W. Ludorff published a review of the existing science and research called "Der indisch Teepilz" (Indian Tea Mushroom) for the highly regarded *Journal of Food Research*.

Prof. Dr. N. Lakowitz published "Tea Mushroom and Tea Kvass" in 1928, suggesting that the "tea fungus be broadly spread to make tea kvass as a remedy for indigestion and all sorts of age-related complaints in all sectors of the population, as well as be grown and dispensed through pharmacies and drug stores."

Dr. Maxim Bing published three brief articles between 1928 and 1929 that identified kombucha as a "very effective means to combat arteriosclerosis" as well as high blood pressure, anxiety, irritability, pain, headaches, vertigo, constipation, and improving the elasticity of brain capillaries.

Dr. L. Mollenda, in an article titled "Kombucha, Its Medical Importance and Breeding" written for *Deutsche Essiginindustrie* (German Vinegar Industry) (1927/28), echoed the digestion, gout, and arteriosclerosis recommendations of others while also specifying his successful use of kombucha, via gargling and consumption, against angina.

Dr. E. Arauner, in an article ("Der japanische Teepilz," 1929) for the same publication, reports that kombucha is an excellent treatment for conditions such as diabetes, anxiety, arteriosclerosis, hemorrhoids, and more, noting that the "mushroom" had been in use for centuries by Asian people.

## An Era of Russian Research

In 1915, following on the heels of the Latvian connection of 1913 made by Germans Lindau and Linder (see page 336), Prof. Stephan Bazarewski wrote in the *Korrespondenzblatt Naturforscher-Vereins zu Riga* (Correspondence of the Nature Researchers Society in Riga) that a Latvian folk remedy known as "wonder mushroom" was credited with considerable healing capabilities for residents of the Livland and Kurland provinces, where it was consumed regularly.

Dr. D. Scherbachov re-sparked Russian interest in kombucha with his 1931 article in a soviet pharmacy journal that recounted international research showing kombucha to be helpful with reducing blood pressure and inhibiting atherosclerosis. In 1938, writings by T. E. Boldyrev established kombucha's therapeutic effect for digestion-related issues as well as dysentery and dyspepsia. His work also affirmed the safety of kombucha for children. Scientists initiated the idea that kombucha could be used to produce gluconic acid specifically for refinement or sale as a therapy.

Researcher K. Doubrovsky led a lengthy, in-depth period of study from 1942 to 1955, attempting to understand the effects of the tea and the culture on acute and chronic diseases. Working from the Kazakh Institute of Epidemiology and Microbiology, Doubrovsky created an extract of the mushroom and tea, called meduzomintin (or "MM" — later known as meduzin), that had highly effective antimicrobial and therapeutic properties. MM demonstrated a bactericidal effect toward *Staphylococcus aureus*, dysentery, typhoid, pneumococcus, and diphtheria bacilli.

Tests on MM conducted over many years with the cooperation of L. T. Danielian of the Yerevan Veterinary Institute and many specialists from the Yerevan's Children's Hospital provided a base of knowledge for many researchers all over the world. By 1949, E. K. Naumov was testing the new concentrate on a variety of animals infected with these diseases and finding positive results in almost all cases. In 1950, Danielian conducted more advanced testing to identify the active ingredients.

In 1950, after receiving numerous inquiries about the efficacy of this popular homebrew, three doctors at Omsk Hospital, V. S. Tinditnik, S. E. Funk, and E. Sabine, engineered an outpatient observation program of the effects of the tea on all kinds of acute inflammation, angina, digestive problems, and more. The results of the study, published in local newspapers such as *Omsk Pravda*, prompted a deluge of mail from all over the country that reaffirmed the researchers' results.

These letters emboldened more doctors to join the research. Additional studies were published in 1953 by A. Matinjan and G. Markarjan regarding kombucha's effectiveness when used with infectious and open-wound healing. The following year, studies released by A. Nurazjan and E. Porichij confirmed kombucha's assistance with intestinal diseases and typhus.

Between 1953 and 1957, G. F. Barbanchik and research partners conducted clinical studies on 52 human patients that confirmed that consuming kombucha reduced atherosclerosis and high blood pressure. They simultaneously tested and treated 75 patients with acute tonsillitis and found more rapid recovery, localized pain relief, and reduced fevers, indicating antibacterial activity toward pathogenic actors.

A study conducted by E. S. Zlatopolskaya and partners at the Second Medical Institute of Moscow in 1955 demonstrated relief from severe stomatitis (mouth sores or inflammation) in 20 two-year-old children treated with meduzin. Another study by the same team showed relief in 17 cases of dysentery as well.

N. M. Ovichinnikov showed in 1956 that animals with tuberculosis benefited from consuming the tea, resulting in inhibition and sometimes elimination of the condition. In 1957, additional studies and presentations poured in: T. Adzjan demonstrated effectiveness against toxic dyspepsia; G. Sakaran published about kombucha working against paratyphus and brucellosis; A. Mihajlova studied pediatric dysentery; and N. Joirisi affirms the effects on cholesterol and high blood pressure.

In 1958, G. F. Barbancik, who first authored a pamphlet-style publication in 1954 recounting research already done on kombucha, reported on his own studies on the significant antimicrobial effects of the tea. I. N. Konovalow confirmed that research just a year later, and more extensive studies by Danielian and associates confirmed kombucha's assistance with dysentery in infants. The Cold War is said to be to blame for the lack of research available after 1960, though whether that was due to lack of funding, a decline in interest, or both, is unclear.

# The Modern Research Movement

After decades of relative absence from the world research stage, the modern kombucha movement has sparked a major uptick in scientific interest in both the tea and the SCOBY. Scientists at universities all over the world have been conducting studies with animal and human subjects for almost two decades, with significant investigations made to determine the mechanisms of kombucha's efficacy. In 2000, Cornell University became the first major U.S. university to publish a study about kombucha, highlighting its antimicrobial benefits and citing Michael Roussin's 1995 study (see page 352) among others as source material.

The body of research conducted since 2000 has proven many long-held beliefs about kombucha to be true. In general, kombucha's fermentation process enhances the benefits of tea — vitamins, polyphenols, catechins, and so on — and reduces those less healthful constituents that the bacteria and yeast use for energy, namely sugar and caffeine.

Perhaps the most important research development is proving the existence of

## STALIN SEEKS CURE FOR CANCER

Like other leaders throughout history, Joseph Stalin used every resource at his disposal to seek the secrets to long life. When the scourge of cancer began spreading across Russia, the deeply paranoid dictator sent teams of doctors in search of causes or, better yet, cures. Moving methodically from city to city, the doctors carefully recorded cancer rates, household habits, and environmental factors.

Two districts emerged as nearly cancer-free despite their comparatively toxic environmental conditions; residents also reported fewer missed workdays, less public drunkenness, and better overall health. Further interviews revealed that most households brewed kombucha tea and residents attributed their health to its consumption.

This data inspired research with the aim of developing a pharmaceutical formula. Conducted at both the Moscow Central Bacteriological Institute and the Biological-Biochemical Central Institute, led by Stalin's personal physician, Dr. Vladimir Vinogradov, and Lavrentiy Beria, minister of internal affairs and chief of the secret service (KGB), along with a board of doctors and KGB agents. The goal was to develop a pharmaceutical formula. These scientists were the first to discover that the SCOBY was a symbiosis of various bacteria and yeast species.

A convinced Stalin began drinking the tea on his doctor's advice, but, sensing an opportunity to grab power, two KGB agents on the research board convinced him that Beria and Vinogradov were actually attempting to poison him. Stalin, already suspicious of Beria, imprisoned Vinogradov and his team of Jewish doctors, coercing confessions via torture. After Stalin's death in 1953 the doctors were exonerated and released, and the agents were sentenced to death for their role in the plot, but research on kombucha in Russia was effectively ended until the 1980s.

glucuronic acid in kombucha. While some studies, including Roussin's, initially disputed its presence, greatly improved testing methods have led to study after study showing that it is present in appreciable amounts. Research is building the case for this versatile acid (see page 361) being responsible for many of kombucha's purported detoxifying and system-rebuilding effects. Other major clusters of studies center on the antimicrobial and anticancer potential of the SCOBY and kombucha tea; both seem to be natural toxin sponges that help organisms either excrete toxins after exposure or avoid absorbing the toxins in the first place.

## International Collaboration

A couple of researchers in particular have conducted repeated studies on the components of kombucha. Since 2001 Radomir V. Malbaša of Serbia has conducted well over a dozen experiments on SCOBYs and kombucha using a variety of substrates, testing for different antioxidant levels and examining which variations yield the greatest nutrient density.

Since 2007 Rasu Jayabalan of India has conducted at least seven studies that focus on not only the potential curative and anticancer properties of kombucha but also the basic biochemical characteristics of kombucha's specific fermentation process, including the improvement of free-radical scavenging.

In 2014, these prolific researchers collaborated with a team of other investigators to release a review of the current literature of Kombucha studies. (For more on modern research, see appendixes 1 and 2.)

*WORD NERD:* **Is This How Kombucha Got Its Name?**

*In Japan, kombucha tea is called kōcha kinoko, or "red tea mushroom." However, the Japanese also make a beverage of brown seaweed steeped in hot water, kombucha, which translates as "seaweed tea." Coincidence? In fact, the natural brown yeast strands that form in our kombucha tea look very much like brown seaweed. Our theory is that the origin of kombucha's name may perhaps have been as simple as confusion based on the look of that yeast!*

## Going Forward

Because kombucha cannot be patented and monetized as a drug, most of these studies involve animal subjects and many are conducted at universities outside the United States. However, newer studies have involved human subjects and many more are using human cells, especially cancer cells, and the work is promising.

Multimillion-dollar, double-blind trials like those used for pharmaceuticals may not be likely anytime soon, but some U.S. universities are launching fermentation courses and even offering degree programs that will open the door to much wider research into how fermented foods work with our bodies. As science continues to catch up with thousands of years of "gut instinct" and tradition, perhaps fermented foods will finally recover from the challenges of pasteurization and germ theory to regain their rightful place as the incredibly important nutritional tools they have always been.

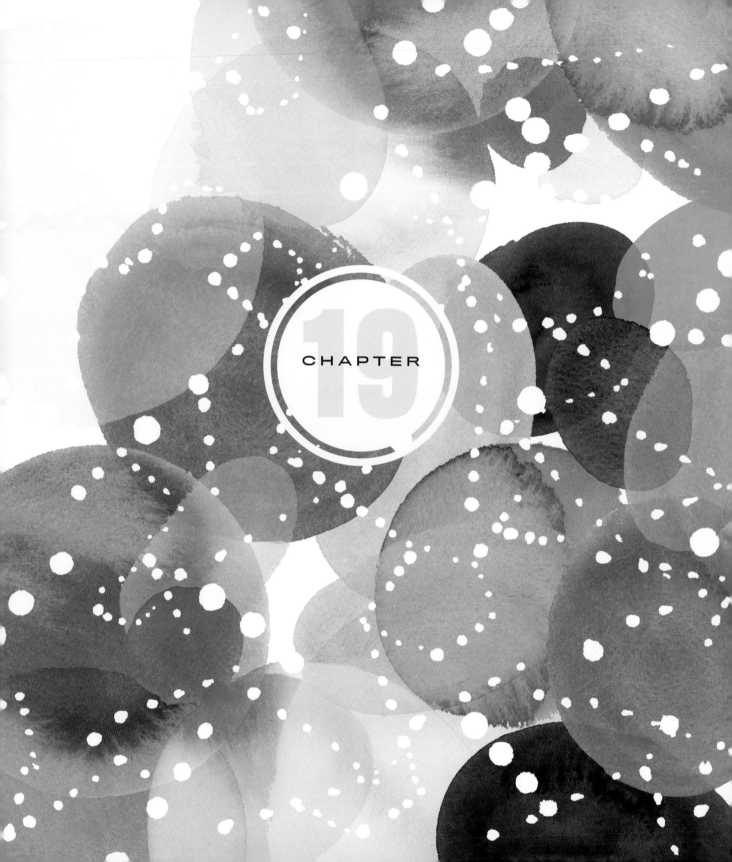

CHAPTER

19

# Taking It out of the Kitchen

Something magical often happens when kombucha comes into people's lives. That moment of Kombucha Kismet is often a bright dividing line between a life ruled by inertia and a path of conscious choice. Once compelled to make their own, many homebrewers find themselves supplying kombucha for friends, neighbors, loved ones, and even sometimes annoying coworkers, because they just won't stop drinking it and keep asking for more!

Requests start pouring in (no pun intended), and sometimes a love of brewing suddenly becomes a labor of love (emphasis on the labor!) as the dedicated homebrewer scales up to a commercial operation. This is how nearly every single kombucha brewery started, even GT's Kombucha, the founder of the modern industry (see page 354). A powerful pull is exerted when you create food that nourishes your community and people express their gratitude for that nutrition. That satisfaction has led directly to the establishment of many a profitable, thriving kombucha business.

The story of how kombucha has emerged from folk remedy to commercial sensation is also the story of the needs of a generation. In this increasingly toxic world, kombucha can help us "clean the filter," so to speak, so that our engines can run smoothly and we can continue to contribute to our local and global communities.

In this new century, traditional career paths no longer exist for many people, and for some, the only way to find a job you love is to create it yourself. If you have been bitten by the kombucha brewing bug, who knows, maybe you could be the local kombucha brewer for your community!

As rewarding as it can be, however, every opportunity comes with challenges. The main concern for commercial brewers involves either maintaining accurate testing to comply with artificially low alcohol percentage requirements, or becoming certified to sell kombucha as an over-21 beverage, which brings its own set of challenges in terms of product placement, distribution, and taxes.

## Is Kombucha a Soft Drink?

One barrier to full acceptance of kombucha in American culture has to do with the fact that it contains a negligible amount of alcohol. The current legal definition of an alcoholic beverage in the United States is one that contains 0.5 percent alcohol by volume (ABV) or more. This limit was defined by the Volstead Act, which established Prohibition in 1919. Even though Prohibition was repealed more than 80 years ago, that limit remains, without any consideration of what it actually means.

"Soft" drinks by definition contain less alcohol than "hard" drinks, but how much exactly? For many thousands of years humans consumed all manner of alcoholic beverages regardless of their age. Into the early twentieth century children were served diluted wine and naturally fermented ginger "ales" and root "beers," as well as small beers containing 2% ABV or less.

Because a small amount of alcohol is a by-product of the fermentation process, kombucha naturally contains 0.2 to 1.0 percent, potentially above the legal limit, which presents an unfortunate challenge for commercially produced living health beverages.

Coupled with testing methods not sophisticated enough to handle such low levels of alcohol without complicated and expensive machinery and education, this creates problems for commercial brewers — namely, they have to choose whether to file for a beer brewing license (or wine, depending on the state) or whether to implement measures to reduce the potential alcohol content of their product, often living in constant fear of being over the limit.

A few select brands, including GT's, offer an over-21 version of their product as well as a less-alcoholic one. Understandable consumer confusion about the differences between these two offerings is compounded by the fact that in some states they have to be sold in completely different sections of the store or even in different stores!

Confounding the issue is the fact that other products on shelves today, including sodas, juices, coconut waters, and energy drinks, can contain more than the legally prescribed limit of alcohol. Since these drinks are not perceived to be alcoholic, those trace amounts have been largely ignored. In fact, all raw juice and fermented beverages contain trace amounts of alcohol ranging from 0.3 to 2% ABV, depending on of the type of beverage and fermentation process. The noninebriating nature of kombucha and the number of other beverages that might slip above the allowed limit without penalty indicate that when we take a component such as a nutrient, toxin, or even alcohol, out of context, our entire perception may end up skewed.

# The Kombucha Crisis of 2010

In 2010 Whole Foods, the top purveyor of kombucha, asked kombucha companies to voluntarily remove their product from shelves due to a labeling discrepancy. The situation began with letters from a couple of state inspectors in different locations. Each had independently become concerned about kombucha products they had seen stored on shelves without refrigeration. When tested with the best machines available at the time, these samples were over the 0.5% ABV legal limit for nonalcoholic beverages, which put legal pressure on the retailer to act. Without an industry association to represent their needs, the companies were left to figure it out for themselves. The ordeal was expensive and scary for most brands, though eventually almost all came back stronger.

To get their products back in its stores, Whole Foods required companies to buy back stock and either reformulate their kombucha or update their labels to sell as an over-21 beverage. The ensuing few months were market anarchy as the scramble for suddenly available shelf space began in earnest.

Reformulation meant changing the fermentation process or removing elements of the brew to artificially lower the alcohol content. Most brands eventually put a compliant product back on the shelf as an under-21 beverage, while some sought beer or wine licenses to make a "traditional brew." Others, like GT's, decided to produce both over- and under-21 products.

What the withdrawal highlighted most clearly is our country's hangups (and hangover) regarding alcohol, many of them left over from Prohibition. Although several brands now offer an over-21 "alcoholic" kombucha, it is misleading to think of kombucha as being in the same class as beer or wine. As we've established, having low levels of alcohol in the diet is actually healthy (see page 15). Naturally fermented soft drinks are not inebriating, and the trace amounts of alcohol they contain contribute to feelings of well-being and decrease stress. Studies have linked moderate alcohol consumption to a decreased risk of heart disease, stroke, diabetes, gallstones, dementia, and even the common cold.

The main problem with the current legal definition for nonalcoholic beverages (0.5% ABV) is that this arbitrary number, not based on any scientific study and not in line with human experience, has inadvertently ensnared an entire category of healthy, nutritious beverages — traditional low-alcohol ferments — in a tangle of unintended consequences. Does anyone believe they can get drunk by downing a six-pack of kombucha? Good luck, you'll be in the bathroom before any buzz hits.

Is society served by preventing a 15-year-old from purchasing a naturally fermented health beverage with noninebriating levels of alcohol? Obviously not. And even more problematic, we have a policy not to tax healthy foods in this country, so why should a health beverage ever be taxed? If it's an "over-21" kombucha, it will be.

Any kombucha manufacturer could easily comply with a 1 percent alcohol limit without having to drastically change its brewing process or compromising the final product. Since the formation of Kombucha Brewers International (see page 354), new testing methodologies are demonstrating that kombucha may have been the victim of unsophisticated protocols that did not take into account the symbiotic fermentation process or healthy acids that look similar to alcohol unless subjected to more rigorous testing.

In hindsight, it is possible that the withdrawal was an overreaction founded on inappropriate testing methods. Still, while there was no safety threat posed to kombucha consumers, Whole Foods acted as responsibly as they could with the information available. And until the law changes or kombucha receives an exemption, commercial producers in the United States must meet compliance laws, although doing so may require altering the final product and adhering to strict handling standards. Even so, commercial kombucha is still a superior beverage choice for those who don't brew their own or, as we like to enjoy it, while traveling.

# National, Regional, Local, and Micro Brands

The kombucha industry is made up of brands that vary widely according to their own particular goals. Some kombucha companies want to sell their product everywhere in the United States. Other companies prefer a regional approach that allows them to remain sustainable and grow at a slow, steady pace. Some of the companies in this category are able to reduce the environmental footprint of their brand with regional programs such as buying back bottles or selling their product only in kegs.

Local brands can be found at farmers' markets, sold by passionate people who are connecting to their local community through food. As the fermentation reevolution continues to expand, more people are waking up to the benefits of reclaiming more natural and healthier foods, creating opportunities to start small-scale local companies to meet the increasing demand. Consumers get healthier options and fermenters boost the health of their communities.

## Starting Your Own Brand

As a fast-growing industry with relatively low barriers to entry, kombucha is an attractive small business opportunity that appeals to many entrepreneurs with an interest in health and food. Nearly every kombucha company in business today started out in a private kitchen, so for those who enjoy hard work, serving their community, and hard work (did we say that already?), kombucha may be an opportunity.

It's one thing to brew small batches for yourself or family, but when it comes to scaling up, learning to do it correctly and safely without appropriate resources can be a challenge. Sanitation, testing standards, and best practices are critical to a successful kombucha venture. A good way to start learning is to join Kombucha Brewers International, an organization dedicated to promoting the commercial kombucha industry worldwide.

# Modern Kombucha Pioneers

As interest in kombucha continues to grow and the community of brewers expands, we acknowledge those who introduced this ancient elixir into the lives of so many who needed a healthful, homemade option for themselves and their families. They have been the original inspiration for our mission as Kombucha Kamp, for they have truly changed the world one gut at a time.

## Colleen Allen and the Original Kombucha List

In the early 1990s, when the Internet was just born, many people joined listservs, where questions could be posed and conversations conducted with others who subscribed to the list. It was through these listservs that many people exchanged information and first learned about how to brew kombucha safely. Colleen Allen founded the Original Kombucha (OK) listserv in February 1995. So it's thanks to her and those who participated on the listserv that kombucha gained a certain level of fame in the nineties.

## HOW TO START A KOMBUCHA BUSINESS IN 10 STEPS

1. Practice brewing recipes and techniques at home in small batches.
2. Share kombucha with friends and note their feedback to refine your recipes.
3. Scale up your kombucha production to develop a feel for how the culture, brewing time, and flavor change with larger batches.
4. Track pH, sugar levels, and brewing conditions as you work to create a consistent product batch after batch.
5. Look for commercial brewing space or shared commercial kitchen space.
6. Source bottles and ingredients in bulk, design labels, and develop and finalize flavors.
7. Sell at farmers' markets, CSAs, and other small outlets to grow initial interest in your brand.
8. Apply for business licenses and permits.
9. Join trade associations and business leagues to network with others in the industry.
10. Sell kombucha to local markets, yoga studios, and food trucks as a way to finding larger outlets.

Although she suffered from physical ailments, Colleen never let them suppress her spirit and quest for true knowledge, which endeared her to those active in that community. Before her death in 2000, she compiled a lot of information about kombucha into a website, the Kombucha Center, based on questions and responses generated by the OK list.

## Michael Roussin

As a youth soccer referee, Michael Roussin spent a lot of time running, so when sore and stiff knees started slowing him down, his sister-in-law passed him a SCOBY (Kombucha Kismet!) and told him to get brewing. Michael credited the booch with gradually eliminating pain, restoring flexibility, and lowering his blood pressure.

Wanting to learn more, he read everything he could find about kombucha, which wasn't much at that point. In 1995 Michael sent a few samples of kombucha, with a list of what he was looking for, to a lab to be analyzed. Eighteen months and over 1,100 samples of kombucha later, he had accumulated more than 14 boxes of documents, subsequently published for sale as the stand-alone study *Analyses of Kombucha Ferments,* which he believed to be the most comprehensive study to that date.

These findings were a huge boon at the time and inspired many modern researchers, although some of the initial conclusions have been disproven based on research completed since. Most notably, Michael concluded that kombucha did not contain glucuronic acid. It turned out that the lab he used did not have the ability to properly test for glucuronic acid, which explains why many studies have since confirmed its presence (see appendix 2).

However, Michael and his researchers were able to identify a parallel explanation for kombucha's detoxifying properties involving glucuronic acid. Study samples consistently showed the presence of a powerful enzyme

## KOMBUCHA BEER

When forced to either restrict themselves to the over-21 market or reformulate their product, some companies chose to get a beer-brewing license. In addition to their regular kombucha tea offerings, Unity Vibration Living Tea in Michigan has won accolades for their line of kombucha/beer hybrids (see more about making kombucha beer and wine on page 152).

Many craft beer breweries have experimented with small batches of kombucha beer — a blend of kombucha fermentation technology with different strains of higher-alcohol yeasts, hops, and other elements — while others offer kombucha as a mainstay alongside their standard brews. Kombucha taprooms, opened by brands at their facilities or by independent entrepreneurs, are growing in popularity, and most also feature low-alcohol brews that people of any age can enjoy, so look around your community for a taproom to visit!

inhibitor, D-saccharic acid-1,4-lactone (DSL) that assists the body in releasing toxins (see page 363).

For Michael, the presence of DSL explained increased levels of glucuronic acid found in the urine of people who drank kombucha. Though researchers before and after Michael have repeatedly proven that glucuronic acid is present in kombucha, his incomplete theory is sometimes quoted as fact. The good news for kombucha drinkers is that both are true: glucuronic acid is present in kombucha, and DSL acts as a glucuronidase inhibitor to help the body expel more toxins.

## Len Porzio

Len Porzio first heard about kombucha from a friend in the mid-1990s. A slender long-distance runner, Len was not feeling well and had inexplicably lost 20 pounds. Shortly after, he found a vendor at a farmers' market selling kombucha cultures. Since his health issues had stumped his doctor, he decided to give brewing a try. About a week after he started drinking kombucha, Len's symptoms began to recede, and after three months, he felt cured of what he later figured to be an overgrowth of *Candida* in his system. Over the years, as he and his wife have kept up their kombucha regimen, he claims his seasonal allergies and his wife's gallstone symptoms (for which she refused surgery) have decreased.

Len also coined the term SCOBY. The OK listserv was having some difficulty distinguishing between kombucha tea and kombucha culture in discussions. Len says that he "suggested to the group that [they] come up with some kind of acronym like SCOBY

(symbiotic culture of bacteria and yeast)." He expected someone else would come up with a better name, "but it stuck."

As the listserv group grew, Len found himself answering the same questions over and over. At the suggestion of the listserv administrator, he designed an answer sheet that has morphed into his internationally read "Balance Your Brew" Web page. With his passion for kombucha, his contributions to the kombucha lexicon, and the body of knowledge he makes available to all, Len Porzio is truly a kombucha legend.

## Betsy Pryor

An outspoken advocate, author, and kombucha lover, Betsy first encountered kombucha while visiting a meditation and spiritual center in Hollywood. After spending time in Liberia reporting on the emerging AIDS epidemic, she felt compelled to help people with their health in some way. Though she was skeptical about the brew at first, kombucha became the answer to her prayers, as she eventually fell in

**KOMBUCHA MAMMA SEZ**

### Kismet in Action

"When Betsy Pryor first began handing out cultures to friends in her neighborhood in Los Angeles, one was given to David Otto, owner of Beverly Hills Juice. Soon after, he passed one on to his friend, who just happened to be the father of GT Dave. Such is the way of Kombucha Kismet!"

love with the process and how it made her feel. Later she shipped cultures all over the country (from Laurel Farms) and cowrote a book, *Kombucha Phenomenon*. Her appearance on *The Today Show* in 1995 helped spread the word about kombucha.

## Laraine and GT Dave of GT's Kombucha

GT Dave was a teenager when his folks first started brewing kombucha in the mid-1990s. The Daves were vegetarians and always enjoyed a health-conscious, spiritual lifestyle. While GT drank kombucha from time to time, he didn't really care for the vinegary flavor and left it for his folks. His mother, Laraine, loved kombucha but became truly inspired by it during a bout with a rare and aggressive form of cancer. Given a year to live, she credits her kombucha consumption with helping her survive surgery and chemotherapy with reduced nausea and quicker recovery. She has been cancer-free ever since.

After his mother's health crisis, GT was inspired to help others by brewing kombucha commercially. A high-school dropout who had fallen in with the wrong crowd, he found in kombucha a creative outlet and a business challenge. In order to give the appearance of having a larger company, GT would play various roles on the telephone, acting as sales rep, business owner, and account manager. He sold his first case of brew to the local health food store, Erewhon. That case turned into 10 cases, and eventually into an entire business.

Within 10 years, the brand was nationally distributed and had two competitors, High Country Kombucha, founded by Ed Rothbauer and Steve Dickman in Eagle, Colorado, and Kombucha Wonder Drink, founded by Steve Lee (a veteran of both Stash and Tazo tea companies). Both brands persist today, among hundreds of companies nationwide.

In a scant 20 years, GT helped elevate a traditional folk remedy into a health phenomenon, while putting kombucha on the commercial beverage map. He has inspired countless homebrewers to start companies and maintains fierce consumer loyalty with a commitment to consistency (he still tastes every batch, which means he drinks quite a lot of kombucha!). Laraine, who tirelessly helped grow the business by giving demos and passing out cultures, continues to offer inspiration and vital support to GT's Kombucha.

## Kombucha Brewers International (KBI)

Following the 2010 kombucha withdrawal and subsequent boom of new companies, an already chaotic industry began growing more quickly than anyone had anticipated as small brands popped up in every corner, while local and regional brands, emboldened by the loyalty of their consumers and ever increasing demand, expanded their reach.

Of course, every industry is made up of competing companies who very often work together to solve common problems, but for an immature industry that had just been badly shaken up, that kind of trust was in short supply. Fearing a repeat of the alcohol-level problem, most commercial brewers avoided communicating with anyone, let alone their competitors, about the challenges of making a delicious yet compliant beverage.

After years of working with a variety of companies as consultants or on marketing and awareness campaigns for kombucha, and even putting a boutique brand on shelves in Los Angeles (Hannah's Homebrew, 2010–2013), we ended up in the unique position of being personally friendly with a large portion of the industry and intimately understanding their problems. When discussions of a trade association would come up, we were repeatedly nominated to get it up and running.

It took a couple of years of prodding, but we accepted the challenge, and in 2014, with the participation of more than 40 companies from around the world, we founded Kombucha Brewers International, a trade association dedicated to promoting and protecting the kombucha industry through education, best practices recommendations, and marketing initiatives.

The future of the commercial bottling industry is very bright, as more and more consumers search for alternatives to sodas and juices. Any growing industry faces emerging issues, but kombucha companies have made the smart move emulating their mother culture to work in symbiosis to create standards, offer member training, and educate consumers, retailers, and wholesalers.

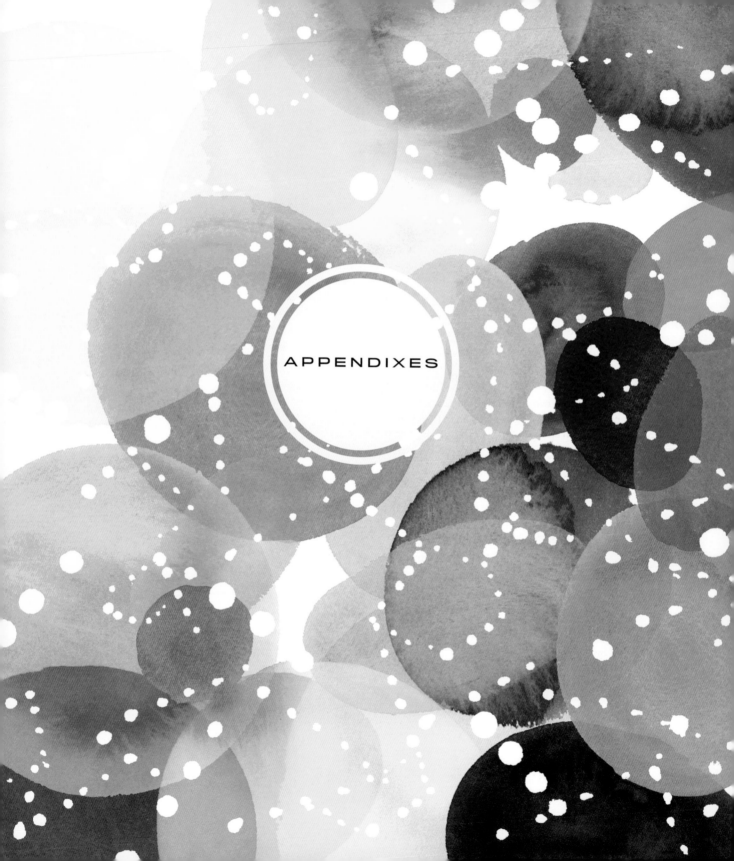

APPENDIXES

# Appendix 1: What's in Kombucha

"The more we know, the less we know." Keeping that approach in mind when it comes to nutrition means being open to the notion that there are likely to be elements inherent in the foods we eat that we have not yet identified or fully understood. The acids, vitamins, and antioxidants enhanced or created by the fermentation process are listed here not to prove kombucha's efficacy but merely to demonstrate some of the potential underlying mechanisms of the health benefits ascribed to this ancient elixir based on the most up-to-date research available.

To fixate on a single bacteria species or nutritional element, however, is to home in on the wrong thing. Bacteriosapiens (see page 4) are complex organisms that derive nourishment at microscopic levels. As such, microdoses of nutrients may be sufficient for supplying what our bodies need, provided it is bioavailable and easily assimilated. Using kombucha as a tonic by drinking small, frequent doses serves the organism best by supplying nutrition in the format we've evolved to utilize most efficiently.

Not every kombucha brew at every stage of brewing contains all of these constituents, as some specific bacteria or yeast may be more likely to produce certain components, while choices of tea, sugar, timing, and temperature, among many others, will change what is present and how much at any one moment. Nor is this list necessarily unabridged. Other amino acids or enzymes or vitamins or varieties of yeast can be present in the untold millions of brews currently in process around the world today. As the research on kombucha continues, and more detailed and effective studies are completed, these lists will grow.

## Primary Constituents Present in Kombucha

Despite hundreds of studies and millions of anecdotal testimonials from kombucha consumers around the world over hundreds (if not thousands) of years, clinical trials of the same rigor as those conducted for pharmaceutical drugs have yet to be conducted. It's important to note that the statements herein have not been evaluated by the FDA. Kombucha and SCOBYs are not intended to diagnose, treat, cure, or prevent any disease.

In lieu of such clinical data, we offer this body of knowledge with the caveat that kombucha be taken for what it is — not a panacea, but simply a tasty, tea-based tonic enhanced by the process of fermentation to provide nutrition in a living form. (See also Bacteria and Yeast Found in Kombucha Cultures, page 33.)

### AMINO ACIDS

Amino acids are the building blocks of protein, and as the SCOBY contains all nine of the essential amino acids (as well as some amino acids not considered essential), it is itself a complete protein. Kombucha contains these amino acids (* denotes the essential ones):

- Alanine
- Arginine
- Aspartic acid
- Cysteine
- Glutamic acid
- Glycine
- Histidine*
- Isoleucine*
- Leucine*
- Lysine*
- Methionine*
- Phenylalanine*
- Proline
- Serine
- Threonine*
- Tryptophan*
- Tyrosine
- Valine*

Quantities of amino acids in kombucha increase as the fermentation period progresses, yielding the highest amounts at 21 days of fermentation in a black tea substrate, according to the study listed below. Lysine, isoleucine, leucine, glutamic acid, alanine, aspartic acid, and proline were found to be present in the highest concentrations.

### *Related study:*

Jayabalan, Rasu, Kesavan Malini, Muthuswamy Sathishkumar, Krishnaswami Swaminathan, and Sei-Eok Yun. Biochemical characteristics of tea fungus produced during kombucha fermentation. *Food Science Biotechnology* 19, no. 3 (2010): 843–47.

## ORGANIC ACIDS

Because organic acids are generally weak and do not fully dissolve in water, they impart their characteristic sour taste to many foods, including the tart punch of a well-fermented kombucha. The total balance of all of these acids contributes to the titratable acidity of the brew (see Testing Tools and Protocols, page 175).

## Acetic Acid

The primary acidic flavor component of properly brewed kombucha, acetic acid boasts a range of positive attributes: boosting energy, aiding digestion, assisting the absorption of calcium and magnesium in the gut, reducing cholesterol, lowering blood triglyceride levels, and reducing blood sugar levels, all while increasing feelings of satiety.

**Related studies:**

Liu, C. H. Liu, C. H., W. H. Hsu, F. L. Lee, and C. C. Liao. The isolation and identification of microbes from a fermented tea beverage, Haipao, and their interactions during Haipao fermentation. *Food Microbiology* 13, no. 6 (1996): 407–15.

Shade, Ashley (Gordon and Betty Moore Foundation Fellow of the Life Sciences Research Foundation – Yale University). The Kombucha Biofilm: A Model System for Microbial Ecology. Final report on research conducted during the Microbial Diversity course, the Marine Biological Laboratory, Woods Hole, Mass., 2011.

Steinkraus, K. H., K. B. Shapiro, J. J. Hotchkiss, and R. P. Mortlack. Investigations into the antibiotic activity of tea fungus/kombucha beverage. *Acta Biotechnologica* 16, no. 2–3 (1996): 199–205.

Sreeramulu, Guttapadu, Yang Zhu, and Wieger Knol. Kombucha fermentation and its antimicrobial activity. *Journal of Agricultural Food Chemistry* 48 (2000): 2589–94.

## 5-keto-gluconic Acid (5KGA)

A by-product of the conversion of sugar to acetic acid, 5KGA is a precursor to vitamin C and tartaric acid among other healthy constituents. Tartaric acid produces a tart flavor while lowering the pH, which prevents spoilage.

## Butyric Acid

A short-chain fatty acid found in butter, milk, and anaerobic ferments, butyric acid also manifests in body odor and is the main acid present in the smell of human vomit. While unpleasant, that smell reflects the important role butyric acid serves in suppressing colonic inflammation, counteracting ulcerative colitis, and inhibiting colonic cancer cells while promoting healthy epithelial cells in the colon.

## Capric Acid (Decanoic Acid)/Caproic Acid (Hexanoic Acid)/Caprylic Acid

This family of acids helps increase good cholesterol (HDL) while decreasing bad cholesterol (LDL) and has antiviral and antitumor properties as well. Taken internally, it is commonly used to treat bacterial infections. Topically, it is used as a disinfectant and antimicrobial in food-contact surface sanitizers. These acids have also been shown effective at disrupting the cell membrane of various strains of *Candida*, including *Candida albicans* (see page 369).

## Citric Acid

This alpha-hydroxy acid is primarily found in citrus fruits. It has a pleasing sour taste and functions as a natural preservative. In culinary uses it adds flavor to marinades, and in beauty products it removes dead skin. As a chelating agent, it gradually eliminates the buildup of toxins in the body and can also be used to dissolve mineral deposits on sinks and faucets.

# ACIDS FOUND IN KOMBUCHA

| | |
|---|---|
| Acetic | Glucuronic |
| Benzoic | Hyaluronic |
| Butyric | Lactic |
| Capric (decanoic) | Malic |
| Caproic (hexanoic) | Nucleic |
| Caprylic | Oxalic |
| Citric | Usnic |
| Gluconic | |

### Related study:

Malbaša, Radomir V., Eva S. Lončar, Jasmina S. Vitas, and Jasna M. Čanadanović-Brunet. Influence of starter cultures on the antioxidant activity of kombucha beverage. *Food Chemistry* 127, no. 4 (2011): 1727–31.

## Lactic Acid

Lactic acid fuels both brain and muscle, allowing them to utilize carbohydrates more efficiently while also catalyzing liver glycogen formation. Commercially, lactic acid is an environmentally safer option for descaling, soap-scum remover, and antibacterial agent. Amounts present in kombucha vary widely due to differences in culture, substrate, and brewing environment.

### Related study:

Malbaša, Radomir V., E. S. Lončar, and L. J. A. Kolarov. L-lactic, L-ascorbic, total and volatile acids contents in dietetic kombucha beverage. *Romanian Biotechnological Letters* 7, no. 5 (2002): 891–96.

## 4-ETHYLPHENOL

This phenolic compound is produced by *Brettanomyces*, a common yeast found in kombucha as well as many wines and some sour beers. By itself, it has been described as having a "barnyard" or "medicinal" aroma, but within a well-balanced brew it adds levels of delicious, earthy flavor. 4-ethylphenol is created from p-coumaric acid, a powerful antioxidant found in wine and vinegar that reduces the formation of carcinogens in the stomach. Its presence in kombucha lends a unique flavor profile and may account for some of kombucha's anticarcinogenic properties.

## ETHYL ACETATE

This by-product of acetic-acid production has a sweet, fruity smell yet produces a sharp acidic flavor that helps create the sweet/tart signature taste of kombucha. Commercially, it is used as a solvent and perfume base and to decaffeinate tea and coffee.

## PHENETHYL ALCOHOL

This aromatic alcohol is found in a variety of essential oils and is used as a flavor and perfume additive. It has antimicrobial activities and is specifically a natural antibiotic for *Candida albicans* (see page 369).

## ANTIOXIDANTS

Antioxidants prevent diseases by combating oxidative stress. Tea is already a rich source of antioxidants, and the fermentation process increases them.

### Related studies:

Bhattacharya, Semantee, Prasenjit Manna, Ratan Gachhui, and Parames C. Sil. Protective effect of kombucha tea against tertiary butyl hydroperoxide induced cytotoxicity and cell death in murine hepatocytes. *Indian Journal of Experimental Biology* 49 (2011): 511–24.

Chen, Chinshuh, and Sheng-Che Shu. Effects of origins and fermentation time on the antioxidant activities of kombucha. *Food Chemistry* 98, no. 3 (2006): 502.

Dipti, P., B. Yogesh, A. K. Kain, T. Pauline, B. Anju, M. Sairam, B. Singh, S. S. Mongia, G. I. Kumar, and W. Selvamurthy. Lead induced oxidative stress: beneficial effects of kombucha tea. *Biomedical and Environmental Sciences* 16 (2003): 276–82.

Gharib, Ola Ali. Does kombucha tea attenuate the hepato-nepherotoxicity induced by a certain environmental pollutant? *Egyptian Academic Journal of Biological Science* 2, no. 2 (2010): 11–18.

Gharib, Ola Ali. Effects of kombucha on oxidative stress induced nephrotoxicity in rats. *Chinese Medicine* 4 (2009): 23.

Ibrahim, Nashwa Kamel. Possible protective effect of kombucha tea ferment on cadmium chloride induced liver and kidney damage in irradiated rats. *World Academy of Science, Engineering and Technology* 5 no. 7 (2011).

Jayabalan, Rasu, P. Subathradevi, S. Marimuthu, M. Sathishkumar, and K. Swaminathan. Changes in free-radical scavenging ability of kombucha tea during fermentation. *Food Chemistry* 109, no. 1 (2012): 227–34.

Jayabalan, Rasu. Effect of kombucha tea on aflatoxin B1 induced acute hepatotoxicity in albino rats — prophylactic and curative studies. *Journal of the Korean Society for Applied Biological Chemistry* 53, no. 4 (2010): 407–16.

Malbaša, Radomir V., Eva S. Lončar, Jasmina S. Vitas, and Jasna M. Čanadanović-Brunet. Influence of starter cultures on the antioxidant activity of kombucha beverage. *Food Chemistry* 127, no. 4 (2011): 1727–31.

Murugesan, G. S., M. Sathishkumar, R. Jayabalan, A. R. Binupriya, K. Swaminathan, and S. E. Yun. Hepatoprotective and curative properties of kombucha tea against carbon tetrachloride-induced toxicity. *Journal of Microbiology & Biotechnology* 19, no. 4 (2009): 397–402.

Velianski, Aleksandra S., Dragoljub D. Cvetković, Siniša L. Markov, Vesna T. Tumbas, and Slađana M. Savatović. Antimicrobial and antioxidant activity of lemon balm kombucha. *Acta Periodica Technologica* 38 (2007): 1–190.

Yang, Zhi-Wei, Bao-Ping Ji, Feng Zhou, Bo Li, Yangchao Luo, Li Yang, and Tao Li. Hypocholesterolaemic and antioxidant effects of kombucha tea in high-cholesterol fed mice. *Journal of the Science of Food and Agriculture* 89 (2008): 150–56.

## Vitamin C

An essential nutrient for the growth and repair of all tissues in the body, vitamin C is a powerful antioxidant that removes excess free radicals, keeping the body in balance and disease-resistant. Increased fermentation times lead to increased vitamin C content in kombucha. In one study (Malbaša, 2011), fermentation increased the vitamin C content from near 0 to almost 25 mg/L with significant increases in $B_2$ as well.

### Related studies:

Djuric, M., E. Lončar, R. Malbaša, L. J. Kolarov, and M. Klašnja. Influence of working conditions upon kombucha conducted fermentation of black tea. *Food and Bioproducts Processing* 84, no. 3 (2006): 186–92.

Bauer-Petrovska, Biljana, and Lidija Petrushevska-Tozi. Mineral and water-soluble vitamin content in kombucha drink. *International Journal of Food Science and Technology* 35 (1999): 201–5.

Malbaša, Radomir V., Eva S. Lončar, Mirjana S. Djurić, Ljiljana A. Kolarov, and Mile T. Klašnja. Batch fermentation of black tea by kombucha: a contribution to scale-up. *Acta Periodica Technologica* 36 (2005): 221–29.

Malbaša, Radomir V., Eva S. Lončar, Jasmina S. Vitas, and Jasna M. Čanadanović-Brunet. Influence of starter cultures on the antioxidant activity of kombucha beverage. *Food Chemistry* 127, no. 4 (2011): 1727–31.

## B VITAMINS

These water-soluble vitamins that play crucial roles in cell metabolism are synthesized by the yeast in kombucha as they break down the sugar. Fermentation has been shown to increase B-vitamin content, with one study (Malbaša, 2004) finding between 161 and 231 percent more present in kombucha versus just the tea.

### Related studies:

Bauer-Petrovska, Biljana, and Lidija Petrushevska-Tozi. Mineral and water-soluble vitamin content in kombucha drink. *International Journal of Food Science and Technology* 35 (1999): 201.

Malbaša, Radomir V., Milan Z. Maksimović, Eva S. Lončar, and Tatjana I. Branković. The influence of starter cultures on the content of vitamin $B_2$ in tea fungus beverages. *Central European Journal of Occupational and Environmental Medicine* 10, no. 1 (2004): 79–83.

$B_1$ — *thiamine.* An essential nutrient that is quickly depleted from the body through a variety of metabolic and neurological functions including the conversion of carbohydrates to energy, production of neurotransmitters, and lipid metabolism for myelin production, it keeps the heart pumping and muscles and nervous system functioning properly.

$B_2$ — *riboflavin.* Required by all parts of the body for proper functioning, it has also been found to help reduce rates of cervical cancer, migraines, and ocular conditions such as cataracts and glaucoma. Like all B vitamins, it boosts energy levels and immune system function while slowing the aging process. Other uses include treating liver disease and preventing memory loss and Alzheimer's, as well as lactic acidosis.

$B_6$ — *pyridoxine.* Vitamin $B_6$ is involved in dozens of enzymatic reactions that digest macronutrients, as well as in the body's synthesis of neurotransmitters and hormones such as serotonin and melatonin. It is critical to brain development and normal daily function. $B_6$ supplements have been used to treat morning sickness since the 1940s and have been shown to alleviate the symptoms of premenstrual syndrome.

$B_{12}$ — *cobalamin or cyanocobalamin.* Tea leaves are considered to be a viable source of $B_{12}$, especially for those who do not consume animal products, which are the most common source of $B_{12}$. The most complex of all the B vitamins, $B_{12}$ is involved in the metabolism of every cell in the human body, and especially DNA synthesis. It plays a key role in brain and nervous system functioning as well as the formation of blood. $B_{12}$ deficiency can cause irreparable damage to the brain and nervous system as well as anemia.

## Catechins

Catechins are chemical messengers that regulate plant physiology and act as powerful antioxidants. They are pretty much antieverything, including anti-inflammatory, antifungal, antiallergenic, anticancer, antiviral, antimicrobial, and antidiarrheal. The following catechins are present in tea:

· Epicatechin (EC)
· Epicatechin gallate (ECG)
· Epigallocatechin (EGC)
· Epigallocatechin gallate (EGCG)
· Theaflavin (TF)

Catechins, like many nutritional elements, are increased significantly by the fermentation process, which may be due to their increased stability in acid environments. Concentrations of catechins in kombucha tend to be higher in green tea than in black and peak on the 12 day of fermentation, according to one study (Jayabalan, 2008).

### Related studies:

Chen, Chinshuh, and Sheng-Che Chu. Effects of origins and fermentation time on the antioxidant activities of kombucha. *Food Chemistry* 98, no. 3 (2006): 502–7.

Jayabalan, Rasu, S. Marimuthu, K. Swaminathan. Changes in content of organic acids and tea polyphenols during kombucha tea fermentation. *Food Chemistry* 102, no. 1 (2007): 392–98.

Jayabalan, Rasu, Subbaiya Marimuthu, Periyasamy Thangaraj, Muthuswamy Sathishkumar, Arthur Raj Binupriya, Krishnaswami Swaminathan, and Sei Eok Yun. Preservation of kombucha tea: effect of temperature on tea components and free radical scavenging properties. *Journal of Agricultural Food Chemistry* 56 (2008): 9064–71.

## ENZYMES

Enzymes are protein molecules that act as catalysts for innumerable physical processes. At the most basic level enzymes in kombucha, such as invertase, amylase, or any of the hexokinases, break down sugar bonds to provide fuel for fermentation. Markers of enzymatic action, such as residual phytase activity proteins, have been found in dried SCOBY, indicating the presence of many other enzymes acting at different phases of kombucha fermentation whenever they are needed, then ceasing activity while others begin their work.

Researchers will need a lot of time and money to untangle and identify every enzymatic machination of the various kombucha brews worldwide. Until then, the following enzymes have been found:

- Amylase
- Carbohydrase
- Catalase
- Hexokinases
- Invertase
- Lipase
- Phytases

- Protease
- Sucrase

## FRUCTOSE

The sweetest of the naturally occurring sugars, fructose fuels several biological processes. In kombucha, yeast metabolize sucrose by breaking it into fructose and glucose in order to fuel cellular respiration, which creates carbon dioxide. Of the low residual sugar levels present in kombucha, fructose makes up the majority rather than glucose, which may be one reason many diabetics consume it without issue (see pages 65 and 367).

## GLUCOSE

The primary energy source for nearly all forms of life, glucose is stored in the body as glycogen, ready to activate whenever fuel is needed. When glycogen stores are depleted, we experience fatigue, and a glycogen imbalance often manifests as diabetes. In the fermentation process, it is metabolized into gluconic and glucuronic acids, which are responsible for many of kombucha's unique health benefits.

## GLUCONIC ACID

As they metabolize glucose, bacteria synthesize several healthy acids, one of which is gluconic acid. This acid is found in many foods including honey, fruit, wine, and, of course, kombucha. In mammals, it plays an important role in carbohydrate metabolism, thereby aiding digestion. Several commercial applications for gluconic acid in the food industry point to why kombucha is effective as an acidity

regulator, chelator, and meat tenderizer with debittering properties. The presence of this acid not only balances the bite created by the acetic acid but also bonds with other elements to boost antioxidant and healing properties — for example, by increasing iron and calcium absorption.

### *Related studies:*

Bhattacharya, Semantee, Prasenjit Manna, Ratan Gachhui, and Parames C. Sil. Protective effect of kombucha tea against tertiary butyl hydroperoxide induced cytotoxicity and cell death in murine hepatocytes. *Indian Journal of Experimental Biology* 49 (2011): 511–24.

Chen, C., and B. Y. Liu. Changes in major components of tea fungus metabolites during prolonged fermentation. *Journal of Applied Microbiology* 89 (2000): 834–39.

Talawat, Sulak, Pimpan Ahantharik, Sajeena Laohawiwattanakul, Apinya Premsuk, and Sunanta Ratanapo. Efficacy of fermented teas in antibacterial activity. *Kasetsart Journal: Natural Science* 40 (2006): 925–33.

## GLUCURONIC ACID

Glucuronic acid, naturally produced in the liver, is the body's toxin patrol. It helps the body eliminate drugs, dietary pollutants, environmental toxins, and bodily wastes like bilirubin, oxidized fatty acids, excess cholesterol, and excess hormones. Once glucuronic acid molecules bond to them, offending toxins are excreted from the body.

Glucuronic acid also readily converts into glucosamine, the very basis of our skeletal system, providing strength and lubrication to our joints, building cartilage, increasing collagen density, and lubricating the whole system to keep it moving smoothly. While the body produces glucuronic acid, it does not make as much as it can use for detoxification and healing.

Recent studies conclusively demonstrate kombucha's synthesis of glucuronic acid in appreciable amounts, though the exact quantity varies greatly depending on what bacteria/yeast are present in the SCOBY, brewing conditions, and the substrate used (type of tea or sugar).

In one study (Vīna, 2013) kombucha cultures fermented on grape juice and black tea yielded very high amounts of glucuronic acid, likely due to the increased amount of glucose from the grapes. Most studies show that the highest levels of glucuronic acid are created by black tea after at least two weeks of fermentation.

### Related studies:

Jayabalan, Rasu, S. Marimuthu, and K. Swaminathan. Changes in content of organic acids and tea polyphenols during kombucha tea fermentation. *Food Chemistry* 102, no. 1 (2007): 392–98.

Suhartatik, Nanik, M. Karyantina, Y. Marsono, Endang S. Rahayu, and Kapti R. Kuswanto. Kombucha as anti-hypercholesterolemic agent. In *Proceedings of the 3rd International Conference of Indonesian Society for Lactic Acid Bacteria (3rd IC-ISLAB). Better Life with Lactic Acid Bacteria: Exploring Novel Functions of Lactic Acid Bacteria* (Gadjah Mada University, Bulaksumur, Yogyakarta, Indonesia, January 21–22, 2011).

Vīna, Ilmāra, Pāvels Semjonovs, Raimonds Linde, and Artūrs Patetko. Glucuronic acid containing fermented functional beverages produced by natural yeasts and bacteria associations. *International Journal of Research and Reviews in Applied Sciences* 14, no. 1 (2013).

Vīna, Ilmāra, Raimonds Linde, Artūrs Patetko, and Pāvels Semjonovs. Glucuronic acid from fermented beverages: biochemical functions in humans and its role in health

protection. *International Journal of Research and Reviews in Applied Sciences* 14, no. 2 (2013).

Yavari, Nafiseh, Mahnaz Mazaheri Assadi, Mohammad Bamani Moghadam, and Kambiz Larijani. Optimizing glucuronic acid production using tea fungus on grape juice by response surface methodology. *Australian Journal of Basic and Applied Sciences* 5, no. 11 (2011): 1788–94.

Yavari, Nafiseh, Mahnaz Mazaheir Assadi, Kambiz Larijani, and M. B. Moghadam. Response surface methodology for optimization of glucuronic acid production using kombucha layer on sour cherry juice. *Australian Journal of Basic and Applied Sciences* 4, no. 8 (2010): 3250–56.

## CAFFEINE (THEINE)

Caffeine, a xanthine alkaloid, is sometimes called *theine* when found in tea. A neurotoxin that acts as a pesticide to protect plants, in humans it is a stimulant, increasing the heart rate and opening the airways by relaxing the smooth muscles of the bronchi. It is a necessary nutrient for kombucha fermentation, but its levels are reduced during the brewing process (see page 55).

## THEOBROMINE AND THEOPHYLLINE

These twin alkaloids are present in trace amounts in tea. Both offer relaxation properties and help soothe smooth muscle tissue in the bronchioles, making it easier to breathe (see Asthma, page 365).

# Other Elements Found in Kombucha

Numerous organic acids and biological components contribute to the vibrancy and flavor of

kombucha. The following elements are often cited as being present in kombucha but have not been as closely studied as the ones discussed above.

## BENZOIC ACID

Found in plants, where it acts as a growth regulator, defensive compound, and pollinator attractor, benzoic acid has antifungal and preservative properties. It has been used to treat skin conditions such as ringworm and athlete's foot and is included in some cancer medications. In the early twentieth century it was used as an analgesic, expectorant, and antiseptic, and it is still included in traditional cures for fungal conditions.

## BENZONITRILE

A solvent, it has also been shown effective in preventing the cold virus from replicating.

## HYALURONIC ACID

This long-chain mucopolysaccharide, similar in quality to gelatin, lubricates joints and other moving parts of the body. It is added to beauty products as a natural moisturizer.

## ITACONIC ACID

This antimicrobial inhibits the growth of pathogenic bacteria such as *Salmonella enterica* and *Mycobacterium tuberculosis*.

## OXALIC ACID

Organically present at healthy levels in leafy greens, nuts, tea, and chocolate, oxalic acid as part of the diet inhibits tumor formation and growth. Manufactured versions

# METABOLITES OF GLUCURONIC ACID

The body derives the following components from glucuronic acid via metabolism, so while they may or may not be present in some kombucha brews, they will be present in the person who consumes the kombucha, as shown through urine samples.

## D-glucaric acid

This metabolite shows similar properties to glucuronic acid such as helping the liver to detoxify the body by removing carcinogens and excess steroid hormones. It also helps regulate estrogen, lower fats in the blood, and has been shown to be chemopreventive. While the body does make some glucaric acid, most of it comes from food sources like fruits and cruciferous vegetables.

## D-saccharic acid-1,4-lactone (DSL)

A derivative of D-glucaric acid, DSL assists the body with toxin removal by inhibiting the production of glucuronidase. This preserves the bonds formed when a molecule of glucuronic acid grabs onto a toxic molecule. If that bond is broken by the glucuronidase enzyme, both the glucuronic acid and the toxin (which becomes fat soluble when unbonded) are released into the bloodstream separately, and no detoxification occurs.

But if the DSL does its job, the toxin is water soluble and can be flushed out of the body by urination. Several studies have demonstrated DSL's prophylactic and protective effects against metabolic disorders such as diabetes, high cholesterol, cancer, and liver dysfunction.

## Chondroitin sulfate

An important structural component of cartilage that is prescribed as a supplement to treat osteoarthritis, chondroitin sulfate is a complex chain of alternating sugars, one of which is glucuronic acid. It has anti-inflammatory properties and stimulates the products of hyaluronic acid while inhibiting the synthesis of substances that damage cartilage.

## Heparin

Heparin is a naturally occurring anticoagulant, but its full role in the body is not understood. Theories center around it being used at the site of wounds to prevent bacterial infection and being stored within mast cells, which reside in several types of tissue specifically to protect against pathogens and speed wound healing. In the pharmaceutical form, heparin is used to treat heart- and lung-related issues such as cardiopulmonary bypass surgery and deep-vein thrombosis.

*Related studies:*

Bhattacharya, Semantee, Prasenjit Manna, Ratan Gachhui, and Parames C. Sil. Protective effect of kombucha tea against tertiary butyl hydroperoxide induced cytotoxicity and cell death in murine hepatocytes. *Indian Journal of Experimental Biology* 49 (2011): 511–24.

Kan Wang, Gan Xuhua, Tang Xinyun, Wang Shuo, and Tan Huarong. The effect of nutrients on the concentrations of DSL and gross acid in kombucha. *Food and Fermentation Industries*, 2007.

Wang, Yong, Baoping Ji, Wei Wu, Ruojun Wang, Zhiwei Yang, Di Zhang, and Wenli Tian. Hepatoprotective effects of kombucha tea: identification of functional strains and quantification of functional components. *Journal of the Science of Food and Agriculture* 94, no. 2 (2014): 265–72.

Yang, Zhi-Wei, Bao-Ping Ji, Feng Zhou, Bo Li, Yangchao Luo, Li Yang, and Tao Li. Hypocholesterolaemic and antioxidant effects of kombucha tea in high-cholesterol fed mice. *Journal of Scientific Food Agriculture* 89 (2009): 150–56

---

Formation of glucuronic acid and gluconic acid by oxidation of glucose can be toxic in large amounts, but the low levels naturally present in kombucha may assist with digestion, regular elimination, and colon health.

### SUCCINIC ACID

Historically derived from amber, it acts as an acidity regulator that also adds flavors of saltiness, bitterness, and acidity to ferments.

### USNIC ACID

Found almost exclusively in lichen but also in trace amounts in kombucha tea, usnic acid exhibits anti-inflammatory and analgesic properties, among others. It is also a potent antibiotic against a variety of pathogenic gram-positive bacteria such as *Staphylococcus* and *Streptococcus* as well as some pathogenic fungi. (See Immunity, Infections, and Infectious Diseases, page 367, for more on kombucha's antimicrobial effects.)

# Appendix 2: Highlights of Kombucha Benefits Research

Once again, to be absolutely clear, kombucha does not *cure* anything. It is an effective detoxifier that helps bring the immune system back into balance so that the body can heal itself. As outlined in appendix 1, kombucha contains acids, vitamins, minerals, and compounds that research shows may mitigate some symptoms, but many of its nutritional components are present only in trace amounts. Those with severely compromised immune systems are advised to consume kombucha or any fermented food cautiously and under the supervision of a primary care physician.

Researchers around the world have conducted studies using either kombucha or SCOBYs, testing them for a variety of components and properties, but a couple of recent papers have synthesized the modern research in very helpful ways.

In the survey paper "Current Evidence on Physiological Activity and Expected Health Effects of Kombucha Fermented Beverage" (*Journal of Medicinal Food*, 2014),

Ilmāra Vīna and colleagues at the Institute of Microbiology and Biotechnology in Latvia concluded that kombucha tea has the "four main potencies necessary for numerous biological activities: a detoxifying property, protection against free-radical damage, energizing capabilities and promotion of immunity."

Additionally, "A Review on Kombucha Tea — Microbiology, Composition, Fermentation, Beneficial Effects, Toxicity, and Tea Fungus," authored by leading kombucha researchers Rasu Jayabalan, Radomir V. Malbaša, and others (*Comprehensive Reviews in Food Science and Food Safety*, 2014), shows the extent to which recent research has begun to establish the connection between the anecdotes and the science. As more research is conducted, we anticipate that the anecdotal evidence that has been mounting for centuries, if not millennia, will continue to be supported by additional studies.

What follows is a summary of research on kombucha's efficacy in treating or relieving a variety of illnesses.

## Arthritis/Rheumatism/Joint Pain

Glucuronic acid (see page 361), perhaps kombucha's most important weapon, aids the body in a number of processes and also can be converted in the human body into several different essential acidic mucopolysaccharides, such as hyaluronic acid, chondroitin sulfate, and glucosamine, all of which relate to building and maintaining healthier joints.

### *Related studies:*

Danielian, L. T. *Kombucha and Its Biological Features*. Moscow: Meditsina, 2005.

Jayabalan, Rasu, S. Marimuthu, and K. Swaminathan. Changes in content of organic acids and tea polyphenols during kombucha tea fermentation. *Food Chemistry* 102, no. 1 (2007): 392-98.

Vīna, Ilmāra, Pāvels Semjonovs, Raimonds Linde, and Artūrs Patetko. Glucuronic acid containing fermented functional beverages produced by natural yeasts and bacteria associations. *International Journal of Research and Reviews in Applied Sciences* 14, no. 1 (2013).

Vīna, Ilmāra, Pāvels Semjonovs, Raimonds Linde, and Artūrs Patetko. Glucuronic acid from fermented beverages: biochemical functions in humans and its role in health protection. *International Journal of Research and Reviews in Applied Sciences* 14, no. 2 (2013).

Yavari, Nafiseh, Mahnaz Mazaheir Assadi, Kambiz Larijani, and M. B. Moghadam. Response surface methodology for optimization of glucuronic acid production using kombucha layer on sour cherry juice. *Australian Journal of Basic and Applied Sciences* 4, no. 8 (2010): 3250–56.

## Asthma

According to the studies listed below, kombucha brewed with black tea increased levels of theophylline, a bronchodilator, amounting to a therapeutic dose for those using it as treatment for asthma. Both caffeine (page 362) and heparin (page 363) can also potentially relieve asthma symptoms.

### *Related studies:*

Rosales, Manuel Cortes, Esther Albarrán Rodríguez, Guillermo Nolasco Rodríguez, Raúl Leonel de Cervantes Mireles, Leticia Ávila Figueroa, Jesus Jonatan Iñiguez Orozco, and Erika Rizo de la Peña. Evaluation of the properties of healing of the extract of kombucha in sheep growth with malnutrition, parasitocis and respiratory problems. *Open Journal of Veterinary Medicine* 4, no. 8 (2014).

Vīna, Ilmāra, Pāvels Semjonovs, Raimonds Linde, and Ilze Denina. Current evidence on physiological activity and expected health effects of kombucha fermented beverage. *Journal of Medicinal Food* 17, no. 2 (2014): 179–88.

## Cancer

It is often impossible to pinpoint an exact cause of cancer, as a host of factors both genetic and environmental may combine to contribute to the disease. Doctors throughout the twentieth century, including Dr. Rudolf Sklenar and Dr. Veronica Carstens, former First Lady of Germany, have included kombucha in their cancer protocols, relying on its systemic balancing effects to assist with the overall healing process.

In a study by R. Jayabalan et al. (2011), kombucha tea was fractionated (a process of isolating components in a mixture), and the effects of those components on human cancer cells was studied in vitro. The study showed that the mechanism by which kombucha's anticancer properties function may be due to the inhibition of metastasis (the spread of cancer from one organ to another), as shown through the presence of dimethyl malonate and vitexin, both of which have known cytotoxic and anti-invasive effects on cancer cells.

Another study, by M. Deghrigue et al. (2013), found that while black tea kombucha was effective against one of two types of human lung cancer cells, green tea kombucha was more effective against both in vitro. While the researchers weren't sure by what mechanism the anticancer properties were achieved, attributing it potentially to polyphenols and other antioxidants, others have speculated that it could be due to metabolites (e.g., alcohol, organic acids, vitamins, amino acids) produced by the symbiosis of the bacteria and yeast.

Other elements of kombucha that have chemopreventive or antitumor properties are butyric acid, oxalic acid, 4-ethylphenol, saccharic acid, heparin, antioxidants, and catechins. Polyphenols present in tea are also generally recognized to have cancer-inhibition properties, and kombucha's effectiveness could be linked to not only those polyphenols but also other elements that appear after they are fermented.

### *Related studies:*

Cetojevic-Simin, D. D., G. M. Bogdanovic, D. D. Cvetkovic, and A. S. Velicanski. Antiproliferative and antimicrobial activity of traditional kombucha and *Satureja montana* L. kombucha. *Journal of the Balkan Union of Oncology* 13, no. 3 (2008): 395–401.

Deghrigue, Monia, Jihene Chriaa, Houda Battikh, Kawther Abid, and Amina Bakhrouf. Antiproliferative and antimicrobial activities of kombucha tea. *African Journal of Microbiology Research* 7, no. 27 (2013): 3466–70.

Jayabalan, Rasu. Effect of solvent fractions of kombucha tea on viability and invasiveness of cancer cells — characterization of dimethyl 2-(2-hydroxy-2-methoxypropylidine) malonate and vitexin. *Indian Journal of Biotechnology* 10, (Jan. 2011), 75–82.

Sriharia, Thummala, Ramachandran Arunkumar, Jagadeesan Arunakaran, and Uppala Satyanarayana. Down regulation of signaling molecules involved in angiogenesis of human prostate cancer cell line (PC-3) by kombucha (lyophilized). *Biomedicine & Preventive Nutrition* 3, no. 1 (2013): 53–58.

## AMELIORATING THE SIDE EFFECTS OF CHEMOTHERAPY AND RADIATION EXPOSURE

Radiation exposure can lead to mutations in DNA that increase the risk of cancer. Yet the most common cancer treatment involves radiation therapy in conjunction with chemotherapy. Anecdotally, people who drink kombucha while receiving chemotherapy have reported reduced nausea and improved appetite, though no research has yet been done to confirm these reports. However, some recent studies have explored how kombucha might help with deeper issues caused by radiation.

The authors of the first study (Cavusoglu, 2010) injected blood cells of healthy humans with kombucha, and then exposed them to high doses of radiation. The blood cells injected with the highest doses of kombucha demonstrated the lowest rate of aberrant metaphases ("broken" DNA) and higher rates of cell proliferation. According to the study, kombucha does provide a "radioprotective effect against ionizing radiation." It's important to note that increased dosages of kombucha provided increased protection.

The second study (Ibrahim, 2013) focused on rats that were exposed to cadmium chloride (a carcinogen) and gamma radiation. When they were injected with cadmium chloride or dosed with radiation (or both), rats consuming a steady diet of kombucha tea absorbed lower levels of toxins than those who were not. Daily kombucha consumption appeared to limit the effects.

### Related studies:

Cavusoglu, K., and P. Guler. Protective effect of kombucha mushroom (KM) tea on chromosomal aberrations induced by gamma radiation in human peripheral lymphocytes in-vitro. *Journal of Environmental Biology* 31, no. 5 (2010): 851–56.

Ibrahim, Nashwa Kamel. Possible protective effect of kombucha tea ferment on cadmium chloride induced liver and kidney damage in irradiated rats. *International Journal of Biological and Life Sciences* 9, no. 1 (2013).

## Cholesterol Issues/ Arteriosclerosis

As far back as 1890, numerous studies, including many papers from the 1920s' research boom, linked kombucha consumption to improvements in cholesterol and arteriosclerosis issues. A series of studies conducted in Russia in the 1950s claimed to demonstrate effectiveness. One study that followed 52 atherosclerotic patients exhibiting high levels of plasma cholesterol showed that after regular kombucha tea consumption their total serum cholesterol decreased to normal levels. (See pages 342–43 for more on that era of Russian research.)

Several animal studies have explored kombucha's potential efficacy at regulating cholesterol. In a study by L. Adriani et al. (2011), researchers found that adding kombucha tea to the ducks' drinking water (totaling 25 percent by volume) decreased low-density lipoprotein (LDL) and increased high-density lipoprotein (HDL) after four weeks of consumption — positive effects that they attributed to the presence of glucuronic acid (page 361).

In another study, by A. Aloulou et al. (2012), rats were fed either unfermented black tea or kombucha. Those consuming the fermented tea exhibited not only lower levels of cholesterol but also greater weight reduction.

In still another study, conducted by N. Suhartatik et al. (2011), in mice fed kombucha, levels of total cholesterol decreased by as much as 52 percent, with LDL dropping by as much as 91 percent and HDL increasing by as much as 27 percent.

Whether these benefits derive from the presence of glucuronic acid (page 361), decanoic acid (also known as capric acid) (page 358) or antioxidant content (page 359), the studies indicate why kombucha seems to be effective at assisting the body with cholesterol regulation.

Consuming the SCOBY itself may also help. Although cellulose is not digestible by the human body (we don't have the enzymes to break it down), it acts as a broom, sweeping waste from the walls of the intestines, including even excretions of cholesterol and sugar, if excess levels are present in the blood.

### Related studies:

Adriani, L., N. Mayasari, and Angga, R. Kartasudjana. The effect of feeding fermented kombucha tea on HDL, LDL and total cholesterol levels in the duck bloods. *Biotechnology in Animal Husbandry* 27, no. 4 (2011): 1749–55.

Aloulou, Ahmed, Khaled Hamden, Dhouha Elloumi, Madiha Bou Ali, Khaoula Hargafi, Bassem Jaouadi, Fatma Ayadi, Abdelfattah Elfeki, and Emna Ammar. Hypoglycemic and antilipidemic properties of kombucha tea in alloxan-induced diabetic rats. *BMC Complementary and Alternative Medicine* 12, no. 63 (2012).

Khaled Bellassouedab, Ferdaws Ghrabc, Fatma Makni-Ayadid, Jos Van Peltb, Abdelfattah Elfekia, and Emna Ammarc. Protective effect of kombucha on rats fed a hypercholesterolemic diet is mediated by its antioxidant activity. *Pharmaceutical Biology* 53, no. 11 (2015).

Semjonovs, P., I. Denina, and R. Linde. Evaluation of physiological effects of acetic acid bacteria and yeast fermented non-alchocolic beverage consumption in rat model. *Journal of Medical Sciences* 14 (2014): 147–52.

Suhartatik, Nanik, M. Karyantina, Y. Marsono, Endang S. Rahayu, and Kapti R. Kuswanto. Kombucha as anti-hyper-cholesterolemic agent. In *Proceedings of the 3rd International Conference of Indonesian Society for Lactic Acid Bacteria (3rd IC-ISLAB). Better Life with Lactic Acid Bacteria: Exploring Novel Functions of Lactic Acid Bacteria* (Gadjah Mada University, Bulaksumur, Yogyakarta, Indonesia, January 21–22, 2011).

Yang, Zhi-Wei, Bao-Ping Ji, Feng Zhou, Bo Li, Yangchao Luo, Li Yang, and Tao Li. Hypocholesterolaemic and antioxidant effects of kombucha tea in high-cholesterol fed mice. *Journal of the Science of Food and Agriculture* 89 (2009): 150–56.

## Diabetes

The antidiabetic properties of kombucha were noted as far back as 1929 by Dr. E. Arauner and others. In the study "Hypoglycemic and Antilipidemic Properties of Kombucha Tea in Alloxan-Induced Diabetic Rats" (2012), diabetic rats fed varying amounts of kombucha over 30 days demonstrated lowered levels of blood glucose, a decrease in plasma cholesterol, and normal levels of liver and kidney toxicity levels compared to the controls. Another study, "Antihyperglycaemic Efficacy of Kombucha in Streptozotocin-Induced Rats" (2013), showed similar beneficial effects.

### Related studies:

Aloulou, Ahmed, Khaled Hamden, Dhouha Elloumi, Madiha Bou Ali, Khaoula Hargafi, Bassem Jaouadi, Fatma Ayadi, Abdelfattah Elfeki, and Emna Ammar. Hypoglycemic and antilipidemic properties of kombucha tea in alloxan-induced diabetic rats. *BMC Complementary and Alternative Medicine* 12 (2012).

Arauner, E. Der japanische Teepilz. *Deutsche Essigindustrie* 33, no. 22 (1929): 11–12.

Chandrakala Shenoy, K. Hypoglycemic activity of bio-tea in mice. *Indian Journal of Experimental Biology* 38 (1999): 278–79.

Srihari, Thummala, Krishnamoorthy Karthikesan, Natarajan Ashokkumar, and Uppala Satyanarayana. Antihyperglycaemic efficacy of kombucha in streptozotocin-induced rats. *Journal of Functional Foods* 5, no. 4 (2013): 1794–1802.

## Gastrointestinal Issues/ Acid Reflux/Ulcers

One of the most commonly claimed benefits of kombucha is improved digestion. For some that means relieving constipation, while for others it calms diarrhea. Many sufferers of irritable bowel syndrome, malabsorption of food, acid reflux, and ulcers have found kombucha helpful. Acid reflux affects an estimated 60 percent of the adult population in the United States.

Kombucha's antimicrobial properties have been well studied and have been shown to kill *H. pylori*, the bacteria that cause ulcers, on contact.

According to a study by D. Banerjee et al. (2010), kombucha was found to be as effective as omeprazole (the generic form of Prilosec) at healing ulceration and reducing acid reflux. The authors speculate that it could be due to kombucha's ability to reduce gastric-acid secretions as well as its high antioxidant levels, with black tea kombucha being the most effective.

### Related studies:

Banerjee, D., Sham A. Hassarajani, Biswanath Maity, Geetha Narayan, Sandip K. Bandyopadhyay, and Subrata Chattopadhyay. Comparative healing property of kombucha tea and black tea against indomethacin-induced gastric ulceration in mice: possible mechanism of action. *Food & Function* 1, no. 3 (2010): 284–93.

Wright, Jonathan V., and L. Lenard. *Why Stomach Acid Is Good for You.* Lanham, MD: M. Evans, 2001.

## Immunity, Infections, and Infectious Diseases

As numerous studies have shown, kombucha possesses superior antioxidant levels compared to unfermented tea. Antioxidants clean up free radicals, keeping them in balance. The antimicrobial effects of kombucha are often attributed to its low pH, which wreaks havoc for pathogenic organisms such as *Bacillus cereus*, *Escherichia coli*, *Helicobacter pylori*, *Listeria monocytogenes*, *Micrococcus luteus*, *Pseudomonas aeruginosa*, *Salmonella typhimurium*, *Staphylococcus aureus*, *Staphylococcus epidermidis*, and *Candida* species.

The weak gluconic and acetic acids in kombucha specifically target and shut down pathogenic organisms by disrupting their cell membranes, inhibiting metabolic actions, changing the pH of the pathogenic cells, and creating an excess of toxic anions to finish the job. Benzonitrile, benzoic acid, and itaconic acid also play a role in boosting the body's immunity and contribute to kombucha's anti-infection properties.

## Related studies:

Battikh, H., A. Bakhrouf, and E. Ammar. Antimicrobial effect of kombucha analogues. *Lebensmittel-Wissenschaft + Technologie* 47, no. 1 (2012): 71–77.

Deghrigue, Monia, Jihene Chria, Houda Battikh, Kawther Abid, and Amina Bakhrouf. Antiproliferative and antimicrobial activities of kombucha tea. *African Journal of Microbiology Research* 7, no. 27 (2013): 3466–70.

Santos, José Rodrigo, Rejane Andrade Batista, Sheyla Alves Rodrigues, Lauro Xavier Filho, and Álvaro Silva Lima. Antimicrobial activity of broth fermented with kombucha colonies. *Journal of Microbial & Biochemical Technology* 1, no. 1 (2009): 72–78.

Velićanski, Aleksandra, Dragoljub D. Cvetković, Siniša L. Markov, Vesna T. Tumbas, and Slađana M. Savatović. Antimicrobial and antioxidant activity of lemon balm kombucha. *Acta Periodica Tecnologica*, no. 38 (2007): 165–72.

## Kidney/Liver Function

A healthy liver filters the blood of xenobiotics, defined as pharmaceutical or natural drugs, alcohol, and parasites. The liver even cleans up excess hormones, bacteria, exhausted blood cells, and other cellular debris. The kidneys filter the blood and excrete toxins from the body through urination. Several studies have indicated kombucha's potential protective effect against environmental toxins.

In a study by O. A. Gharib (2009), rats were exposed to trichloroethylene, a common environmental pollutant that generates oxidative stress and alters antioxidant enzymes in the body, leading to liver and kidney stress. In all the studies listed here, rats that received kombucha tea were found to have improved levels of renal and liver health indicators such as serum creatinine and malondialdehyde. P. Dipti et al. (2003) demonstrated kombucha's protective effect of the liver in rats, while N. K. Ibrahim (2013) showed that administration of kombucha tea to rats with liver damage resulted in recovery from all ill effects. The most commonly credited mechanisms for this effect are the work of glucuronic acid and antioxidants.

## Related studies:

Aloulou, Ahmed et al. Hypoglycemic and antilipidemic properties of kombucha tea in alloxan-induced diabetic rats. *BMC Complementary and Alternative Medicine* 12, no. 63 (2012).

Bhattacharya, S. Hepatoprotective properties of kombucha tea against TBHP-induced oxidative stress via suppression of mitochondria dependent apoptosis. *Pathophysiology* 18, no. 3 (2011): 221–34.

Dipti, P., B. Yogesh, A. K. Kain, T. Pauline, B. Anju, et al. Lead induced oxidative stress: beneficial effects of kombucha tea. *Biomedical and Environmental Sciences* 16, no. 3 (2003): 276–82.

Gharib, Ola Ali. Does kombucha tea attenuate the hepato-nephrotoxicity induced by a certain environmental pollutant? *Egyptian Academic Journal of Biological Sciences* 2, no. 2 (2010): 11–18

Gharib, Ola Ali. Effects of kombucha on oxidative stress induced nephrotoxicity in rats. *Chinese Medicine* 4 (2009).

Ibrahim, Nashwa Kamel. Possible protective effect of kombucha tea ferment on cadmium chloride induced liver and kidney damage in irradiated rats. *International Journal of Biological and Life Sciences* 9 (2013).

Jayabalan, Rasu. Effect of kombucha tea on aflatoxin B1 induced acute hepatotoxicity in albino rats — prophylactic and curative studies. *Journal of the Korean Society for Applied Biological Chemistry* 53, no. 4 (2010): 407–16.

Murugesan, G. S. Hepatoprotective and curative properties of kombucha tea against carbon tetrachloride-induced toxicity. *Journal of Microbiology & Biotechnology* 19, no. 4 (2009): 397–402.

Pauline, T., P. Dipti, B. Anju, S. Kavimani, S. K. Sharma, et al. Studies on toxicity, anti-stress and hepatoprotective properties of Kombucha tea. *Biomedical and Environmental Sciences* 14, no. 3 (2001): 207-13.

Semjonovs, P. Evaluation of physiological effects of acetic acid bacteria and yeast fermented non-alchocolic beverage consumption in rat model. *Journal of Medical Sciences* 14 (2014): 147–52.

## Multiple Sclerosis (MS)

In the 1980s German doctor Reinhold Weisner conducted research on almost 250 patients that suggested drinking kombucha boosts production of interferons, proteins that interfere with a virus's ability to attack cells, thus improving the immune response. Kombucha also contains appreciable amounts of vitamin $B_1$, aka thiamine (page 360), which plays a role in the production of myelin tissue, the fatty substance surrounding the nerve fibers that is degraded by MS.

On an individual level, Dr. Terry Wahls details her personal struggle with and recovery from MS in her book *The Wahls Protocol*; her treatment program includes incorporating kombucha into the diet.

## Related studies:

Marzban, Fatemeh et al. Kombucha tea ameliorates experimental autoimmune encephalomyelitis in mouse model of multiple sclerosis. *Food and Agricultural Immunology* 26, no. 6, 2015.

Wahls, Terry, and Eve Adamson. *The Wahls Protocol: How I Beat Progressive MS Using Paleo Principles and Functional Medicine.* Avery, 2014.

## Skin Ailments

### (BURNS/LESIONS/ECZEMA/ PSORIASIS)

The SCOBY's cellulosic nanofibers nourish the skin and support its own natural healing abilities, while the low pH of the tea softens tissues. A SCOBY or similar sheet of *Acetobacter*-grown culture can also provide a sterile covering for wounds and other sites of inflammation, making SCOBYs and SCOBY-like materials an emerging choice in medicine, as discussed in "Microbial Cellulose — the Natural Power to Heal Wounds" (2006) from the University of Texas at Austin.

*Bacterial NanoCellulose: A Sophisticated Multifunctional Material* (2013) collects the work of nine recent in-depth papers on the medical usefulness and future of bacterial cellulose treatments, including a myriad of current and potential medical uses.

With all of this interest at the research level, it is no surprise that over-the-counter facial masks of bacterial cellulose are available in Asia and South America as beauty enhancements. A variety of mainstream cleansing products also contain kombucha tea or SCOBY as an ingredient. (See page 314 for more.)

#### Related studies:

Barati, Fardin. Histopathological and clinical evaluation of kombucha tea and nitrofurazone on cutaneous full-thickness wounds healing in rats: an experimental study. *Pathology* 8 (2013).

Czaja, Wojciech. Microbial cellulose — the natural power to heal wounds. *Biomaterials* 27 (2006): 145–51.

Gama, Miguel. *Bacterial NanoCellulose: A Sophisticated Multifunctional Material*. Boca Raton, Fla.: CRC Press, 2013.

Parivar, Kazem, et al. Effects of synchronized oral administration and topical application of Kombucha on third-degree burn wounds regeneration in mature rats. *Medical Science Journal of Islamic Azad University Tehran Medical Branch* 22, no. 1 (2012).

Persaud, R. T. Re, and V. Srinivasan. A weight-of-evidence approach for the safety evaluation of kombucha extract in cosmetic products. Study by L'Oreal Research & Innovation at the Society of Toxicology 51st Annual Meeting and ToxExpo, March 11–15, 2012, San Francisco, California.

Rosales-Cortés, Manuel, et al. Healing effect of the extract of kombucha in male Wistar rats. *Open Journal of Veterinary Medicine* 5, no.4 (2015).

## Weight Management

Kombucha contains natural alpha-hydroxy acids (such as malic and lactic acids), the synthetic versions of which are used by both dieters and weight lifters to improve the effectiveness of their regimens. In one study, kombucha consumption was linked to antilipidemic effects in rats, meaning it prevented the body from absorbing too much fat. In another study, green tea kombucha was found to prevent weight gain and improve weight loss in diabetic rats. Many people claim kombucha helps reduce their cravings and improve digestion, which may lead to better nutrient absorption and potentially reduced caloric intake.

#### Related studies:

Aloulou, Ahmed. Hypoglycemic and antilipidemic properties of kombucha tea in alloxan-induced diabetic rats. *BMC Complementary and Alternative Medicine* 12, no. 63 (2012).

Hosseini, Seyed Ahmad, Mehran Gorjian, Latifeh Rasouli, and Saeed Shirali. A comparison between the effect of green tea and kombucha prepared from green tea on the weight of diabetic rats. *Biosciences Biotechnology Research Asia* 12 (Spl. Edn.1), (March 2015): 141–146.

Yang, Zhi-Wei. Hypocholesterolaemic and antioxidant effects of kombucha tea in high-cholesterol fed mice. *Journal of the Science of Food and Agriculture* 89 (2008): 150–56.

## Yeast Infections/*Candida*

*Candida albicans* is a common inhabitant of the human gut; at normally low and manageable levels, it presents no threat to health. But if the gut falls into dysbiosis, these and other usually harmless (or even desirable, at low levels) organisms may overproduce, causing new issues.

Kombucha creates specific healthy acids that are known *Candida*-cides, such as phenethyl alcohol (page 359), decanoic and caprylic acids (page 358), and catechins (page 360). The study "Antimicrobial Effect of Kombucha Analogues" (2012) demonstrated kombucha's antimicrobial activity against six out of seven strains of *Candida*. In experiments using black tea kombucha, kombucha fermented with lemon balm, and kombucha fermented with peppermint, all three kombucha brews proved to be effective against *Candida* strains, with the lemon balm kombucha being the most efficacious.

#### Related study:

Battikh, H., A. Bakhrouf, and E. Ammar. Antimicrobial effect of kombucha analogues. *Lebensmittel-Wissenschaft + Technologie* 47, no. 1 (2012): 71–77.

# Full Citations

**Page 19:** Leclercq, Sophie, et al, Intestinal permeability, gut-bacterial dysbiosis, and behavioral markers of alcohol-dependence severity. *Proceedings of the National Academy of Sciences of the United States of America* 111, no. 42 (2014).

**Page 56:** Djuric, M., et al, Influence of working conditions upon kombucha conducted fermentation of black tea. *Food and Bioproducts Processing* 84, no. 3 (2006): 186–92.

Tu, You-Ying, and Hui-Long Xia. Antimicrobial Activity of Fermented Green Tea Liquid, *International Journal of Tea Science* 7, no. 4 (2008).

**Page 60:** M.A. Heckman, K. Sherry, and E. Gonzalez de Mejia, Energy drinks: an assessment of their market size, consumer demographics, ingredient profile, functionality, and regulations in the United States, *Comprehensive Reviews in Food Science and Food Safety* 9, 2010.

**Page 64:** Chen, C., and B. Y. Liu, Changes in major components of tea fungus metabolites during prolonged fermentation. *Journal of Applied Microbiology* 89 (2000): 834–39.

R. Malbaša, R. E. Lončar, M. Djurić, and I. Došenović. Effect of sucrose concentration on the products of Kombucha fermentation on molasses. *Food Chemistry* 108, no. 3 (2008): 926–32.

Tu, You-Ying, and Hui-Long Xia. Antimicrobial Activity of Fermented Green Tea Liquid, *International Journal of Tea Science* 7, no. 4 (2008)

Kallel, Lina, V. Desseaux, M. Hamdi, P. Stocker, and E. Ajandouz. Insights into the fermentation biochemistry of Kombucha teas and potential impacts of Kombucha drinking on starch digestion. *Food Research International* 49, no. 1 (2012): 226–32.

Lončar, Eva, K. Kanurić, R. Malbaša, M. Đurić, and S. Milanović. Kinetics of saccharose fermentation by kombucha. *Chemical Industry and Chemical Engineering Quarterly* 20, no. 3 (2014): 345–52.

**Page 327:** Afsharmanesh, M., and B. Sadaghi. Effects of dietary alternatives (probiotic, green tea powder, and Kombucha tea) as antimicrobial growth promoters on growth, ileal nutrient digestibility, blood parameters, and immune response of broiler chickens. *Comparative Clinical Pathology* 23, no. 3 (May 2014): 717–24.

Murugesan, G. S., M. Sathishkumar, and K. Swaminathan. Supplementation of waste tea fungal biomass as a dietary ingredient for broiler chicks. *Bioresource Technology* 96, no. 16 (December 2005): 1743–48.

Jayabalan, Rasu, K. Malini, M. Sathishkumar, K. Swaminathan, and S. Yun. Biochemical characteristics of tea fungus produced during kombucha fermentation. *Food Science Biotechnology* 19, no. 3 (2010): 843–47.

Rosales, M. C., A. R. Esther, N. R. Guillermo, R. L. de Cervantes Mireles, L. A. Figueroa, J. J. I. Orozco, and E. R. de la Pena. Evaluation of the properties of healing of the extract of kombucha in sheep in growth with malnutrition, parasitocis and respiratory problems. *Open Journal of Veterinary Medicine* 4, no. 8 (2014).

# Recommended Reading

Buhner, Stephen Harrod. *Sacred and Herbal Healing Beers*. Siris Books, 1998.

Fallon, Sally, and Mary G. Enig. *Nourishing Traditions: The Cookbook That Challenges Politically Correct Nutrition and the Diet Dictocrats*. NewTrends Publishing, 1999.

Frank, Günther W. *Kombucha: Healthy Beverage and Natural Remedy from the Far East: Its Correct Preparation and Use*. Ennsthaler Verlag, 1991.

Heiss, Mary Lou, and Robert J. Heiss. *The Tea Enthusiast's Handbook*. Ten Speed Press, 2010.

Katz, Sandor Ellix. *The Art of Fermentation: An In-Depth Exploration of Essential Concepts and Processes from around the World*. Chelsea Green Publishing, 2012.

———. *Wild Fermentation*. Chelsea Green Publishing, 2003.

Page, Karen, and Andrew Dornenburg. *The Flavor Bible*. Little, Brown and Company, 2008.

Price, Weston A. *Nutrition and Physical Degeneration*. Heritage ed. Price-Pottenger Nutrition Foundation, 1970.

Pryor, Betsy, and Sanford Holst. *Kombucha Phenomenon: The Miracle Health Tea*. Sierra Sunrise Publishing, 1995.

Sklenar, Rudolf, and Rosina Fasching. *Tea Fungus Kombucha: The Natural Remedy and Its Significance in Cases of Cancer and Other Metabolic Diseases*. 6th ed. Ennsthaler Publishing, 1995.

Solzhenitsyn, Aleksandr. *Cancer Ward*. Bodley Head, 1968.

# Appendix 3: Brew Minder Logs

| Brew Date | Recipe Notes (type of tea/sugar) | Harvest Date | Observations and Flavor Notes (pH, taste, etc.) |
|---|---|---|---|
| | | | |
| | | | |
| | | | |
| | | | |
| | | | |
| | | | |
| | | | |
| | | | |

Downloadable versions of these logs can be found at KombuchaKamp.com/DIY.

# PROFESSIONAL BREWING LOG

| Date | Sweet Tea: Brix | pH | Qty | Starter Liquid: Brix | pH | Qty | Temp | SCOBY Qty |
|------|-----------------|----|-----|----------------------|----|-----|------|-----------|
|      |                 |    |     |                      |    |     |      |           |
|      |                 |    |     |                      |    |     |      |           |

| Date | Ending Brix: | pH | % ABV | # Days Brewing | Flavor | Notes | | |
|------|--------------|----|-------|----------------|--------|-------|--|--|
|      |              |    |       |                |        |       |  |  |
|      |              |    |       |                |        |       |  |  |

| Date | Sweet Tea: Brix | pH | Qty | Starter Liquid: Brix | pH | Qty | Temp | SCOBY Qty |
|------|-----------------|----|-----|----------------------|----|-----|------|-----------|
|      |                 |    |     |                      |    |     |      |           |
|      |                 |    |     |                      |    |     |      |           |

| Date | Ending Brix: | pH | % ABV | # Days Brewing | Flavor | Notes | | |
|------|--------------|----|-------|----------------|--------|-------|--|--|
|      |              |    |       |                |        |       |  |  |
|      |              |    |       |                |        |       |  |  |

| Date | Sweet Tea: Brix | pH | Qty | Starter Liquid: Brix | pH | Qty | Temp | SCOBY Qty |
|------|-----------------|----|-----|----------------------|----|-----|------|-----------|
|      |                 |    |     |                      |    |     |      |           |
|      |                 |    |     |                      |    |     |      |           |

| Date | Ending Brix: | pH | % ABV | # Days Brewing | Flavor | Notes | | |
|------|--------------|----|-------|----------------|--------|-------|--|--|
|      |              |    |       |                |        |       |  |  |
|      |              |    |       |                |        |       |  |  |

## ACKNOWLEDGMENTS

First and foremost, this book wouldn't be possible without 10+ years learning from you! Everyone who has ever reached out to Kombucha Kamp or attended a workshop has offered questions, photos, tips, ideas, healing stories and, yes, your mistakes (!), all of which have inspired every part of this book. Spreading this information, our "symbiotic collective wisdom," is the purpose of KombuchaKamp.com, and this book is the manifestation of that mission, inspired by you, the reader. So one more time, thank you!

To all the scientists studying kombucha today, thank you, and please keep going, there's so much more to learn! A debt of gratitude is owed to kombucha authors and researchers who have come before, particularly those whose works are mentioned; you have paved the way for this collection. And as an educator and inspiration to so many fermentationists worldwide, thanks are also due to Sandor Katz; we are fortunate to include your generous words.

The support and friendship of our real food and alternative health blogging, podcasting, and conferencing community have been an invaluable source of wisdom and guidance for many years, professionally and personally. We are deeply grateful to be on this journey with you, and you're helping us spread the word, reaching so many more people than we ever could on our own. A special thank you to Jenny McGruther for her friendship and for introducing us to our agent Sally Ekus and The Lisa Ekus Group, without whom this book would never have come together as it did.

Thank you to the entire team at Storey Publishing, whose hours of dedication and attention to detail forced us to sharpen our efforts and raise our standards; this book would be very different without your efforts — especially those of Lisa Hiley, our editor. Both teams of food photographers, stylists, and assistants brought great skill and joy to the process, capturing the sparkle of living kombucha tea so beautifully for the world to enjoy here. Thank you for your craft and collaboration.

Deep appreciation and love goes to both our families, who cheered us through the process. Valerie Messerall and Keren Crum Jenkins contributed their hands and hearts, and their own kitchens, to help bring recipes and flavor inspirations to life. And when it comes to recipes, the KKamp staff deserves a special round of applause for helping refine and execute hundreds of flavor ideas, dishes, and cocktails, not to mention preparing expertly for two extensive photo shoots. Your work is all over the pages!

To all our friends brewing quality kombucha for the masses, we salute your service to the community. Offering a freshly produced kombucha is hard work, but it sure is needed. Finally, to all those "party planner" bacteria and "party animal" yeast out there, you make the kombucha, we just work for you!

*From Hannah:* This book never could have been written without the steadfast encouragement and support of my partner and husband, Alex LaGory. Whether on the road or in the office, his confidence in my abilities and loving words have seen me through the dark nights when my soul doubted we'd ever glimpse the light at the end of this process. Kismet brought us together, every step of our journey has been evolutionary, and I am eternally grateful to share this life.

*From Alex:* Hannah is the founder and inspiration for everything that is KKamp: optimism, empowerment, education, and fun. She is also both brilliant and dazzling, of mind and personality. But it is her patience, generosity of spirit, kindness, and nurturing nature that have made this life together a reality. We have truly grown together, and her light has made our path visible.

# Index

Page numbers in *italic* indicate photos; numbers in **bold** indicate charts.

# Trust Your Gut *and* Drink to Your Health with More Storey Books

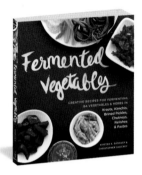

### by Kirsten K. Shockey & Christopher Shockey

Get to work making your own kimchi, pickles, sauerkraut, and more with this colorful and delicious guide. Beautiful photography illustrates methods to ferment 64 vegetables and herbs, along with dozens of creative recipes.

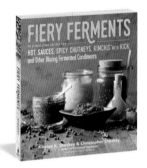

### by Kirsten K. Shockey & Christopher Shockey

Expand your fermented repertoire with more than 70 recipes for spicy sauces, mustards, chutneys, and relishes from around the globe. An additional 40 recipes for breakfast foods, snacks, entrées, and beverages highlight many uses for the hot ferments.

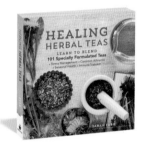

### by Sarah Farr

These 101 original recipes not only offer health advantages like calming nerves, fighting colds, and reducing inflammation; they also taste great! In addition, herb profiles and instruction on the art of tea blending will help you develop your own signature mixtures.

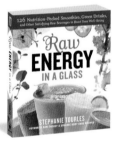

### by Stephanie Tourles

Raise a glass to longevity! Boost your health and energy using just a standard blender and these 126 super-nutritious, super-delicious recipes for smoothies, fruity frappés, vegan shakes, power shots, mocktails, and more.

**Join the conversation.** Share your experience with this book, learn more about Storey Publishing's authors, and read original essays and book excerpts at storey.com. Look for our books wherever quality books are sold or by calling 800-441-5700.